Essentials of Pediatric Urology

Essentials of Pediatric Urology

Third Edition

Edited by

Duncan T Wilcox, MBBS, MD
Surgeon-in-Chief
The Ponzio Family Chair for the Surgeon-in-Chief
Director, Center for Children's Surgery
Professor, University of Colorado School of Medicine
Colorado, USA

David F M Thomas, FRCP, FRCPCH, FRCS
Emeritus Consultant Paediatric Urologist
Leeds Teaching Hospitals NHS Trust
Professor of Paediatric Surgery University of Leeds
Leeds, UK

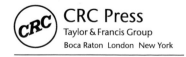

CRC Press
Taylor & Francis Group
Boca Raton London New York

CRC Press is an imprint of the
Taylor & Francis Group, an **informa** business

To our wives: Anne and Marilyn.

Contents

Contributors

Veronica I Alaniz
Department of Pediatric and Adolescent
Gynecology
Children's Hospital of Colorado
Denver, CO, USA

Berk Burgu
Department of Pediatric Urology
Ankara University School of Medicine
Ankara, Turkey

Kevin Cao
Department of Paediatric Urology
Great Ormond Street Hospital for Sick Children
London, UK

David J Chalmers
Department of Pediatric Urology
Maine Medical Center,
South Portland, ME, USA

Alexander Cho
Department of Paediatric Urology
Great Ormond Street Hospital for Sick Children
London, UK

Christopher S Cooper
Department of Pediatric Urology
University of Iowa
Iowa City, IA, USA

Nicholas G Cost
Department of Pediatric Urology
Children's Hospital of Colorado
Denver, CO, USA

Peter Cuckow
Department of Paediatric Urology
Great Ormond Street Hospital for Sick Children
London, UK

Divyesh Y Desai
Department of Paediatric Urology
Great Ormond Street Hospital for Sick Children
London, UK

Patrick G Duffy
(Formerly)
Department of Paediatric Urology
Great Ormond Street Hospital for Sick Children
London, UK

Charlotte Dunford
Department of Adolescent and Reconstructive
Urology
Institute of Urology
University College Hospitals
London, UK

Prasad P Godbole
Department of Paediatric Urology
Sheffield Children's Hospital
Sheffield, UK

Parviz Hajiyev
Department of Pediatric Urology
Ankara University School of Medicine
Ankara, Turkey

Nadia V Halstead
Department of Pediatric Urology
Children's Hospital of Colorado
Denver, CO, USA

Sarah L Hecht
Department of Pediatric Urology
Oregon Health and Science University
Portland, OR, USA

Melanie P Hiorns
Department of Radiology
Great Ormond Street Hospital for Sick Children
London, UK

Patricia Huguelet
Department of Pediatric and Adolescent
Gynecology
Children's Hospital of Colorado
Denver, CO, USA

Kim A R Hutton
(Formerly)
Department of Paediatric Surgery
University Hospital of Wales
Cardiff, UK

Emilie K Johnson
Division of Urology
Ann & Robert H. Lurie Children's Hospital of
Chicago
Chicago, IL, USA

Sara Lobo
Department of Paediatric Urology
Great Ormond Street Hospital for Sick Children
London, UK

Pierre D E Mouriquand
Department of Pediatric Urology
Claude – Bernard University
Debrousse Hospital
Lyon, France

Nicholas P Madden
(Formerly)
Department of Paediatric Urology
Chelsea and Westminster Hospital
London, UK

Stephen D Marks
Department of Paediatric Nephrology
Great Ormond Street Hospital for Sick Children
London, UK

Imran Mushtaq
Department of Paediatric Urology
Great Ormond Street Hospital for Sick Children
London, UK

Stuart J O'Toole
Department of Paediatric Urology
Royal Hospital for Sick Children
Glasgow, UK

Jonathan C Routh
Department of Pediatric Urology
Duke University Medical Center,
Durham, NC, USA

Kyle O Rove
Department of Pediatric Urology
Children's Hospital of Colorado
Denver, CO, USA

Naima Smeulders
Department of Paediatric Urology
Great Ormond Street Hospital for Sick Children
London, UK

Henrik Steinbrecher
(Formerly)
Department of Paediatric Urology
University Hospital of Southampton
Southampton, UK

Douglas J Stewart
Department of Paediatric Nephrology
Great Ormond Street Hospital for Sick Children
London, UK

Rohit Tejwani,
Division of Urologic Surgery,
Duke University Medical Center
Durham, NC, USA

David F M Thomas
(Formerly)
Department of Paediatric Urology
Leeds Teaching Hospitals NHS Trust
Leeds, UK

Vijaya M Vemulakonda
Department of Pediatric Urology
Children's Hospital of Colorado
Denver, CO, USA

Jonathan Walker
Department of Pediatric Urology
Erlanger Children's Hospital
Chattanooga, TN, USA

Duncan T Wilcox
Department of Pediatric Urology
Children's Hospital of Colorado
Denver, CO, USA

Dan Wood
Department of Adolescent Urology
Children's Hospital of Colorado
Denver
CO
USA

Christopher R J Woodhouse
(Formerly)
Department of Adolescent and Reconstructive
  Urology
Institute of Urology
University College Hospitals
London, UK

Elizabeth B Yerkes
Department of Urology
Northwestern University
Feinberg School of Medicine
Chicago, IL, USA

Karly Zaher
Department of Paediatric Urology
Great Ormond Street Hospital for Sick Children
London, UK

Preface

This new edition of *Essentials of Pediatric Urology* has been extensively updated, revised and rewritten to reflect the many advances and innovations in Pediatric Urology since the publication of the second edition. This new edition has also been updated to reflect the valuable information on long-term outcomes now emerging from follow-up studies.

The publication of a new edition and the appointment of an Anglo American Pediatric Urologist co-editor created an exciting opportunity to extend the international reach of *Essentials of Pediatric Urology*. This new edition therefore includes authoritative chapters contributed by leading North American Urologists in addition to chapters by new and existing contributors from the United Kingdom, France and Turkey.

The new, more multinational authorship of chapters created a dilemma regarding the preferred use of spelling and terminology. Pediatric or Paediatric? Ureteric of Ureteral? Ureteropelvic or Pelviureteric? After careful consideration we decided against a standardized policy, opting instead to allow contributors to use the spelling and terminology with which they were familiar. We are grateful to our publisher for endorsing this decision. *Essentials of Pediatric Urology* is not intended to serve as a comprehensive source of reference for specialist Pediatric Urologists. Nevertheless, it provides authoritative coverage of the complex anomalies managed by specialist Pediatric Urologists as well as the urological conditions comprising a substantial part of the everyday workload of Urologists, General Pediatric Surgeons and Pediatricians.

We have strived to retain the accessible, generously illustrated format which proved popular with readers of the first two editions. Throughout the book our over-riding aim has been to provide a concise and up-to-date account of the diagnosis and management of the urological conditions of childhood which is factual and evidence based.

The content of this new edition has been designed to meet the requirements of the Intercollegiate Fellowship examinations in Urology and Paediatric Surgery in the United Kingdom, the Fellowship of the European Academy of Paediatric Urology and the North American Board Examinations. With this in mind, the book includes a self-assessment section of multiple choice questions which is intended to serve as a valuable learning and revision aid.

Finally, we hope that the new edition of *Essentials of Pediatric Urology* will retain the role established by previous editions as a source of easy reference for Pediatricians, Pediatric Nephrologists, Radiologists and Nurse Specialists.

Duncan T Wilcox
David F M Thomas

Acknowledgements

We are indebted to Miranda Bromage at CRC Press/Taylor & Francis for commissioning and overseeing the publication of this new edition of *Essentials of Pediatric Urology*. It would not have happened without her. Samantha Cook played a vital role at various stages in the production of the book and we gratefully acknowledge her important contribution. We would also like to express our sincere thanks to the medical artist Paul Brown for kindly agreeing to provide the new and updated illustrations for this edition. His clear and informative artwork has enhanced all three editions of *Essentials of Pediatric Urology*.

Acknowledgements

Embryology

DAVID F M THOMAS

Topics covered

Genetic basis of genitourinary malformations
Embryogenesis
Upper urinary tract

Lower urinary tract
Genital tracts

INTRODUCTION

This chapter will concentrate predominantly on the clinical aspects of the embryological development of the genitourinary tract but will also refer to relevant advances in scientific methodology.

Techniques such as polymerase chain reaction (PCR), fluorescence in situ hybridisation (FISH) and studies using transgenic "knockout" mice have greatly advanced our understanding of the genes involved in regulating normal embryological development. In addition, innovations in microscopy and three-dimensional (3D) reconstruction are shedding new light on structural development of the human embryo and fetus.

GAMETOGENESIS, FERTILISATION AND THE GENETIC BASIS OF UROLOGICAL ABNORMALITIES

In males, the formation of gametes (spermatozoa) does not commence until puberty whereas in females it commences during fetal life but does not progress beyond prophase of the first meiotic division. At this stage the **primary oocytes** enter a dormant phase until the onset of puberty when a small number of primary oocytes resume the long – arrested meiotic division. Under the influence of follicle-stimulating hormone and luteinising hormone, one or two **secondary oocytes** are extruded from the ovaries at the time of ovulation. Penetration of the protective zona pellucida of the oocyte by a spermatozoon triggers a second meiotic division to create a "**definitive oocyte**".

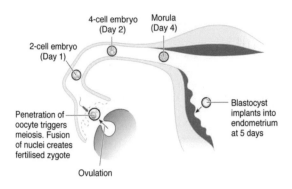

Figure 1.1 **Key stages between fertilisation and implantation of the blastocyst at 5–6 days.**

As a result of the meiotic divisions during gametogenesis, the nuclei of the definitive oocyte and spermatozoon contain a single copy of each of the 22 autosomes and 1 sex chromosome. Fusion of the nuclear DNA of the two gametes during fertilisation creates a **zygote** whose nucleus contains 46 chromosomes – with one copy of each pair of autosomes and one of the two sex chromosome derived from each parent. On its journey along fallopian tube, the newly fertilised zygote undergoes a series of mitotic divisions (termed cleavage) to form a mass of cells termed the **blastocyst** (Figure 1.1).

Major chromosomal abnormalities can arise either during gametogenesis or fertilisation or the early mitotic divisions of the zygote. Most chromosomal abnormalities of this severity lead to spontaneous abortion of the embryo but **trisomy 21** (Down syndrome), **trisomy 13** (Patau syndrome) and **trisomy 18** (Edward syndrome) are compatible with survival. Of these, however, only trisomy 21 is compatible with longer term survival into adult life.

Trisomies can occur as a result of **non-disjunction** (in which a pair of chromosomes fail to separate during gametogenesis) or **translocation** (in which a chromosome, or piece of a chromosome, becomes attached to another chromosome during meiotic division).

The corollary of non-disjunction and translocation is the formation of a gamete which lacks one copy of that particular chromosome. This results in the formation of a zygote whose nucleus contains only a single (unpaired) copy of the particular chromosome. This is termed **monosomy**. Absence of an entire autosome (complete monosomy) invariably leads to spontaneous abortion of the embryo whereas some partial monosomic states are compatible with survival. By contrast to the abnormalities affecting autosomes, major structural abnormalities of the sex chromosomes are not only consistent with survival but are relatively common. Examples include **Klinefelter syndrome** (47XXY) and **Turner syndrome**. Approximately 50% cases of Turner syndrome exist as complete monosomy (45X) whilst 30% of cases occur in mosaic form 45X/46XX) and 20% result from a structural deletion of genetic material on one of the X chromosomes. 45X/46XY mosaicism is known as mixed gonadal dysgenesis. **Mosaicism** is defined as the presence of two genetically distinct cell lines derived from the same zygote. Abnormalities of the sex chromosomes often occur in mosaic form.

Genetic mutations occurring at the level of individual genes can be studied using techniques such as polymerase chain reaction (**PCR**) and fluorescence in situ hybridisation (**FISH**). A number of inherited conditions affecting the genitourinary tract can be ascribed to identifiable mutations, e.g. **autosomal recessive polycystic kidney disease (ARPKD), autosomal dominant polycystic kidney disease (ADPKD), X-linked Kallmann's syndrome and renal coloboma syndrome**. However, attempts to identify specific mutations in common urological conditions with a strong familial tendency such as vesico ureteric reflux, upper tract duplication and hypospadias have been unrewarding. The occurrence of these disorders in members of the same family is more likely to result from the interaction of multiple genes than the effect of a single gene mutation. The possible role of environmental factors in modifying gene expression during embryological development of the genitourinary tract is poorly understood.

EMBRYOGENESIS

Human gestation spans a period of 38 weeks, from fertilisation to birth. The formation of

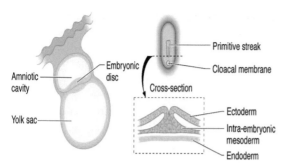

Figure 1.2 Embryonic disc at 16 days with inpouring of cells into the primitive streak to create intraembryonic mesoderm.

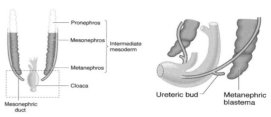

Figure 1.3 Precursors of the upper urinary tract, metanephros and ureteric bud.

organs and systems occurs mainly between the third and tenth weeks with subsequent development being characterised mainly by differentiation, branching, maturation and growth. By the time the blastocyst implants into the primed endometrium (approximately 6 days after fertilisation) it has undergone organisation to form an outer trophoblastic layer and inner cell mass. Over the ensuing 10 days, the amniotic cavity and the yolk sac develop within the blastocyst – with the embryonic disc forming in the interface between them. Ectodermal tissue originates from cells on the amniotic surface of the embryonic disc whereas endodermal tissues are derived from cells adjacent to the yolk sac. Inpouring of cells into the embryonic disc from the amniotic surface via the primitive streak creates a third layer – the intraembryonic mesoderm (Figure 1.2). It is from the intraembryonic mesoderm that much of the genitourinary tract is ultimately derived.

UPPER URINARY TRACT (FIGURE 1.3)

By the fourth week, two blocks of mesoderm have appeared on each side of the midline. Sequential differentiation within this mesoderm gives rise to the pronephros in the most cephalad region, the mesonephros in the midzone and the metanephros in the most caudal region. The pronephros regresses rapidly and serves no function in the human embryo. At around the same time, condensations of mesenchyme lying lateral to the mesonephros undergo canalisation to form the mesonephric ducts, which advance in a caudal direction to merge with the cloaca. Tubular structures within the mesonephros establish a communication with the mesonephric duct to fulfil a transient excretory role until around 10 weeks. These tubules then regress in the female but in the male they persist as precursors of the efferent tubules of the testis.

At around 28 days, the ureteric bud develops as a protrusion from the mesonephric duct. The ureteric bud then advances towards the metanephros to penetrate the metanephric mesenchyme at around 32 days. The formation of nephrons by interaction between the ureteric bud and metanephros occurs by a process of reciprocal interaction between the two tissues – a phenomenon which occurs in the embryological development of a number of systems. Sequential budding and branching of the ureteric bud gives rise to the renal pelvis, the major calices, the minor calices and the collecting ducts whilst the glomeruli, convoluted tubules and loop of Henle are derived from the metanephric mesenchyme (Figure 1.4). The cortex and medulla are discernible by 15 weeks and new generations of nephrons continue to be added to the cortex up until 36 weeks. In humans, the process of nephrogenesis ceases at 36 weeks and the total number of nephrons remains fixed thereafter at approximately 1 million per kidney. Nephron numbers are reduced in the kidneys of preterm and low-birth-weight infants. Almost 3000 different genes have been identified as being involved in ureteric bud

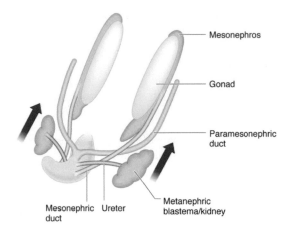

Figure 1.4 Embryonic urinary tract at 6–8 weeks.

formation and nephrogenesis. The roles played by many of these genes have been studied in transgenic mice and in clinical genetic studies. Of these, the gene encoding for glial cell line-derived neurotophic factor (GDNF), Wilms tumour suppressor gene (WT1) and RET proto-oncogene have been shown to play key roles.

Renal Dysplasia

Although "dysplastic" is often used loosely to refer to any congenitally small kidney, the term "dysplasia" refers more accurately to kidneys demonstrating certain characteristic histological features. These include disordered renal architecture, immature "primitive" undifferentiated tubules, small cysts and the inappropriate (metaplastic) presence of cartilage and fibromuscular tissue. Renal dysplasia can arise from faulty interaction between the ureteric bud and metanephric tissue or the effects of insults to the developing kidney – notably severe obstructive uropathy.

A hypoplastic kidney is one which is reduced in size but retains normal internal architecture – although with fewer nephrons.

Cystic Anomalies

The patterns of cystic renal disease and their aetiology are considered in Chapter 10.

Abnormalities of Renal Ascent and Fusion

These anomalies date from the sixth to tenth weeks of gestation, when the embryonic kidney is ascending in its relative position on the posterior abdominal wall before adopting its definitive position. Examples include, horseshoe kidney (Figure 1.5), pelvic kidney (Figure 1.6) and crossed fused renal ectopia (Figure 1.7).

Fetal Renal Function

Although the kidneys excrete urine into the amniotic cavity from around the ninth week onwards, the homeostatic role which is normally played by the kidneys is fulfilled by the placenta – which effectively "dialyses" the fetus until birth. The kidneys nevertheless serve an important function by producing urine – which is a major constituent of the amniotic fluid surrounding the fetus. In addition to providing a protective environment for the fetus, amniotic fluid also promotes normal lung development. Reduced amniotic fluid

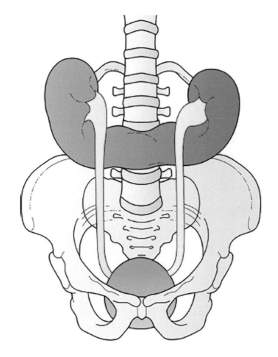

Figure 1.5 Abnormality of ascent and fusion-horseshoe kidney.

volume (oligohydramnios) is associated with pulmonary hypoplasia as well as "moulding deformities" of the fetus such as "Potter's facies" and limb deformities.

LOWER URINARY TRACT (FIGURE 1.8)

The lower urinary tract is derived from the cloaca, a single cavity comprising the primitive hindgut and allantois. Between the fourth and seventh weeks the cloaca subdivides to form the urogenital sinus anteriorly and anorectal canal posteriorly. Historically, this subdivision was ascribed to a process of active descent of the urorectal septum (Tourneux fold) aided by lateral ingrowth of (Rathke) folds from the side walls of the cloaca. However, this explanation has been largely refuted by more recent studies which have demonstrated that subdivision of the cloaca occurs as a predominantly "passive" process resulting from spatial realignment, differential dorsoventral growth of the cloaca and unfolding of the caudal body axis.

As the bladder develops, the mesonephric ducts migrate caudally to merge with the upper urethra, whereas the ureters retain a more fixed position in relation to the bladder (Figure 1.9).

Clinical Considerations

Persistent cloacal malformations represent the female equivalent of high anorectal malformations in males and are characterised by confluence of the urethra, vagina and rectum to form a common channel with a single opening on the perineum. Cloacal malformations originate from abnormalities occurring during subdivision of the cloaca between 4 and 7 weeks. The origins of bladder exstrophy and epispadias are less clear. Complete upper tract duplication occurs when two (rather than one) ureteric buds develop on the mesonephric duct. A bifid ureteric bud gives rise to incomplete ureteric duplication.

The Meyer-Weigart law describes the paradoxical anatomy of the ureters observed in cases of complete duplication whereby the upper pole

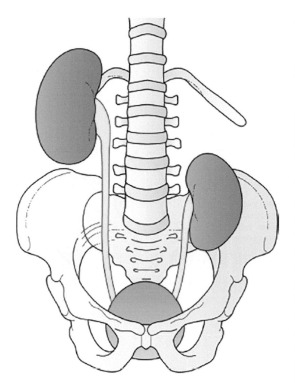

Figure 1.6 **Abnormality of ascent-pelvic kidney.**

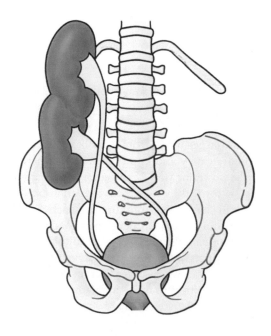

Figure 1.7 **Abnormality of ascent and fusion-crossed fused renal ectopia.**

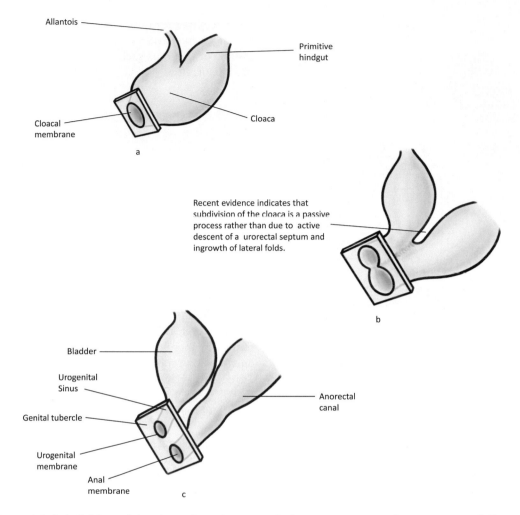

Allantois

Primitive
hindgut

Cloacal
membrane

Cloaca

a

Recent evidence indicates that
subdivision of the cloaca is a passive
process rather than due to active
descent of a urorectal septum and
ingrowth of lateral folds.

b

Bladder

Urogenital
Sinus

Genital tubercle

Urogenital
membrane

Anal
membrane

Anorectal
canal

c

Figure 1.8 Subdivision of the cloaca into the urogenital compartment and anorectum at 4–7 weeks.

ureter enters the urinary tract in a more caudal position than the lower pole ureter. This phenomenon is explained by the pattern of early development in which the mesonephric duct descends towards the developing posterior urethra taking the upper pole ureter with it whilst the lower pole ureter remains anchored on the trigonal region of the bladder.

GENITAL TRACTS

Differentiation and development of the gonads and genital tracts is initiated by the migration of primordial germ cells from the yolk sac, across the coelomic cavity and into primitive mesenchyme on the posterior wall of the embryo. The genital ridge is formed by reciprocal induction between the germ cells and surrounding mesenchyme. The paramesonephric ducts develop as condensations of coelomic epithelium lying lateral to the mesonephric ducts. At 6 weeks the structures which represent the precursors of the reproductive tract are identical in males and females. With the exception of the gonads these structures are destined to differentiate passively down a "default" female pathway unless actively switched down a male pathway by the genetic information carried by the testis-determining gene (SRY).

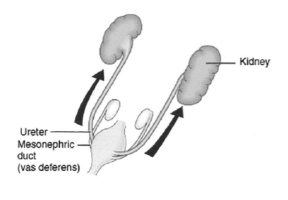

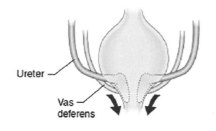

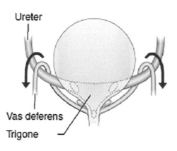

Ureter

Vas deferens

Trigone

Figure 1.9 Changing anatomical configuration of the ureters and mesonephric duct derivatives.

Internal Genitalia

Female (Figure 1.10)

Within the genital ridge, primordial germ cells and mesenchymal support cells interact to form ovarian follicles within the developing ovary. Because they are not exposed to testosterone, the mesonephric ducts regress spontaneously, to leave only vestigial remnants (epioophoron, paroophoron and Gartner's cysts). In the absence of exposure to anti-Müllerian hormone (AMH), the paramesonephric ducts in females persist to give rise to the fallopian tubes and lower genital tract.

It has become apparent that differentiation and development of the ovary is not a purely passive ("default") process determined solely by the absence of the SRY gene. The Dax1 ovarian promoting factor gene encoded on the X chromosome has been shown to act in conjunction with other genes to actively promote ovarian development and inhibit expression of the SRY gene. At around the tenth week, the caudal extremities of the paramesonephric ducts fuse and attach to the urogenital sinus. Over the ensuing weeks the uterus forms from the fused paramesonephric ducts. In the conventional account of the development of the vagina, the fused paramesonephric ducts attach to the urogenital sinus to create a condensation of tissue (sinu vaginal bulb) which advances downwards to the perineum as a solid vaginal plate which then canalises to create the vaginal lumen. The upper two-thirds of the vagina have been conventionally described as being of paramesonephric origin with the lower

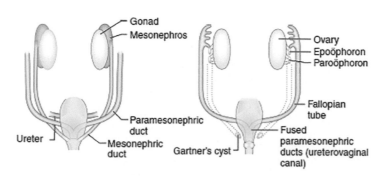

Figure 1.10 The undifferentiated genital tract is genetically programmed down a pathway of female differentiation unless directed down a male pathway by the presence of the SRY gene.

third of the vagina and introitus being derived from urogenital sinus and ectoderm, respectively (Figure 1.11). However, recent studies have cast doubt on this model and it has become apparent that the development of the human vagina is more complex than was previously thought.

Male (Figure 1.12)

Differentiation of the male genital tract is ultimately dependent on the presence of the testis-determining gene (SRY) located on the short arm of the Y chromosome. However, the role of the SRY gene is mediated by a cascade of other downstream genes. The testis determining factor encoded by the SRY gene is a transcription factor which promotes upregulation of SOX9 and other transcription factors.

Anti-Müllerian Hormone (AMH), also termed Müllerian Inhibitory Substance (MIS) substance, is secreted by the Sertoli cells of the testis from the seventh week onwards.

- AMH is responsible for causing regression of the paramesonephric ducts (with the exception of vestigial remnants such as the testicular appendage and utriculus).
- AMH stimulates the Leydig cells of the fetal testis to secrete testosterone from the ninth week onwards.
- AMH promotes the first stage of testicular descent.

Under the influence of testosterone the mesonephric ducts differentiate to form the epididymis, rete testis, vas deferens, ejaculatory ducts and seminal vesicles. Development of the prostate gland between 12 and 19 weeks commences with the emergence of buds from the urogenital sinus.

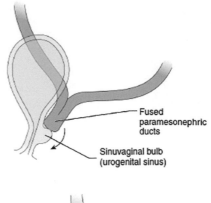

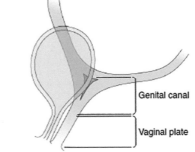

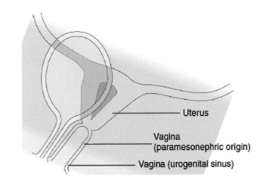

Figure 1.11 Development of the female lower genital tract between 10 and 12 weeks.

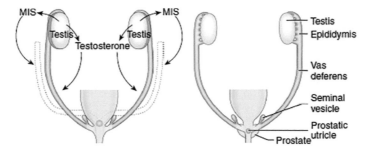

Figure 1.12 Differentiation of the male genital tract in response to anti-Müllerian hormone and testosterone.

These undergo branching morphogenesis to form the ducts and glandular acini of the prostate gland whilst the capsule and stroma are derived from surrounding mesenchyme. Development of the prostate relies on reciprocal inductive signalling between urothelium and mesenchyme and is highly dependent on androgenic stimulation.

External Genitalia (Figure 1.13)

Unless they are exposed to androgens, the external genitalia of both males and females are destined to differentiate passively down a female pathway.

Female

The external genitalia differentiate passively to create the normal female genital phenotype. The genital tubercle gives rise to the clitoris and the urogenital sinus contributes to the vestibule of the vagina. The urogenital folds persist as the labia minora and the labio scrotal folds form the labia majora.

Male

Until 12 weeks the male external genitalia share the same undifferentiated morphology as the female (Figure 1.14). Thereafter, the urethral plate in the male advances further onto the genital tubercle, expands in width and opens out to create the urethral groove. Formation of penile urethra has been likened to the action of a zip, with the "closing zipper" drawing the lateral margins of the urethral groove together in the midline in a proximal to distal direction. Formation of the penile urethra is complete by 15 weeks, with the terminal portion being formed by in-growth of ectoderm from the tip of the glans. Virilisation of the male genitalia is highly dependent on exposure to androgens and the presence of the appropriate androgen receptors within the target tissues. The enzyme 5-alpha reductase plays a key role in promoting virilisation by converting testosterone to its more potent derivative, dihydrotestosterone.

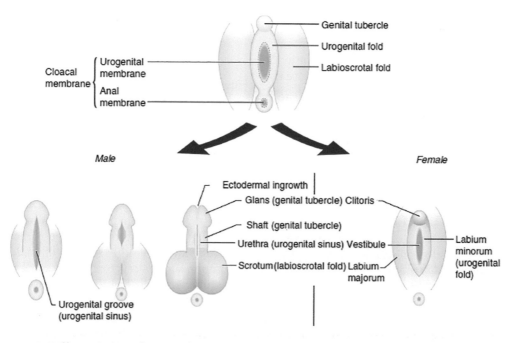

Figure 1.13 Differentiation of external genitalia determined by androgenic stimulation in the male.

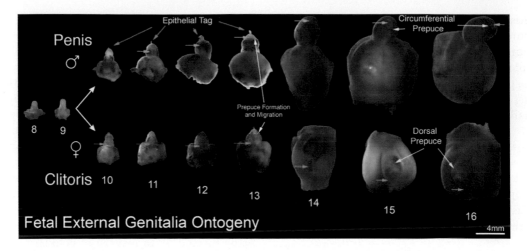

Figure 1.14 Diverging pathways of differentiation from 12 weeks onwards. (Reproduced by kind permission of Lawrence Baskin.)

Testicular Descent

Anti-Müllerian Hormone initiates the first stage of testicular descent by stimulating contraction of the gubernaculum and anchoring the testis in the inguinal region. The second stage is testosterone dependent and occurs around 25–30 weeks when the gubernaculum draws the testis down the inguinal canal into its final scrotal position. Descent of the testis is preceded by a protrusion of the peritoneum (processus vaginalis). This normally closes spontaneously before birth or in the first few weeks of life but may persist to give rise to a communicating hydrocele or inguinal hernia.

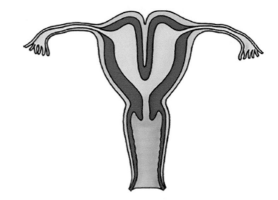

Figure 1.15 Fusion defect – bicornuate uterus.

Clinical Considerations

Female

Abnormalities originating from defective development of the paramesonephric ducts include: absence of a Fallopian tube and hemiuterus, absence (agenesis) of the upper vagina (Rokitansky syndrome) septate vagina and bicornuate uterus (Figure 1.15). Virilisation of the external genitalia occurs in females with congenital adrenal hyperplasia who are exposed to high levels of circulating androgens *in utero*. By contrast to the external genitalia, the ovaries and internal reproductive tract develop normally.

Male

Persistent Müllerian duct syndrome is characterised by bilateral undescended testes and the presence of persistent paramesonephric duct structures. Proximal and mid-shaft forms of hypospadias arise from incomplete closure of the urethral groove and proximal hypospadias may be accompanied by other features of inadequate virilisation such as cryptorchidism and a persistent Müllerian utriculus. Virilisation defects can result from a number of different mechanisms; defects in androgen synthesis pathways, 5-alpha reductase deficiency and insensitivity of the genital tissues to androgens due to receptor and post receptor defects. Intrauterine exposure to environmental "endocrine disruptors" has also been suggested as a possible factor but the evidence is still largely lacking.

KEY POINTS

- The genitourinary tract is commonly affected in children with chromosomal abnormalities.
- The ureteric bud plays a pivotal role in nephrogenesis and the embryological development of the upper tract.
- With the exception of the gonads, the genital tracts of both sexes differentiate passively down a female pathway unless actively switched down a male pathway by the testis-determining gene (SRY).
- Single-gene mutations have been identified in some inherited conditions of the urogenital systems. However, the conditions most commonly encountered in paediatric urology are sporadic or result from the interaction of multiple genes.

FURTHER READING

Baskin L. Basic science of the genitalia (Chapter). In: Docimo SG, Canning D, Khoury A, Pippi Salle JL (eds), Textbook of Clinical Paediatric Urology, 6th Edition. Boca Raton, FL: Taylor & Francis, 2019: 1141–1149.

Baskin L, Shen J, Sinclair A, Cao M, Liu X, Liu G, Isaacson D, Overland M, Li Y, Cunha GR. Development of the human penis and clitoris. Differentiation. 2018 Sep–Oct;103:74–85.

Schoenwolf GC, Bleyl SB, Brauer PR, Francis-West PH. Larsens Human Embryology. Philadelphia: Elsevier Saunders, 2015: 375–428.

Thomas DFM. Embryology of cloaca and genitourinary sinus malformations. Asian J Androl. 2020 Mar–Apr;22(2);124–128.

Renal Development and Dysfunction

DOUGLAS J STEWART and STEPHEN D MARKS

Topics covered

Renal physiology in the fetus and neonate
Renal impairment in infancy, childhood and
    adolescence

Complications of chronic kidney disease
Renal replacement therapy

RENAL PHYSIOLOGY IN THE FETUS AND NEONATE

Introduction

Nephron formation (nephrogenesis) commences during the fifth week of gestation. Recognisable glomerular structures are present from the ninth week and glomerular development (glomerulogenesis) is complete by 32–34 weeks. Over 80% of nephrogenesis occurs in the third trimester. Kidney growth continues after 34 weeks' gestation but this is due to maturation of existing nephrons (tubular and vascular growth) rather than formation of new glomeruli or nephrons. In preterm infants, the process of nephrogenesis may continue after birth but the immature kidneys are vulnerable to potential insults during this period. The total number of nephrons in the two kidneys at the time of birth is highly variable, ranging from 200,000 to 2.7 million. Because damaged nephrons are incapable of repair or regeneration anything which impairs nephrogenesis (such as intrauterine urinary tract obstruction), may result in a reduced number of nephrons at birth. This increases the subsequent risk of chronic kidney disease (CKD) and related complications.

The presence of urine in the fetal bladder can be visualised on ultrasound at 9 weeks gestation. Fetal urine is the major constituent of amniotic fluid and the volume of amniotic fluid increases with gestational age. Amniotic fluid is swallowed, absorbed in the gastrointestinal tract and 'recycled' into the amniotic cavity via the kidneys. By 20 weeks gestation, fetal urine constitutes 80% of liquor volume (approximately 800 mL/day). Fetal urine flow rate increases progressively throughout pregnancy to 15–30 mL/hour from 31 weeks onwards. Reduced or absent urinary output (e.g. due to severe outflow obstruction, bilateral cystic disease or bilateral renal agenesis) leads to oligohydramnios-reduced amniotic fluid volume.

After birth, the glomerular filtration rate (GFR) correlates with gestational age, total kidney volume and mean arterial pressure. GFR is approximately 3.5–6 mL/min/1.73 m² in premature infants depending on birth weight, and 13 mL/min/1.73 m² in infants born at term (40 weeks). Postnatally there is a sharp increase in GFR, which doubles by 2 weeks of age and triples by 4 weeks of age. However, it takes approximately 1–2 years for adjusted GFR values to reach adult levels. This increase in GFR is a consequence of greater glomerular surface area as well as renal maturation and growth. At birth, the kidneys only receive a small percentage (2.5–4%) of cardiac output. This increases over the first few weeks of life to 15–18% of cardiac output. For comparison, renal perfusion accounts for 20–25% of cardiac output in adults.

Serum creatinine is an unreliable marker of renal function in neonates because it freely crosses the placental barrier and maternal creatinine is present in the neonate's circulation. Furthermore, there is a variable degree of proximal tubular reabsorption of creatinine in the immature kidneys.

The low GFR in neonates is of considerable relevance to clinical management, especially when interpreting laboratory results and calculating fluid requirements and drug dosages. This is particularly important in sick premature infants. Although the neonatal kidney can cope with many physiological demands, its functional reserve is limited and may be overwhelmed by some of the stresses commonly encountered in the neonatal period.

Fluid and Water Homeostasis

In early fetal life, water constitutes approximately 90% of body weight, and the extracellular fluid (ECF) represents 60% of body weight. During fetal development there is contraction of the ECF volume so that by term, 75% of body weight is composed of water and the ECF volume constitutes 40% of body weight. Preterm infants have much higher body water composition than those born at term.

Following delivery, there may be an early phase of oliguria but after 24–48 hours this is followed by an acute isotonic volume contraction leading to weight loss. A loss of 10% of birth weight is not uncommon. This phenomenon, which is part of the normal physiological adaptation to extrauterine life, is most pronounced and prolonged in premature infants. Most babies regain their birth weight between 7 and 10 days of age. The reduction in pulmonary vascular resistance and increase in pulmonary venous return after birth stimulates release of atrial natriuretic peptide (ANP), thus contributing to diuresis and contraction of the ECF volume. Early and excessive administration of sodium and water before this period of diuresis/natriuresis has occurred may contribute to hypervolaemic (dilutional) hyponatraemia. This poses an increased risk of morbidity and mortality in neonates compared with regimens where water and sodium intake is restricted in the first few days of life.

Due to tubular immaturity, the maximal urine concentrating ability of the kidney in new born infants is impaired (up to 600–800 mOsmo/kg). Neonates therefore produce large volumes of dilute urine, typically at a rate of 2–3 mL/kg/hour. The concentrating ability of the kidneys increases rapidly over the first 2 months and continues to increase at a slower rate thereafter. The limited concentrating ability of the kidney reflects a reduced responsiveness of the kidneys to antidiuretic hormone (vasopressin) and an inability to maintain a corticomedullary osmotic gradient (partially because the tubules themselves are small). Neonates can usually respond to a hypotonic fluid load by initially producing a greater volume of dilute urine but have difficulty in producing more concentrated urine thereafter. Neonates are therefore easily predisposed to dehydration.

Sodium Homeostasis

Total body sodium content is higher in neonates, infants and young children. A positive sodium balance is essential for normal growth. In healthy neonates the sodium requirement is typically 2–3 mmol/kg/day in the first week, rising to 3–5 mmol/kg/day after the first week. In preterm babies, and very low birth weight infants, the sodium requirement can be two to three-fold higher as a result of reduced ability of the immature renal tubules to reabsorb sodium combined with the additional sodium requirements for growth. The use of diuretics may also increase sodium and potassium excretion leading to increased requirement for supplementation.

Potassium Homeostasis

Tubular excretion of potassium in neonates differs from infants and older children. Their renal clearance of potassium is reduced even after correction is made for their lower GFR. The combination of reduced renal clearance and increased intestinal absorption of potassium puts neonates into a net positive potassium balance. In term infants, potassium levels usually fall rapidly in the first week of life whereas preterm infants experience a gradual rise the serum potassium which reaches a maximum around the third to fourth weeks of life. Elevated serum potassium levels may be a consequence of hypoxia, metabolic acidosis, catabolic stress, oliguric renal failure and inadequate excretion by the immature distal nephron. The daily potassium requirement in a healthy neonate is typically 1–2 mmol/kg/day in the first week, rising to 2–3 mmol/kg/day thereafter.

Acid-Base Homeostasis

Due to tubular immaturity, neonates are unable to adequately acidify their urine and their blood is therefore relatively acidotic. This may be a mixed respiratory and metabolic acidosis, and is usually accompanied by cardiopulmonary compensation. The renal threshold for bicarbonate reabsorption is lower in neonates (18–20 mmol/L) but this rises to 24–26 mmol/L by 1 year of age as the renal acidification mechanism develops. Because excessive administration of sodium chloride can contribute to a hyperchloraemic metabolic acidosis the sodium content of total parenteral nutrition (TPN) is therefore often given in the form of sodium acetate, a base, rather than sodium chloride. Prolonged acidosis in the neonate and infant (e.g. secondary to CKD) should be avoided as this can lead to poor

feeding and growth impairment. Bicarbonate supplementation may therefore be required with the aim of maintaining serum bicarbonate level above 17 mmol/L.

RENAL IMPAIRMENT IN INFANCY, CHILDHOOD AND ADOLESCENCE

Introduction and Definitions

Renal impairment may be congenital or acquired, and is classified as either acute kidney injury (AKI) or chronic kidney disease (CKD).

Acute kidney injury (AKI)

AKI has now superseded the term acute renal failure (ARF). It is characterised by a sudden, potentially reversible reduction in kidney function which is typically accompanied by a rise in serum creatinine. AKI is usually associated with a decrease in urine output but polyuria may also occur. Different classification systems exist for AKI including the Kidney Disease Improving Global Outcomes (KDIGO) 2012 (Table 2.1) and pRIFLE (Table 2.2) classification systems. The pRIFLE system is used to identify children with AKI and those at risk of renal impairment. The different categories have been found to correlate

Table 2.1 KDIGO 2012 AKI classification

AKI stage	Measured serum creatinine	Urine ouput (mL/kg/hour)
1	>1.5–1.9 times baseline creatinine	<0.5 for 6–12 hours
2	2–2.9 times baseline creatinine	<0.5 for ≥12 hours
3	≥3 times baseline creatinine	<0.3 for ≥24 hours or anuric for 12 hours

Table 2.2 pRIFLE classification

Category	Estimated GFR	Urine output (mL/kg/hour)
Risk	Decrease by 25% from baseline	<0.5 for 8 hours
Injury	Decrease by 50%	<0.5 for 16 hours
Failure	Decrease by 75% or <35 mL/min/1.73 m^2	<0.3 for 24 hours or anuric for 12 hours
Loss	Renal failure for >4 weeks	
End-stage	Renal failure >3 months	

Table 2.3 CKD staging

Stage	GFR (mL/min/1.73 m^2)	Description
1	>90	Kidney damage but normal renal function
2	60–89	Kidney damage with mild loss of renal function
3a	45–59	Mild to moderate loss of renal function
3b	30–44	Moderate to severe loss of renal function
4	15–29	Severe loss of renal function
5	<15	End-stage kidney disease

with morbidity and mortality outcomes. The management of AKI includes: identifying and avoiding the causative agent(s), avoiding exposure to other potential nephrotoxic agents and careful fluid management with supportive measures to correct electrolyte disturbance. In severe cases, renal replacement therapy may be required to facilitate clearance of waste products and fluid removal.

Chronic kidney disease (CKD)

The Kidney Disease Improving Global Outcomes (KDIGO) guidelines define CKD as the presence of kidney damage, either functional or structural, exceeding 3 months duration. Table 2.3 lists the different CKD stages.

Epidemiology of CKD

The true incidence of CKD in childhood is unknown. Figures of 2 to 16 per million of age-related population (pmarp) per year are quoted depending on different national registry data. However, this is probably an underestimate because the early stages of CKD are usually asymptomatic. Many patients with CKD may not present until later in childhood or adolescence – or until they reach adulthood.

The incidence and prevalence of CKD are higher in males because they have a higher incidence of congenital anomalies of the kidney and urinary tract (CAKUT) – which is the commonest cause of CKD. Congenital anomalies

of the kidney and urinary tract account for around 30% of all congenital anomalies and are more common in certain ethnicities, particularly in African Americans and Australian aboriginals.

Some patients with CKD may have stable renal function for several years and there may even be some improvement in their GFR, particularly over the first 4 years of life. However, they typically experience a decline in GFR with puberty.

Aetiology of CKD

Primary causes of CKD differ significantly in children compared with adults. The main aetiologies are:

- Congenital anomalies of the kidney and urinary tract (CAKUT) (49.1%)
- Steroid-resistant nephrotic syndrome (10.4%)
- Chronic glomerulonephritis – e.g. in lupus nephritis, Henoch–Schönlein nephritis, and Alport syndrome (8.1%)
- Renal ciliopathies such as nephronophthisis (5.3%)

Rarer causes of CKD include haemolytic uraemic syndrome (HUS) and malignancy such as Wilms tumour. Prematurity is being increasingly recognised as a risk factor for CKD and rising rates of childhood obesity are associated with early type 2 diabetes mellitus and consequent diabetic nephropathy.

Renal replacement therapy is usually required once stage 5 CKD (end-stage kidney disease [ESKD]) is reached. Pre-emptive living donor (LD) kidney transplantation is considered the gold standard of treatment for ESKD. Ideally patients should undergo transplantation before they reach the point of requiring dialysis. However, this is challenging and many patients experience deterioration in renal function before a donor can be found. Alternatively, they may present acutely with ESKD which necessitates the need for acute dialysis. The GFR in early childhood is a predictor of the likely requirement for renal replacement therapy by 20 years of age.

- GFR 51–75 mL/min/1.73 m² – 37% likelihood of renal replacement therapy
- GFR 25–50 mL/min/1.73 m² – 70% likelihood of renal replacement therapy
- GFR <20 mL/min/1.73 m² – 97% likelihood of renal replacement therapy

Assessment of Renal Function in Children

Although measurement of serum creatinine is widely used to assess renal function it has several limitations. Creatinine is a breakdown product of creatinine phosphate in muscle and is produced at a rate of 10–25 mg/kg/day (90–210 μmol/kg/day). Serum creatinine values rise with growth and increasing muscle mass. After the neonatal period, creatinine is freely secreted via the renal tubules with only minimal reabsorption. When renal function is impaired, however, the ability of the tubules to secrete creatinine is reduced and serum values rise. Saturation of tubular secretion of creatinine may not occur until GFR has fallen by 50% with the result that reliance on creatinine values may result in an overestimate of GFR. Furthermore, creatinine can only be used to estimate GFR

when it is in steady state and rapid fluctuations in serum creatinine may make it an unreliable way of estimating GFR.

Children with low muscle mass may have low serum creatinine values which are not an accurate reflection of their true GFR.

The gold standard measurement of GFR is by inulin clearance. This requires injection of an intravenous bolus of inulin followed by a continuous infusion with subsequent measurement of serum and urine inulin levels. This test is impractical in the clinical setting, particularly for children who are not toilet trained and for those with voiding difficulties. Clearance of radioactive isotopes, such as ^{51}Cr[EDTA], can be used to measure GFR but this requires serial serum samples to be taken and exposure to radioisotopes – which is undesirable. The use of iohexol serum clearance is a promising alternative to inulin and radioisotopes for GFR determination but remains expensive and is not in widespread use.

Cystatin C measurement may be of use in children with low muscle bulk in whom calculations based on serum creatinine are unreliable. Cystatin C is a small protein produced from all nucleated cells and is readily filtered via the glomeruli. As such, it is not affected by muscle mass.

The modified Schwartz formula is frequently used as a creatinine-clearance estimate of GFR in paediatrics, although the aforementioned considerations need to be taken into account. However, the formula lacks validation the range of GFR values of 15–75 mL/min/1.73m². The formulae, adapted for different units of creatinine, are listed below:

- eGFR (mL/min/1.73 m²) = 0.413 × height (cm)/serum creatinine (mg/dL)
- eGFR (mL/min/1.73 m²) = 36.5 × height (cm)/serum creatinine (μmol/L)

Outcomes for Patients with CKD

CKD is associated with reduced life expectancy, with cardiovascular risk being increased even for patients in the early stages of CKD. Cardiovascular disease is the main cause of death for patients with ESKD. Survival rates for children and young people on dialysis, and post-transplant, continue to increase, albeit at a relatively slow rate. The lifespan of patients on chronic dialysis is reduced by 40–60 years and by 20–30 years for renal transplant recipients.

COMPLICATIONS OF CHRONIC KIDNEY DISEASE

Chronic Kidney Disease-Mineral and Bone Disorder (CKD-MBD)

CKD-MBD (previously referred to as 'renal osteodystrophy') is a systemic disorder which results from impaired vitamin D metabolism and secondary hyperparathyroidism. In CKD, the kidneys produce less 1-alpha hydroxylase, the enzyme required to convert 25-hydroxyvitamin D (calcidiol) to its active form, 1,25 dihydroxyvitamin D_3 (calcitriol). Low calcitriol levels result in reduced calcium absorption from the gut and reduced renal calcium reabsorption. Coupled with hyperphosphataemia (resulting from reduced renal excretion of phosphate) this stimulates increased secretion of parathyroid hormone (PTH) from the parathyroid glands. Secondary hyperparathyroidism results in increased bone resorption and impaired osteoid mineralisation. Bones are weakened and there may be radiological evidence of rickets. If untreated, secondary hyperparathyroidism can cause bone pain and an increased risk of fractures and slipped epiphyses. Measurement of intact PTH levels serves as a marker of active bone disease and can be used to monitor response to treatment. The aims of treatment are to normalise bone metabolism, improve bone strength and growth, reduce the risk of bony deformity, and also reduce the risk of vascular calcification (by maintaining serum calcium levels within a normal range).

Management of CKD-MBD (renal osteodystrophy) includes:

1. Correction of acidosis using medications such as sodium bicarbonate.

2. Dietary phosphate restriction and the use of phosphate binding medications, e.g. calcium acetate, calcium carbonate and Sevelamer. These need to be taken at mealtimes to promote intestinal excretion of phosphate.

3. Supplementation with alfacalcidol (a vitamin D analogue) or calcitriol to suppress PTH if control cannot be achieved by dietary restriction alone.

4. The use of cinacalcet (a calcimimetic agent that mimics the action of calcium on tissues via activation of the calcium-sensing receptors) for patients with refractory secondary hyperparathyroidism and those at risk of tertiary hyperparathyroidism.

Anaemia

Anaemia is common in children with CKD and it may affect their neurocognitive ability, exercise tolerance and cardiovascular status (e.g. increased risk of left ventricular hypertrophy). The ideal haemoglobin level for children with CKD is debated but evidence suggests that outcomes are not improved above a haemoglobin level of 13 g/dL. The reported prevalence of anaemia is 73% for stage 3 CKD, 87% for stage 4 and >93% for stage 5. Anaemia in CKD is caused predominantly by decreased renal erythropoietin production and impaired physiological regulation of iron. Recombinant human erythropoietin (rHuEPO) is almost invariably required in the latter stages of CKD, and can be used safely in children on dialysis. It can be administered either subcutaneously or intravenously. Younger children typically require higher doses of rHuEPO than adults. Iron supplementation, either administered orally or intravenously, is also required and iron stores should be monitored closely to avoid iron overload.

Growth, Nutrition and Development

Growth impairment is a common and visible complication of CKD. In a study of 5000 children with CKD it was found that 35% had a height which was lower than the third percentile (or below a median height standard deviation score [HtSDS] of –1.88). Factors limiting the growth of children with CKD include disorders of mineral and bone metabolism, polyuria, metabolic acidosis, poor nutritional intake, anaemia and fluid and electrolyte disorders. Uraemia may cause anorexia and vomiting with a consequent reduction in nutritional intake. For this reason nasogastric or gastrostomy feeding may be required in order to maximise caloric intake. Protein intake should be maintained above the recommended reference nutrient intake to ensure adequate growth. However, protein intake should be no higher than 120% of daily recommended intake in children with stage 4–5 CKD or 100% of daily recommended intake for children on dialysis.

Recombinant human growth hormone (rhGH) should be considered if the child's height and/or growth velocity remain significantly reduced despite optimal nutritional and dialysis status, correction of metabolic acidosis and reduction of steroid therapy to a minimum.

Standard childhood vitamin supplements should not routinely be prescribed for CKD patients because of adverse effects related to increased intake of Vitamin A. Special multivitamin supplements are available for patients on dialysis.

Hyperkalaemia occurs when GFR has declined to less than 10% of normal. This is mainly related to dietary intake but other contributory factors include: reduced caloric intake, acidosis, and the use of certain antihypertensives (e.g. ACE inhibitors) and potassium-sparing drugs (e.g. spironolactone, amiloride). Hyperkalaemia can often be managed with dietary restriction but treatment with agents such as calcium resonium or sodium resonium may also be required.

RENAL REPLACEMENT THERAPY

Peritoneal Dialysis

Peritoneal dialysis (PD) is usually the best form of renal replacement therapy for children on chronic dialysis. The major benefit of PD is that it can be performed at home. PD relies on the principles of diffusion and osmosis. Sterile dialysate is instilled into the peritoneal cavity. Solutes move along a concentration gradient across the peritoneal membrane via diffusion, and the transfer of water occurs by osmosis. In addition, the 'ultrafiltration' of water across the peritoneal membrane is accompanied by 'solvent drag' which results in the transfer of solutes across the peritoneal membrane even when a concentration gradient is not present.

Commercial dialysate solutions are typically available with dextrose concentrations of 1.5%, 2.5% and 4.25%. By increasing the osmotic gradient across the peritoneal membrane, higher dextrose concentrations usually have a greater ability to remove fluid. However, the long-term use of hypertonic dialysate solutions results can result in peritoneal fibrosis and impaired function due to chronic exposure of the peritoneal membrane to glucose degradation products (GDPs).

The main PD regimens are:

- *Continuous ambulatory peritoneal dialysis (CAPD).* Fluid is manually instilled into the peritoneal cavity and then drained from it – typically up to four times per day. Fluid is also instilled overnight and drained in the morning. In practice, CAPD is rarely used in children
- *Automated peritoneal dialysis (APD)* (Figure 2.1)

An automated PD cycler machine is used to deliver a personalised programme of dialysis over a certain number of cycles and hours. Children receiving this form of dialysis are either managed by nocturnal intermittent PD (NIPD) or continuous cycling PD (CCPD).

- *NIPD*: This consists of an overnight regimen, with PD being performed while the young patient is asleep. The peritoneal cavity is left empty during the day.
- *CCPD*: This involves a combination of overnight PD and day time filling.
- *Adapted APD* (AAPD): Some machines offer more flexible control of dwell times and fill volumes overnight to promote sodium removal.
- *Tidal PD*: In this variant only a proportion of the fill volume (usually 50–80%) is drained with each cycle during the overnight PD regimen. This may be indicated in children who experience discomfort/pain with drainage of PD.

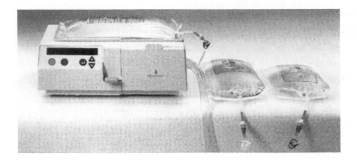

Figure 2.1 Compact peritoneal dialysis machine for automated overnight home dialysis.

The efficiency of PD is dependent on the integrity of the peritoneal membrane and the ease with which the PD catheter allows the instillation and drainage of fluid in and out of the peritoneal cavity.

Infection

If peritonitis is suspected, a PD fluid sample should be collected as soon as possible and be sent for cell count and bacterial/fungal culture. Treatment with intraperitoneal and/or intravenous antibiotics is commenced it there is an elevated white cell count (>100 WBC × 10^6/L) in the PD effluent or the presence of peritonitis is confirmed on positive culture. Appropriate antifungal coverage (usually with oral anti-fungal agent) may also be indicated.

Indications for removal of a PD catheter include:

- Recurrent bacterial peritonitis with the same organism within 4 weeks of stopping therapy (particularly Pseudomonas infection as this is difficult to eradicate)
- Refractory catheter infections
- Exit-site and PD catheter tunnel infections with an organism which is also responsible for concurrent peritonitis, or which then leads to peritonitis
- Fungal peritonitis
- Severe peritonitis leading to septic shock

Haemodialysis

Haemodialysis (HD) is more efficient for solute clearance and can be used in the acute setting to rapidly remove large volumes of fluid (e.g. in patients with pulmonary oedema). HD works on the principles of both diffusion and convection. Removal of water is due mainly to hydrostatic pressure across the dialyser membrane (ultrafiltration) while waste products are mostly removed from the circulation by via diffusion. Convection relies on the principle of solvent drag. It is independent of the concentration gradient across the dialysis membrane but is dependent on both the dialyser and the rate of ultrafiltration.

Patients requiring acute in-centre HD usually attend 3–4 times a week for sessions lasting between 3 and 4 hours. Some centres offer nocturnal in-centre dialysis whereby the dialysis time can be maximised whilst the patient is asleep. The use of home HD is increasing and has been demonstrated to have many benefits including increased opportunities to attend school, improved cardiovascular outcomes, improved blood pressure control and reduced requirement for antihypertensive medications. It also offers improved growth and energy levels, and improved quality of life.

New HD machines have been designed for small infants requiring intermittent HD. One such machine can be used in infants weighing between 2.5 and 10 kg whilst another machine is suitable for use in infants weighing as little as 800 g.

Vascular access for acute HD typically requires the insertion of a temporary double lumen catheter (e.g. Vascath) (Figure 2.2). Chronic HD is performed via a tunnelled double lumen catheter (e.g. Permcath) or an arteriovenous fistula. Fistulas are often preferable because of the lower risk of catheter-related infection. However, the disadvantages of fistulas include the delay of around 6 weeks before they can be used and the requirement for the child to co-operate with repeated needle punctures.

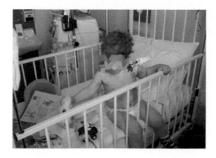

Figure 2.2 Haemodialysis via subclavian vascular access catheter.

Haemodiafiltration (HDF) is a modality which provides more effective removal of middle-sized molecular weight molecules and has been proven to improve long-term cardiovascular outcomes. However, there are a number of limitations to its use and HDF is only provided by a few paediatric nephrology centres at present.

Continuous renal replacement therapy (CRRT) involves an extracorporeal circuit similar to intermittent HD and is typically used in the intensive care setting. CRRT is the modality of choice for patients who are haemodynamically unstable as it generally avoids causing rapid fluid shifts which may precipitate drops in blood pressure or cardiac output.

Kidney Transplantation

Kidney transplantation remains the gold standard for renal replacement therapy. Compared with both PD and HD, renal transplantation provides a better quality of life, improved growth potential and a lower risk of significant complications. Young children receiving a renal transplant have the best long-term outcomes of any age group. The freedom from dietary and fluid volume restrictions, as well as the ability to attend school and live a life independent of a dialysis machine benefits both the child and their family.

A living donor (LD) kidney is preferable because graft survival rates are superior to those obtained with deceased donor (DD) kidneys. To increase the rates of living donation, several countries have introduced living kidney sharing schemes to promote paired donation of kidneys.

An induction regimen of immunosuppression is given at the time of transplantation. This comprises steroids, and either basiliximab (an anti-CD25 monoclonal antibody) or antithymocyte globulin. Following renal transplantation the immunosuppressive regimen usually includes a calcineurin inhibitor (e.g. tacrolimus) and an antiproliferative agent (e.g. mycophenolate mofetil) with or without corticosteroids.

The complications and potential adverse long-term effects of transplantation include:

- *Infection.* Immunosuppression may allow proliferation of Epstein–Barr virus (EBV), cytomegalovirus (CMV) and BK virus (BKV). Screening for EBV should be performed prior to transplantation. Proliferation of EBV may increase the risk of post-transplant lymphoproliferative disorder (PTLD) – which may range in severity from benign enlargement of tissues or an organ to classical Hodgkin lymphoma-type PTLD. Patients are particularly at risk of *Pneumocystis jirovecii* pneumonia in the first 6 months post-transplant and co-trimoxazole prophylaxis is often prescribed during this time period.
- *Immunisation risks.* Any immunisations with live vaccines should be given prior to transplantation. Thereafter, children with a renal transplant should only be immunised with inactivated vaccines because of the risk of vaccine-induced disease secondary to immunosuppression.
- *Acute rejection.* This is an important cause of early graft dysfunction and may be due to either T-cell mediated rejection or antibody-mediated rejection. The diagnosis is made by renal biopsy and identifying donor specific antibodies (DSA) in the recipient's blood.
- *Increased cancer risk.* In addition to post-transplant lymphoproliferative disorder, transplant recipients are known to be at an increased long-term risk of developing skin cancer (particularly squamous cell carcinoma) and Kaposi sarcoma.
- *Recurrent disease.* Certain conditions, such as focal and segmental glomerulosclerosis (FSGS) have a high risk of recurring in the transplant kidney. Other conditions carrying a risk of recurrence include: atypical HUS, C3 glomerulopathy and dense deposit disease.

- *New onset diabetes after transplantation (NODAT)*: Impaired glucose tolerance may be exacerbated by corticosteroids and calcineurin inhibitors, thus leading to a diabetic state requiring treatment with oral antihyperglycaemic agents or insulin. NODAT is known to be associated with poorer graft survival.
- *Transition period.* The transition period from paediatric to adult health care services is recognised to be a high-risk period for graft loss, primarily due to poor medication adherence and risk-taking behaviours. Many centres now offer counselling and education to patients and families and provide specialised transition services and clinics.

In the absence of a pre-emptive kidney transplant, patients typically require a period of dialysis.

- Kidney transplantation does not offer a cure for renal failure and an allograft will have its own life expectancy. Patients with chronic kidney disease are involved in a cycle of dialysis and transplantation for the remainder of their lives.

KEY POINTS

- The developing kidney has a limited capacity to respond to physiological insults and damaged nephrons are incapable of repair or regeneration. Careful management of fluid and electrolyte balance is particularly important in sick or compromised infants.
- Chronic kidney disease in children is rare and may not be diagnosed until it is relatively advanced because the early stages are typically asymptomatic. Its management is complex and demands the expertise of a skilled multidisciplinary team.
- Chronic kidney disease is associated with many complications that may have an adverse impact on quality of life. Skilled nutritional and medical management are important in helping to reduce morbidity.
- Renal transplantation is the treatment of choice for end-stage kidney disease in children as it confers improved survival and better quality of life. Living donation is preferred over deceased donation for the same reason.

FURTHER READING

Abitbol CL, DeFreitas MJ, Strauss, J. Assessment of kidney function in preterm infants: lifelong implications. Pediatr Nephrol. 2016;31(12):2213–2222.

Becherucci F, Roperto RM, Materassi M, Romagnani P. Chronic kidney disease in children. Clin Kidney J. 2016;9(4):583–591.

Chesayne NC, van Stralen KJ, Bonthuis M, Harambat J, Groothoff JW, Jager KJ. Survival in children requiring chronic renal replacement therapy. Pediatr Nephrol. 2018;33:585–594.

Mumford L, Maxwell H, Ahmad N, Marks SD, Tizard J. The impact of changing practice on improved outcomes of paediatric renal transplantation in the United Kingdom: a 25 years review. Transpl Int. 2019;32(7):751–761.

North American Paediatric Renal Trials and Collaborative Studies. NAPRTCS 2014 Annual Transplant Report. 2014. http://naprtcs.org/system/files/2014_annual_transplant_report.pdf

Rees L, Bockenhauer D, Webb NJA, Punaro MG. Paediatric Nephrology, 3rd Edition. Oxford: Oxford University Press; 2019.

Watson AR, Harden P, Ferris M, Kerr PG, Mahan J, Ramzy MF. Transition from paediatric to adult renal services: a consensus statement by the International Society of Nephrology (ISN) and the International Paediatric Nephrology Association (IPNA). Pediatr Nephrol. 2011;26(10):1753–1757.

Imaging

MELANIE P HIORNS

Topics covered

Ultrasonography (US) including contrast-
enhanced ultrasound (CEUS)
Micturating cystourethrography (MCUG)
Alternative methods of cystography
(IRC and DIC)
DMSA scintigraphy

Dynamic diuresis renography
(MAG3 and DTPA)
Magnetic resonance imaging (MRI)
Computed tomography (CT)
Abdominal X-ray (AXR)
Interventional techniques

INTRODUCTION

Imaging of the urinary tract provides valuable information on anatomy, function, and frequently, both. The imaging techniques described in this chapter are those of greatest relevance to contemporary urological imaging in children in a standard healthcare setting. Some new modalities such as magnetic resonance imaging (MRI) and contrast-enhanced ultrasound (CEUS) are also being used increasingly in specialist centres.

ULTRASOUND AND DOPPLER

Ultrasound (US) is very well tolerated in children and is the investigation of first choice for suspected urinary tract pathology. It offers considerable advantages in this age group, being a painless,

low cost investigation which does not expose the child to ionising radiation. The anatomical resolution provided by US is usually excellent in children because they have less body fat and a smaller body habitus. US is highly sensitive in the detection of renal stones, cysts, and conditions associated with dilatation. However, it is less sensitive for visualising abnormalities in nondilated ureters and provides no information on function. Another drawback is the degree of operator/observer dependence. Contrast-enhanced ultrasound (CEUS) is a dynamic imaging technique which can be used to assess renal perfusion when the contrast is given intravenously, or to study the structure of the urinary tract when it is introduced via a catheter into the bladder.

Technical Aspects

Children are routinely scanned in both the supine and prone positions.

The bladder is scanned first because infants tend to void when their abdomen is exposed and older children who arrive with a full bladder are more comfortable if the bladder is scanned at the outset.

A significant post-void residual volume is defined as one exceeding 10% of normal age-adjusted bladder capacity. If the bladder is very full it may give rise to transient "physiological" upper tract dilatation (hydronephrosis) and when this is present the bladder should be rescanned after voiding.

US is not a reliable means of detecting vesico ureteric reflux – which requires either a micturating cystourethrogram (MCUG), indirect radionuclide cystogram (IRC) or, where available, CEUS.

Measurements in the Lower Urinary Tract

A bladder wall thickness of up to 3 mm is normal. Bladder volume is either calculated automatically by the imaging software, or by reference to standard formulae. This methodology is not suitable for bladders which have been augmented or are irregular in shape. In such cases it is more accurate to directly measure the volume of urine drained from the bladder – for example at the time of intermittent catheterisation.

Measurements in the Upper Urinary Tract

Longitudinal dimensions of the kidneys are usually obtained with the child in a supine position. Values for renal length can be compared with data in standard charts providing 5th and 95th centile values for renal length at different ages. An antero posterior (AP) diameter of the renal pelvis of <7 mm is regarded as normal whereas an AP diameter greater than 10 mm is considered to be abnormal. Normal renal parenchyma should be of lower echogenicity than the adjacent liver or spleen. The term "corticomedullary differentiation" is used to describe the slightly lower echogenicity of the pyramids (or medulla) by comparison with the cortex. The kidneys of children with end-stage chronic renal failure are also echo-bright but lose their normal corticomedullary differentiation.

Indications

The principal indications for performing renal US are for:

- Evaluation of congenital anomalies (including antenatally detected hydronephrosis)
- Investigation of urinary tract infection
- Imaging of stone disease (Figure 3.1) or nephrocalcinosis (Figure 3.2)

US plays an important role in the evaluation of antenatally diagnosed hydronephrosis. It is also valuable for the assessment of ectopic kidneys and duplicated systems (Figure 3.3) and renal cystic disease – although it is important to distinguish the appearances from those of severe hydronephrosis (Figures 3.4, 3.5).

In the acute phase of a urinary tract infection (UTI) ultrasound may reveal evidence of an obstructed or dilated urinary tract, calculi or debris within the collecting system or features of focal pyelonephritis. The US findings may contribute to acute management, including the possible need for intervention.

Even when the US findings do not influence acute management they may be helpful in identifying congenital abnormalities predisposing the child to further UTIs. Although US can detect pyelonephritic scarring, Tc 99m dimercaptosuccinic acid (DMSA) and magnetic resonance imaging (MRI) with contrast are more sensitive examinations for this purpose.

Ultrasound can visualise calculi as small as 1–2 mm in diameter and it is a more worthwhile investigation than plain radiography for the initial investigation of suspected renal colic (Figure 3.1).

Unlike renal stones, mid ureteric stones are often difficult to visualise with US because of overlying bowel gas and bowel contents. Ultrasound (usually in conjunction with micturating cystourethrography (MCUG) can also be used for the investigation of urethral abnormalities such as syringocele, posterior urethral valves, or stone disease. In suspected renal tumours US

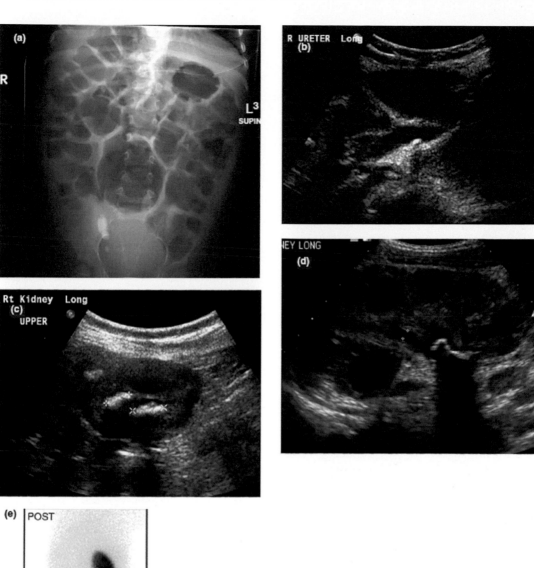

Figure 3.1 Urinary calculi. (a) Abdominal X-ray demonstrating stones in the right ureter. (b) Ultrasound demonstrating the same stones in the distal ureter. (c) Ultrasound demonstrating further stones in the kidney with characteristic acoustic shadowing. (d) Ultrasound in a different patient showing a staghorn renal calculus. (e) DMSA demonstrating complete loss of function in this kidney.

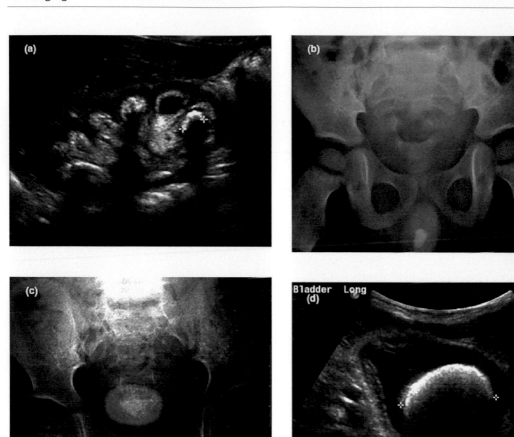

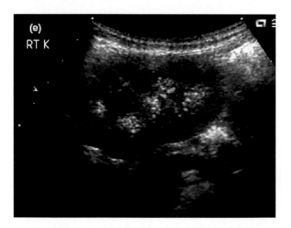

Figure 3.2 Other examples of calcification in the urinary tract. (a) Ultrasound showing nephrocalcinosis and calculi occurring together in the same kidney. The nephrocalcinosis shows the typical arching calcification around the renal pyramids and the stone casts an acoustic shadow. (b) Stone in the urethra demonstrated on plain X ray. (c) Bladder stone on abdominal X-ray. (d) Ultrasound appearances of the same stone. (e) Ultrasound in a different patient showing the specks of echogenicity in medullary calcinosis.

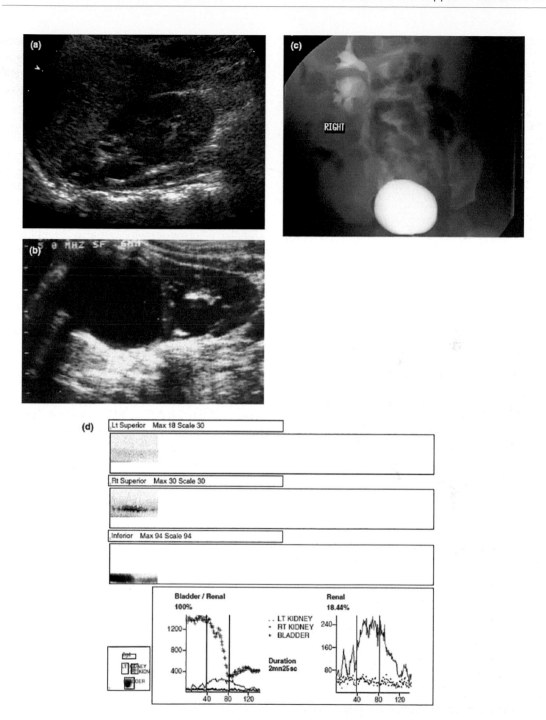

Figure 3.3 Imaging of duplex kidneys in different patients. (a) Ultrasound showing a scarred upper pole in the right upper moiety. (b) Ultrasound in another patient demonstrating marked dilatation of the upper pole due to distal ureteric obstruction by a ureterocele and moderate lower pole dilatation associated with lower pole reflux. (c) Micturating cystourethrogram (MCUG) in a different patient showing reflux into both the upper and lower moiety on the right. (d) Reflux demonstrated in the same patient by indirect MAG3 cystogram showing an increase in activity over the right kidney during voiding.

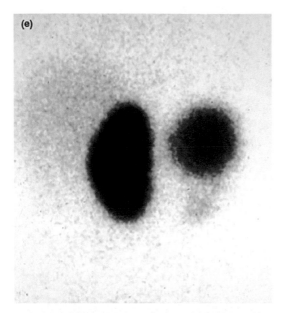

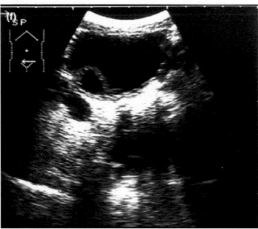

Figure 3.3 (Continued) Imaging of duplex kidneys in different patients. (e) DMSA scan in another patient demonstrating near total loss of function in the lower pole of duplex kidney due to scarring/dysplasia. (f) Dilated distal ureter and associated ureterocele visualised on US.

provides information on the contralateral kidney, the integrity of the capsule of the affected kidney and whether there is tumour thrombus within the renal vein or the inferior vena cava (IVC).

Finally, US plays an important role in the initial imaging of renal trauma by providing information about the integrity of the kidney and the renal capsule and the presence of haematoma. It can also provide some information on renal blood flow and perfusion – which can be augmented by CEUS (Figure 3.6).

Doppler Ultrasonography

Doppler US is used to assess renal blood flow in transplant kidneys and in cases of renal artery stenosis or arteriovenous malformations. It is also used in the investigation of hypertension. Doppler ultrasonography can also be applied to venous flow to assess tumour extension within the renal vein or IVC and suspected renal vein thrombosis.

Contrast-Enhanced Ultrasound (CEUS)

This technique utilises the differing characteristics of US waves when they are reflected by interfaces within structures and tissues. The contrast medium used for CEUS consists of a solution of gas-filled microbubbles which can either be injected intravenously or introduced into the bladder via a catheter. Tissues or structures containing the microbubbles appear echogenic on US scanning. Contrast-enhanced ultrasound can be used to demonstrate areas of perfusion in a kidney or renal tumour or haemorrhage from a renal laceration (Figure 3.6). When the contrast is introduced into the bladder CEUS can be used for the dynamic assessment of vesico ureteric reflux and has the advantage that several filling cycles can be performed. CEUS can also be used to visualise the urethra during voiding to facilitate the detection of obstructive and nonobstructive urethral pathology. It is also a useful technique for the evaluation of ambiguous genitalia and cloacal malformations because the solution of microbubbles may demonstrate unexpected connections between cavities which may be less apparent on conventional contrast examinations.

However, CEUS requires availability of a high quality modern US scanner and a suitably trained sonographer or radiologist.

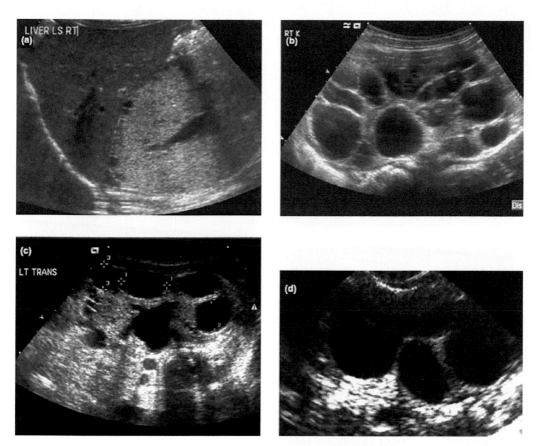

Figure 3.4 Cystic disease. US appearances of (a) Autosomal recessive polycystic kidney disease with bright parenchyma and multiple tiny cysts. (b) Autosomal dominant polycystic kidney disease with multiple large hypoechoic cysts. (c) Cystic dysplasia with scattered cysts. (d) Multicystic dysplastic kidney with multiple cysts and septa containing no intervening renal parenchyma.

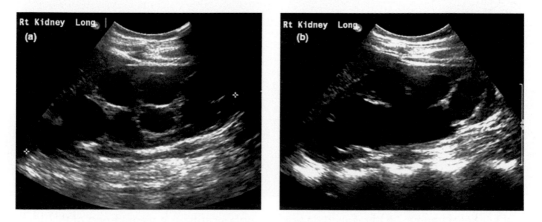

Figure 3.5 Renal ultrasound in a patient with (a) Autosomal dominant polycystic kidney disease compared with a different patient with (b) Marked hydronephrosis. The initial appearances are very similar but a skilled sonographer can demonstrate that in the hydronephrotic kidney (b) the 'cysts' all interconnect because they are in fact, calyces in a dilated collecting system.

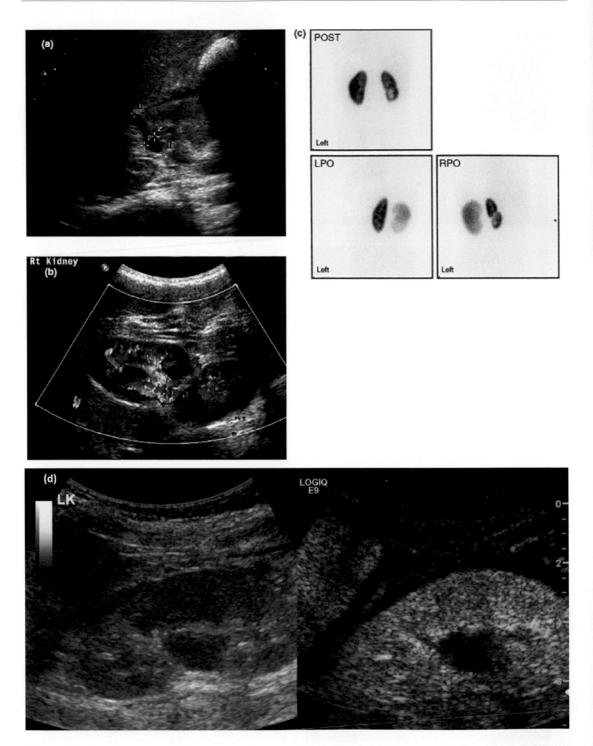

Figure 3.6 Renal trauma. (a) Ultrasound demonstrating a laceration in the mid-part of the right kidney. (b) Repeat ultrasound 3 months later showing shrinkage of the lower pole and reduction in blood flow on Doppler. (c) DMSA appearances at 3 months in this patient. (d) Contrast-enhanced ultrasound (CEUS) demonstrating active haemorrhage (visualised as a stream of 'bubbles') from a traumatic injury to the upper pole of a kidney.

MICTURATING CYSTOURETHROGRAPHY (VOIDING CYSTOURETHROGRAPHY)

Indications

The MCUG – or voiding cystourethrogram (VCUG) remains the most widely used and readily available examination for detecting and grading vesicoureteric reflux (VUR). However, it is important to be aware that VUR sometimes occurs as an intermittent phenomenon and it is possible to "miss" reflux if it does not occur during the course of the study. MCUG is the only form of imaging which can provide detailed anatomical information on the urethra (Figure 3.7). For this reason it remains the key investigation for excluding or confirming the presence of an obstructing urethral abnormality in boys with bilateral hydronephrosis. Other indications include; bladder wall thickening, poor urinary stream and incomplete emptying – all of which may be indicative of an underlying urethral obstruction. MCUG (sometimes supplemented by retrograde urethrography) is also widely used for the evaluation of urethral trauma in males. A principal limitation of MCUG is the burden of ionising radiation. However, the radiation dose can be significantly reduced by using "grabbed" digital images and removing the grid on the image intensifier.

Technical Aspects

A micturating cystourethrogram (MCUG) is routinely performed under antibiotic cover. If the child is suffering from an active (or suspected) UTI or is generally unwell the MCUG should be deferred until 4–6 weeks after the infection has been eradicated.

Following urethral catheterisation (typically with a 6F feeding tube) the bladder is filled with water soluble contrast. Imaging during the voiding phase is important because in some children (including those with an ectopic ureter) reflux may only occur when they void. Conversely, very early filling views are required to visualise ureteroceles (Figure 3.8).

Steep oblique or true lateral views are needed to demonstrate posterior urethral valves (PUV) and it is important that the entire urethra is visualised to avoid missing rare anterior urethral lesions or meatal stenosis.

Alternatives to MCUG

CEUS voiding ultrasonography

This is described above in section titled Contrast-Enhanced Ultrasound.

Isotope cystography

Direct isotope cystography (DIC) requires catheterisation to introduce the isotope into the bladder whereas in the technique of indirect cystography (IRC) the isotope (Tc-99m labelled dimercaptoacetyltriglycine) — MAG3 is injected intravenously and is then excreted into the urine. In addition to being a more "physiological" investigation, the radiation burden of IRC is lower than MCUG. It also provides information on differential renal function when combined with conventional renography. Good hydration is essential to promote an adequate diuresis and ensure that the isotope does not accumulate in the kidneys and prevent adequate visualisation of the rest of the urinary tract. In the absence of reflux, activity over the kidneys decreases as the study progresses but when reflux is present, isotope which has already drained into the bladder is transported back to the kidney- giving rise to a detectable increase in activity in the renal region. IRC can only be used to detect reflux during the voiding or resting phases of bladder function and not during bladder filling.

The limitations of IRC include poor sensitivity for the detection of lower grades of VUR and unsuitability for use in infants or in children of any age who are uncooperative or not toilet trained. In addition, the reliability of IRC for the detection of VUR is reduced when there is stasis of urine in a dilated upper tract. Nevertheless, IRC can be a useful investigation for excluding clinically significant VUR in older girls with recurrent UTIs, and for following up of known reflux in children of either sex.

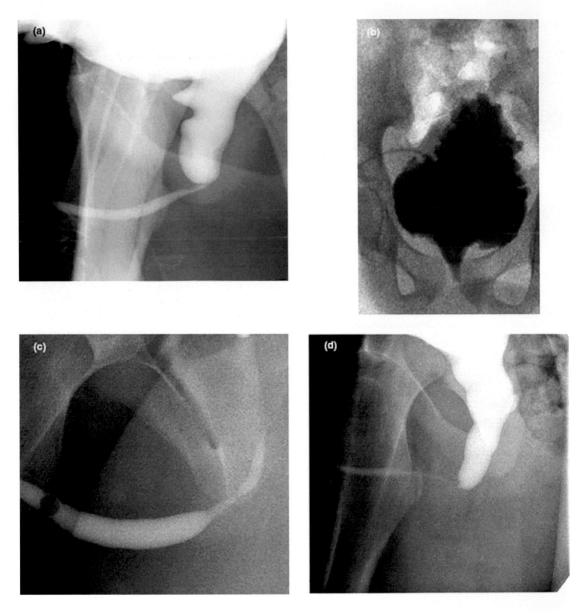

Figure 3.7 Examples of urethral abnormalities demonstrated by MCUG. (a) Typical appearance in posterior urethral valves with an abrupt change in calibre of the urethra at the level of the valve leaflet. (b) Heavily trabeculated bladder indicating long standing outflow obstruction. (c) Urethral stricture – best demonstrated with a simultaneous retrograde urethrogram. (d) MCUG alone does not delineate the distal extent of the stricture.

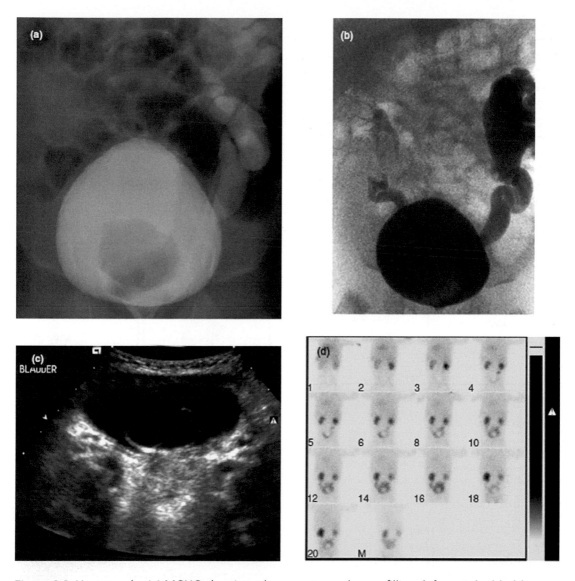

Figure 3.8 Ureterocele. (a) MCUG showing a large ureterocele as a filling defect at the bladder base with (b) Associated reflux into the dilated lower moiety of a duplex kidney. (c) US demonstrating the ureterocele at the bladder base. (d) MAG3 renogram demonstrating reflux on the left and the photopenic area of the ureterocele in the bladder.

DMSA SCINTIGRAPHY (STATIC RENOGRAPHY)

Technical Aspects

Technetium-99m DMSA binds to the proximal convoluted tubules with only 10% of the injected dose being excreted in the urine.

The injected dose of Tc99m DMSA is calculated according to body surface area – which is estimated from the child's age and weight. Static images are acquired approximately 2–3 hours after the injection of isotope tracer.

Indications

A DMSA scan provides static images of functioning tissue and can be used to quantify relative (differential) function between two kidneys. Normal values for differential renal function are in the range 45%–55%. It is important to note, however, that values for differential function are comparative rather than absolute measures of renal function. Despite significant impairment of overall renal function DMSA can therefore yield misleadingly "normal" values for differential function if both kidneys are equally affected by renal damage.

DMSA is a sensitive modality for documenting the presence and progression of renal scarring. It is also very useful for identifying small and/or ectopic kidneys and cryptic or occult duplication anomalies (Figures 3.9, 3.10). By demonstrating an "isthmus" of functioning tissue crossing the midline, DMSA can play a useful role in the diagnosis of horseshoe kidneys (Figure 3.11). It can also be used to confirm the diagnosis of multicystic dysplastic kidney (MCDK) by demonstrating that it is entirely non functioning. During the acute phase of a UTI, DMSA can demonstrate photopenic areas

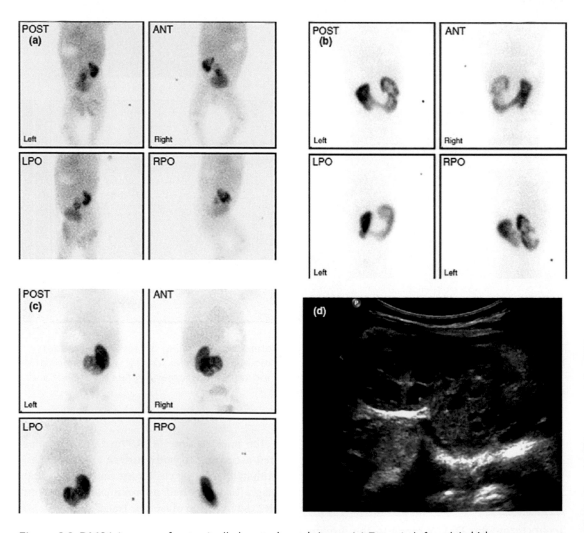

Figure 3.9 DMSA images of ectopically located renal tissue. (a) Ectopic left pelvic kidney. (b) Horseshoe kidney with functioning tissue crossing the midline. (c) Crossed fused ectopic kidney with (d) US demonstrating the two fused moieties in this patient.

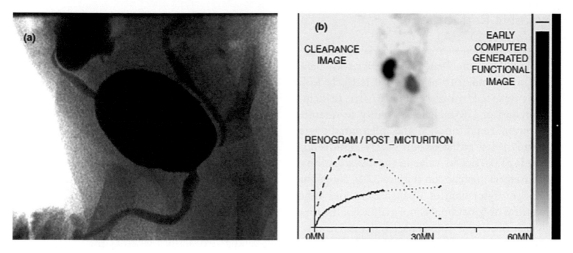

Figure 3.10 Pelvic kidney. (a) MCUG showing reflux into an abnormally sited kidney. (b) MAG3 demonstrating functioning parenchyma in an abnormal pelvic position with rising renogram curve.

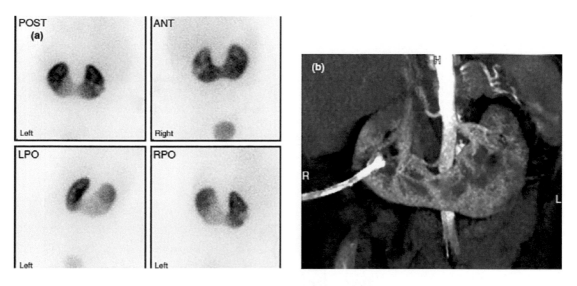

Figure 3.11 Horseshoe kidney. (a) DMSA demonstrates the presence of functioning renal tissue crossing the midline. (b) Coronal reconstruction from a CT angiogram for vascular anatomy pre surgery also demonstrates the configuration of the kidney (a nephrostomy tube is in place in the right moiety).

of renal parenchyma affected by pyelonephritis. However, the changes seen during or shortly after acute pyelonephritis may be transient and in order to demonstrate areas of permanent renal scarring the scan should be delayed until at least 8 weeks (preferably longer) after the infection has been eradicated. DMSA can also be used to delineate areas of renal tissue which are still functioning in cases of renal trauma (Figure 3.6). Disadvantages include the requirement for venous cannulation, the limited yield of anatomical information and the reduced image quality in neonates with immature renal function. DMSA also imposes a higher radiation burden than dynamic renography (DR) with Tc-99m labelled MAG3.

Dynamic Renography (MAG3 or DTPA)

Although Dynamic Renography (DR) is still being used in the majority of centres it is likely to be largely replaced by functional MRI. The principal advantages of DR include its ability to quantify differential renal function and differential drainage and the low radiation burden. Dynamic renography is of particular value in the investigation of pelviureteric obstruction (Figure 3.12), congenital drainage abnormalities (megaureters and other structural or functional abnormalities of the renal pelvis or ureters) and in duplex systems. However, it is of more limited value in children with reduced renal function and in those under 2 years of age – especially infants under 6 months.

Technical Aspects

Differential renal function is usually acquired at about 1 to 2 minutes after the injection of the iso-tope. Drainage from the kidney is estimated by assessing the renogram curve, with the normal pattern being an early peak followed by a rapidly descending phase. A continually ascending curve suggests a delay in excretion. In this situation the administration of a diuretic may help to distin-guish between stasis and obstruction. (See also Chapter 7.)

The most commonly used isotope is Tc99m dimercaptoacetyltriglycine (MAG3) (which relies on tubular extraction) whereas the use of Tc99m diethylentriaminepentaacetic acid (DTPA) - which relies on filtration is declining.

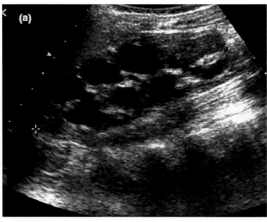

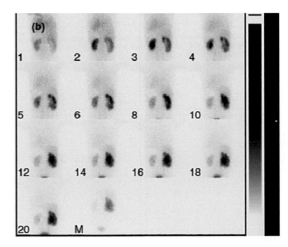

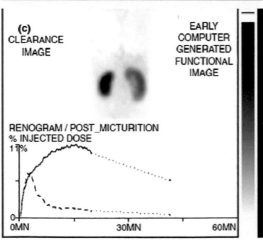

Figure 3.12 Pelviureteric junction obstruction. (a) US showing hydronephrosis (b) MAG 3 in the same case demonstrating delayed transit of isotope with poor drainage after micturition and (c) Rising excretion curve in the right kidney indicating accumulating isotope and poor drainage.

Cross-Sectional Imaging

This term is most commonly applied to computed tomography (CT) and magnetic resonance imaging (MRI). CT plays only a limited role in children because of the high ionising radiation dose. MRI does not involve any exposure to radiation but has the disadvantage that sedation or general anaesthesia are often required to ensure the child remains absolutely still during the scan.

Magnetic Resonance Imaging (MRI)

Unlike CT, MRI provides multiplanar images and also offers superior delineation of different types of tissue (both before and after contrast media). For imaging of the urinary tract MRI offers the additional advantage of providing excellent delineation of urine-containing structures.

Indications

MR is now the examination of choice for the assessment of malignant and benign renal tumours (Figures 3.13, 3.14). In this context, MR angiography can yield particularly useful information on tumour vasculature prior to surgery. The role of preoperative MR angiography is not confined to malignant conditions and, for example, it can demonstrate the presence of aberrant "crossing vessels" prior to a pyeloplasty or vascular hitch procedure for pelviureteric junction (PUJ) obstruction (Figure 3.15). Because many paediatric urological procedures are now being performed laparoscopically, MR is playing an increasingly important role by providing the surgeon with anatomical information which could previously only have been obtained at the time of open surgery.

MR is also a very valuable means of defining complex upper tract anatomy – notably in duplex systems with ectopic insertion of ureters.

MR angiography forms an important part of the work-up for renal transplantation by delineating vasculature within the abdomen prior to surgery (Figure 3.16).

Technical Aspects

Scan times can be up to 30 minutes or even longer, and the patient must remain absolutely still for the duration of the scan. Infants under 6 months can be immobilised using a "feed and wrap" technique in which they sleep throughout the study. Older infants can be scanned with sedation but between the ages of 18 months and 5 years general anaesthesia is usually required.

The child must be well hydrated and venous access is necessary for the administration of furosemide (to promote diuresis) and a gadolinium-based contrast medium.

The term "sequence" is applied to a selected group of different technical parameters which determine the characteristics of the resulting image. T1 weighted images provide anatomical detail whereas T2 weighted images are a better guide to pathology. On T2 images, water returns a high signal (white) and therefore T2 weighted sequences are very useful for imaging structures such as the renal pelvis, ureters and bladder. The use of gadolinium intravenous MRI contrast medium is very useful for assessing tumour vascularity and in demonstrating kidney function and excretion.

MR urography (MRU) is being increasingly used to provide accurate anatomical evaluation of abnormalities of both the upper and lower urinary tract. Heavily weighted T2 sequences are generally used for this purpose because of their ability to clearly delineate urine-containing structures. MRU has the added advantage of providing high resolution images of the renal parenchyma and collecting system during all phases of kidney function – vascular, filtration, and excretion. It is capable of providing detailed images of the ureters and any part of the urinary tract which is dilated. The use of MRI is also being extended to include the acquisition of the same type of functional information which is provided by a MAG3 or DMSA scan.

In summary, MR is rapidly becoming regarded as a standard "mainstream" form of diagnostic imaging in paediatric urology.

Computed Tomography (CT)

CT is not regarded as a "front line" investigation in paediatric urology because many of the roles fulfilled by CT in adults can be fulfilled by US in children. Nevertheless, CT remains an important

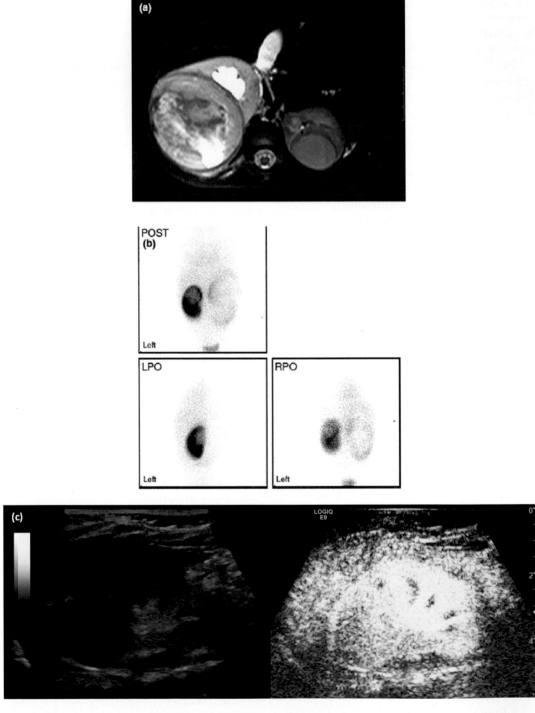

Figure 3.13 Renal tumours. (a) MRI with intravenous contrast. Coronal plane image showing bilateral Wilms tumour in a horseshoe kidney. (b) DMSA in the same patient demonstrating the bilateral tumours as photopenic areas which do not contain normally functioning renal tissue. (c) CEUS showing poor washout of a hypoechoic lesion at the upper pole of a lesion confirmed as mesoblastic nephroma.

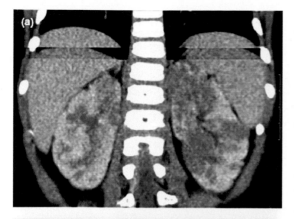

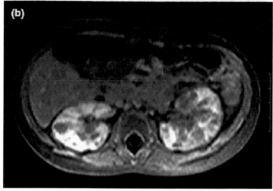

Figure 3.14 Nephroblastomatosis. (a) CT with intravenous contrast reconstructed in the coronal plane showing extensive nephroblastomatosis in both kidneys (the misregistration at the level of the diaphragm is due to the patient taking a breath during the scan). (b) MRI in the same patient demonstrates the same finding (in the transverse plane).

investigation for the evaluation of major trauma because of its high sensitivity for the detection of contusions, lacerations, perinephric fluid collections, areas of avascularity, bladder rupture, extra or intra peritoneal leakage of urine, and injury to other organs. CT also retains a role in the investigation of stone disease (including colic) – particularly in children with physical features such as marked scoliosis or obesity which limit the usefulness of US. MRI is a vastly superior technique for assessing tumours and has therefore superseded CT for this purpose. However, chest CT still plays a role for the assessment of pulmonary metastases.

Technical Aspects

Intravenous access is required for the administration of contrast medium – with the exception of scans being performed to visualise calcification (calculi) for which contrast is not required. Because modern multidetector CT scanners acquire images very rapidly (typically in 5–10 seconds after the start of the scan) most children can be successfully scanned without requiring sedation or anaesthesia. Contrast is usually administered as a "split bolus", typically with two boluses given 30–40 seconds apart. In this way both portal venous and arterial enhancement are obtained in a single scan. For a delayed scan in cases of trauma or suspected bladder rupture the two boluses are given 3–5 minutes apart. Every effort is made to keep the radiation dose to a minimum but even with ultramodern CT scanners the radiation dose from a combined abdominal and pelvic CT examination is significantly higher than that of a chest X-ray.

Abdominal X-Ray (AXR)

AXR is no longer regarded as a routine investigation in paediatric urology and its role is now largely limited to the detection of urinary tract calculi, spinal anomalies, abdominal or pelvic mass lesions and constipation. US can provide most of the information previously sought by AXR.

Arteriography

Arteriography may be indicated when renal artery stenosis is suspected. However, this is usually investigated by US (including Doppler) in the first instance and then by MRI. Conventional arteriography does, however, have the advantage that it can be combined with renal artery angioplasty under the same anaesthetic. Arteriography is also useful in middle aortic syndrome, and again angioplasty may be used. Some renal and bladder arteriovenous malformations are treatable by embolisation.

Venography

Selective sampling of renal veins (for renin) and the IVC may be indicated in children whose

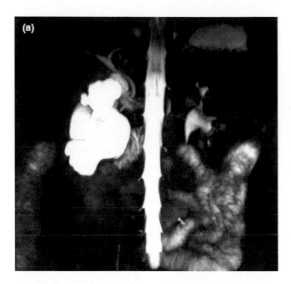
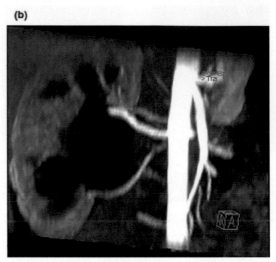

Figure 3.15 Pelviureteric junction obstruction. MRI in a patient with a 'crossing vessel' causing pelviureteric junction obstruction. (a) Heavily T2 weighted sequence showing marked hydronephrosis of the right kidney. (b) T1 weighted sequence after intravenous gadolinium. This demonstrates both the main right renal artery and the accessory artery 'crossing' the distended renal pelvis (and causing the PUJ obstruction. This example demonstrates the ability of MRI to delineate both the renal pelvic anatomy and the dynamic vascular anatomy in the same examination.

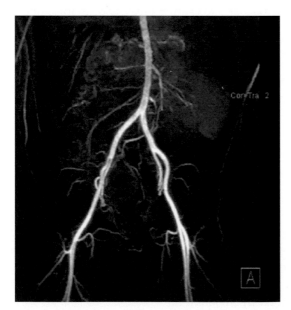

Figure 3.16 Pre-transplant "work-up" MR angiography: coronal images following intravenous gadolinium performed in the work-up for renal transplant showing a normal aorta, iliac and femoral arteries

hypertension is thought to arise from excessive renin production by a scarred or dysplastic kidney. Venography and embolisation are a widely accepted technique for the treatment of varicoceles.

Antegrade Pyelography

The principal indication lies in the investigation of distal obstruction in the upper urinary tract. Antegrade pyelography via percutaneous renal puncture can be performed by an interventional radiologist or by a urologist.

Percutaneous Nephrostomy

This is often performed under ultrasound control but may be combined with fluoroscopy. The procedure is usually performed under general anaesthesia in children. Percutaneous nephrostomy is generally preferred to open surgical nephrostomy and drainage. Its main use is in the decompression and drainage of acutely obstructed or infected hydronephrosis – usually due to PUJ obstruction.

Renal and Tumour Biopsy

Although ultrasound guided procedures can generally be performed using sedation and local anaesthesia in compliant older children, general anaesthesia is required for the younger age group. Multiple cores are obtained. Whenever possible these undergo immediate microscopic examination to confirm that adequate tissue has been obtained so as to minimise the possible need for a repeat procedure and further anaesthetic.

KEY POINTS

- Congenital abnormalities of the urinary tract account for many of the conditions encountered in paediatric urology. A combination of imaging techniques is usually required to provide the degree of anatomical and functional information needed to plan open or minimally invasive surgical management.
- Ultrasound is invariably the initial urological investigation of choice in children. The scope of ultrasound is being extended by the introduction of contrast-enhanced ultrasound (CEUS) using microbubble contrast media.

- Dynamic and/or static renography is still widely used to assess functional parameters across a broad range of paediatric urological conditions. However, MR urography is being increasingly used for this purpose.
- MR provides excellent anatomical detail of normal and abnormal anatomy of the urinary tract without exposure to radiation. The principal limitation is the requirement for sedation or general anaesthesia in younger children.
- The use of CT in children is limited by the high radiation dosage. However, it retains an important role in the evaluation of major abdominal trauma.

FURTHER READING

Dickerson EC, Dillman JR, Smith EA, DiPetro MA, Lebowitz RL, Darge K. Paediatric MR urography: indications, techniques, and approach to review. Radiographics. 2015;35:1208–1230.

Duran C, Beltran VP, Gonzalez A, Gomez C, del Riego J. Contrast-enhanced voiding uro-sonography for vesicoureteral reflux diagnosis in children. Radiographics. 2017;37:1854–1869.

Prenatal Diagnosis

SARAH L HECHT and VIJAYA M VEMULAKONDA

Topics covered

Prenatal imaging	Initial management
Hydronephrotic anomalies	Non-hydronephrotic anomalies
Classification	Fetal intervention
Diagnoses	Counseling

INTRODUCTION

Since its inception in the 1970s, prenatal screening with fetal ultrasonography has become nearly ubiquitous. Abnormalities of the urogenital system are among the most commonly prenatally detected congenital anomalies because of their relatively high incidence and the fact that dilatation of the fetal urinary tract (hydronephrosis) is readily detected on ultrasound. The overwhelming majority of prenatally detected urologic abnormalities are associated with some degree of hydronephrosis. In most cases, prenatally detected hydronephrosis is a mild and/or transient ultrasound finding. While most infants with prenatally detected hydronephrosis have a very favorable outcome, a small but significant minority will prove to have significant renal disease. Depending on prevailing attitudes to termination of pregnancy a small proportion may survive to term but then die shortly after birth. Researchers and consensus panels have invested substantial effort into trying to distinguish between those ultrasound findings which denote clinically significant urologic disease and ultrasound appearances which are essentially innocent findings of little or no clinical significance. Many studies have been undertaken with the aim of defining reliable criteria to guide the postnatal investigation and management of infants with prenatally detected hydronephrosis. However, this remains a source of controversy.

PRENATAL IMAGING

Ultrasonography

Ultrasonography is the primary imaging modality during pregnancy. First trimester ultrasound is frequently obtained to confirm a viable intrauterine pregnancy, estimate conception date, and assess nuchal pad translucency to screen for aneuploidy. However, this is of limited value in screening for most congenital anomalies. The World Health

Organization recommends a single ultrasound prior to 24 weeks gestation. In the United States, the primary anatomic survey is obtained at 18–22 weeks gestational age, with additional scans being performed in high risk pregnancies or if a congenital anomaly is suspected. The second trimester scan usually provides sufficient anatomical detail to screen for major congenital anomalies. Additional information includes the position, size and movement of the fetus, heart rate, placental position, and the volume of amniotic fluid. The sensitivity and specificity of prenatal ultrasonography for the detection of congenital anomalies depends on many factors including maternal obesity, fetal position, sonographic equipment, and experience of the person performing the scan. Most of the serious, potentially lethal genitourinary anomalies, such as posterior urethral valves and bilateral renal agenesis are detected in the second trimester. However more common anomalies such as vesicoureteral reflux, ectopic ureters, and ureteroceles are not reliably detected at this stage in gestation and may not be detected prenatally unless further scans are performed later in pregnancy.

Magnetic Resonance Imaging

During the last two decades, prenatal magnetic resonance imaging (MRI) has been gaining popularity as a means of providing more detailed information on fetal abnormalities detected by prenatal ultrasound. MRI has higher soft tissue contrast resolution and is not limited by maternal habitus, fetal position, ossified structures or oligohydramnios. MRI does not use ionizing radiation and poses no known risk to the fetus. Common applications in urological diagnosis include distinguishing hydronephrosis from cystic abnormalities, delineating ureteral anatomy including duplication, ectopia, and ureteroceles, and clarifying the anatomy of complex anomalies such as cloacal anomalies and exstrophy-epispadias complex.

HYDRONEPHROSIS

Dilatation of the fetal urinary tract (fetal hydronephrosis) is the most common genitourinary abnormality identified on antenatal screening.

The reported incidence of fetal hydronephrosis ranges from 0.5% to 5% but this figure varies according to the gestational age at which scans are performed. Mild prenatally detected hydronephrosis is usually an innocent ultrasound finding which represents a transient physiologic state of no clinical significance. The overall incidence of antenatally detected hydronephrosis associated with a clinically significant uropathy is approximately 0.2%. It is important to minimize unnecessary investigation and repeated scans so as not to exacerbate parental anxiety. There is a broad correlation between the degree of hydronephrosis and the probable severity of the abnormality affecting the kidneys and/or urinary tract. Several classification systems have been developed to grade the severity of fetal hydronephrosis and guide further investigation but there is no consensus on which is the best for this purpose.

Classification Systems

Anterior-posterior renal pelvic diameter

This system classifies the severity of hydronephrosis based solely on the degree of dilatation of the renal pelvis. It is based on measurements of the anterior-posterior (AP) diameter of the renal pelvis in the transverse plane at the level of the renal hilum (within the confines of the parenchyma). The AP renal pelvic diameter varies according to gestational age. Therefore, the value chosen as the upper limit of normality strongly influences the specificity and sensitivity of AP diameter as a predictor of genitourinary pathology at different stages in pregnancy. Although there is no universal consensus, a renal pelvic diameter of greater than 10 mm in the second trimester is generally regarded as a significant finding, with an AP diameter of greater than 15 mm being regarded as the upper threshold in the third trimester.

Society for Fetal Urology (SFU) classification

The SFU developed a grading system for neonatal and infant hydronephrosis based on a combination of dilatation of the renal pelvis, calyceal dilatation and a subjective assessment of parenchymal thickness. Though originally devised for grading hydronephrosis postnatally, the SFU classification is also commonly applied to antenatal hydronephrosis. The SFU grading is based on the following criteria:

Grade 0: Normal ultrasound findings with no dilatation

Grade I: Dilatation confined to the renal pelvis

Grade II: Dilatation of the renal pelvis accompanied by dilatation of the major calyces

Grade III: Dilatation of the renal pelvis accompanied by dilatation of the major and minor calyces

Grade IV: As for Grade III plus thinning of the renal cortex (Figure 4.1)

Urinary Tract Dilation (UTD) classification

The UTD classification was devised by a multidisciplinary consensus panel with the aims of unifying different grading systems, introducing consistency into the terminology applied to antenatal and postnatal classification of hydronephrosis and correlating the antenatal grading with the clinical significance of the underlying genitourinary abnormality. The classification encompasses the following ultrasound findings:

1. Anterior-posterior renal pelvic diameter
2. Calyceal dilation
3. Renal parenchymal thickness
4. Renal parenchymal appearance (echogenicity, corticomedullary differentiation, cortical cysts)
5. Ureteral dilation
6. Bladder pathology (ureterocele, wall thickening, dilated posterior urethra)
7. Oligohydramnios (antenatal classification only)

This is the only classification to take account of ureteral and lower urinary tract abnormalities and the only one to offer clinical guidance according to risk. Patients are allocated to different risk categories by a combination of ultrasound findings (with the most severe findings taking precedence) and gestational or postnatal age. Antenatal and postnatal risk categories are denoted by A or P, respectively. There are two antenatal risk categories: A1 (low risk) and A2-3 (intermediate/high risk) and three postnatal risk categories: P1 (low risk), P2 (intermediate risk), and P3 (high risk). (Figure 4.2)

Each risk category has associated clinical recommendations to guide the clinician (Figure 4.3). The physiological reduction in urine output which normally occurs during the first 48 hours after birth may reduce the sensitivity of ultrasound for the detection of hydronephrosis during this period. Decision-making should therefore be based on ultrasound findings after 48 hours.

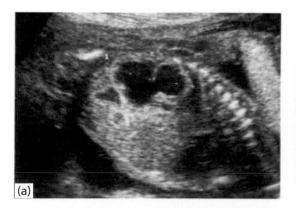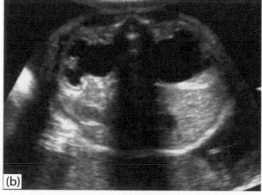

Figure 4.1 (a) Unilateral SFU grade 4 hydronephrosis with blunted calyces and thinned, echogenic renal cortex at 22/40 weeks. (b) Bilateral SFU grade 4 hydronephrosis at 22/40 weeks.

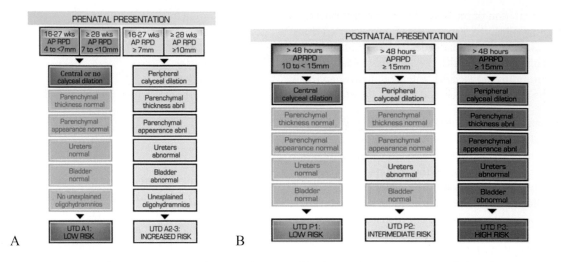

Figure 4.2 UTD risk-based sonographic classification of hydronephrosis. **(A)** Prenatal classification. Central and peripheral calyceal dilation may be difficult to evaluate early in gestation. Oligohydramnios must be suspected to result from a genitourinary cause. **(B)** Postnatal sonographic classification of hydronephrosis.

Postnatal investigation

Prenatally detected hydronephrosis is a non-specific finding and, where appropriate, further imaging investigations are required to establish the urological diagnosis. Postnatal diagnostic imaging always begins with a renal and bladder ultrasound. Depending on the initial ultrasound findings and other factors, further investigations typically comprise a voiding cystourethrogram (VCUG) and functional isotope renography.

Mild hydronephrosis

Dilatation of the renal pelvis corresponding to Grade I on the SFU scale is a common finding which is present in 1:100 pregnancies. It is often a self-limiting physiological phenomenon – which resolves spontaneously by the third trimester in more than 50% of cases. There is now general agreement that this finding can usually be disregarded if the dilatation is confined to the renal pelvis and the AP diameter is less than 10mm. Follow up studies of children born with mild hydronephrosis have found that their incidence of UTIs and bladder symptoms in childhood is no higher than in age matched normal controls. Nevertheless, the discovery of mild

hydronephrosis on routine antenatal ultrasonography can cause considerable parental anxiety and it is important that parents are given appropriate reassurance. It is also important that newborn infants with mild hydronephrosis are not submitted to unnecessary, invasive investigations. Mild hydronephrosis may be a marker of underlying VUR but when this is the case it usually low grade and of doubtful clinical significance. SFU and AUA guidelines do not advocate routine VCUG in infants with mild (SFU Grade I) prenatally detected hydronephrosis but recommend that VCUG is used more selectively on the basis of additional ultrasonographic criteria.

Ureteropelvic junction (UPJ) obstruction

The most common underlying cause of clinically significant hydronephrosis is UPJ obstruction, which occurs in approximately 1 in 500 live births. UPJ obstruction is characterized by partial or intermittent occlusion of the lumen of the UPJ. Dilatation is confined to the renal collecting systems unless the UPJ obstruction is associated with other urinary tract abnormalities – in which case ureteral dilatation and/or bladder abnormalities

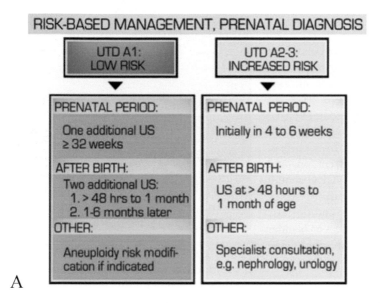

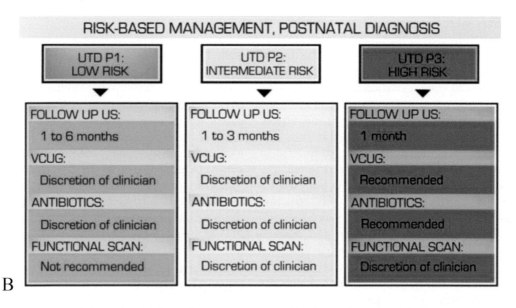

Figure 4.3 UTD risk-based guidelines for management of hydronephrosis. **(A)** Follow-up recommendations for prenatally diagnosed hydronephrosis. **(B)** Management recommendations based on postnatal ultrasound.

may also be present. Boys are affected more commonly than girls, and approximately 10% of cases are bilateral. There is usually a good correlation between the degree of hydronephrosis and the severity of obstruction and impact on renal function (as demonstrated by isotope renography). The indications for pyeloplasty and the arguments surrounding conservative or surgical management of prenatally detected UPJ obstruction are reviewed in greater detail in Chapter 7. In brief, it is generally agreed that early pyeloplasty is indicated for infants with severe hydronephrosis and/or reduced differential function. Pyeloplasty remains the surgical "gold standard" and has a very high success rate for the correction of UPJ obstruction.

Vesicoureteral reflux

As noted already, VUR is one of the conditions which may give rise to prenatal hydronephrosis. However, there are no pathognomonic ultrasonographic features and the diagnosis of VUR can only be reliably established on a postnatal VCUG. At one time this was performed routinely in all infants with prenatally detected hydronephrosis, regardless of severity. However, current SFU and AUA guidelines recommend that VCUG should be limited to infants with higher grades of hydronephrosis (III–IV on the SFU scale) and/or those with ureteral dilatation (hydroureter) or bladder abnormalities. This is considered in more detail in Chapter 6.

Other urological conditions

Primary megaureter accounts for around 5–10% of cases of fetal hydronephrosis. On ultrasound, the degree of ureteral dilatation may be disproportionally greater than the degree of renal dilatation. After 30 weeks gestation a ureteral diameter of greater than 7 mm is regarded as an abnormal finding constituting a diagnosis of megaureter. The postnatal investigation, classification, and management of megaureters are considered in Chapter 7. **Ureteroceles** may be detected prenatally and are characterized by appearances of a thin septum or thin walled cystic structure within the bladder. This finding may be accompanied by upper tract dilatation and bilateral hydronephrosis if the ureterocele has prolapsed into bladder outlet or urethra to cause outflow obstruction. Similarly, ureteroceles which are associated with an **ectopic ureter** associated with the upper pole of a duplex kidney may be accompanied by ureteral dilatation and abnormal ultrasound appearances of the kidney itself. The postnatal assessment and management of ureteroceles and upper tract duplication is addressed in Chapter 8.

Posterior urethral valves (PUV)

Bilateral hydronephrosis in a male fetus is highly suggestive of posterior urethral valves and the diagnosis is strongly supported by additional

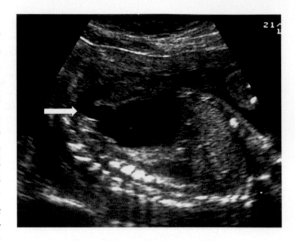

Figure 4.4 Prenatal ultrasound showing a distended bladder and dilated posterior urethra (arrow) in a fetus with posterior urethral valves.

ultrasound findings such as a distended, thick walled bladder and dilated posterior urethra (keyhole sign) (Figure 4.4). Other ultrasound findings may include changes in the renal parenchyma denoting dysplasia, bladder diverticula, patent urachus, or rupture of a renal fornix or calyx with a perinephric urinoma or urinary ascites. Oligohydramnios and pulmonary hypoplasia are indicative of severe renal dysplasia and predictors of a poor prognosis. The role of fetal intervention is described later in this chapter and the postnatal investigation and management of PUV is reviewed in Chapter 9.

Postnatal Management: General Considerations

The UTD guidelines leave much to the discretion of the clinician. There is significant variation in the empirical use of prophylactic antibiotics and indications for VCUG and isotope renography.

Prophylactic antibiotics

The published evidence provides limited support for the use of antibiotic prophylaxis in infants born with prenatally detected hydronephrosis. A randomized controlled trial comparing trimethoprim to placebo in infants with prenatally detected SFU Grade III–IV hydronephrosis is ongoing. The antibiotics used most commonly for urinary prophylaxis in neonates include amoxicillin (10–20 mg/kg/day), cephalexin (10 mg/kg/day), and trimethoprim (2 mg/kg/day). Trimethoprim-sulfamethoxazole and nitrofurantoin are contra-indicated because of the risks of kernicterus and hemolytic anemia, respectively. The following pre-natally detected urological conditions are gener-ally regarded as indications for postnatal antibiotic prophylaxis:

- Lower urinary tract obstruction (e.g. poste-rior urethral valves, urethral atresia)
- Ureterovesical junction obstruction (e.g. obstructing megaureter, ectopic ureter, or ureterocele)
- Moderate to high grades of vesicoureteral reflux in girls

Voiding cystourethrogram (VCUG)

The generally accepted indications for postnatal VCUG include:

- Abnormal bladder (e.g. thick wall, keyhole sign, diverticula)
- Bilateral hydronephrosis in boys (a VCUG should always be performed prior to dis-charge from the hospital to investigate for posterior urethral valves)
- Multicystic dysplastic kidney with an abnor-mal contralateral kidney
- Ureteral dilation
- Duplex kidney with hydronephrosis in either moiety
- Large ureterocele (to investigate possible prolapse)

Renography

The most widely used radionuclide scan is the technetium-99 m-mercaptoacetyltriglycine (MAG-3) diuretic renogram. This has the advantage of com-bining information on drainage with an assess-ment of differential renal function. The technical aspects are detailed in Chapter 3. Radionuclide scans are less reliable and the results are more

difficult to interpret in neonates because of the functional immaturity of their kidneys. For this reason radionuclide scans should be deferred until 6–8 weeks. of age. The indications for diuretic renography include:

- Moderate to severe hydronephrosis (anterior-posterior renal pelvic diameter >10mm, SFU Grade III–IV) with absence of vesicoureteral reflux
- Establishing baseline function prior to sur-gery to relieve obstruction (e.g. UPJ obstruc-tion, UVJ obstruction)
- Confirming poor function in a kidney prior to nephrectomy

NON-HYDRONEPHROTIC ANOMALIES

Urological abnormalities which are associated with hydronephrosis are more readily detected on prenatal ultrasonography than those which are not. Nevertheless, other urologic abnor-malities can be identified by prenatal ultra-sound – and genital anomalies are occasionally diagnosed prenatally. The finding of a urologi-cal anomaly may also lead to the diagnosis of a more severe, complex congenital abnormality, or syndrome.

The anatomical features and clinical aspects of abnormalities of ascent and fusion are described in Chapter 14. Renal ectopia is fre-quently associated with other congenital anom-alies and may be a component of more complex syndromes such as VACTERL and agenesis of the corpus callosum.

A simple **ectopic kidney** may be located any-where along the embryological path of ascent to the lumbar renal fossa. Pelvic kidneys are the most common form of simple ectopia-accounting for 60% of all cases. In addition to its abnormal location, a pelvic kidney is frequently malrotated, hypoplastic, and irregular in shape. A **horseshoe kidney** is formed by fusion of the left and right kidneys which, in the major-ity of cases are joined at their lower poles by an isthmus of renal parenchyma or dysplastic or fibrous tissue. Horseshoe kidneys are commonly found in association with other abnormalities or syndromes, notably Turner's syndrome and abnormalities of the central nervous system, the gastrointestinal tract, and the skeletal and cardiovascular systems. **Crossed renal ectopia** is a rare form of renal ectopia in which both kidneys are located on the same side of midline. In most cases the kidneys are fused but the kidney which is abnormally located retains its vessels and ureters from the contralateral side. The abnormality may either be visualized directly by prenatal ultrasonography or may be identified indirectly when a kidney cannot be visualized in the contralateral renal fossa. Further investigation is usually indicated after birth because of the relatively high incidence of VUR and other abnormalities. **Unilateral renal agenesis** occurs in 1 in around 1300 pregnancies and is more common in twins. On ultrasound, the lumbar fossa is empty and the adrenal gland appears elongated. The contralateral kidney may demonstrate compensatory hypertrophy. Unilateral renal agenesis is typically a sporadic anomaly but can occur in association with chromosomal or developmental defects such as DiGeorge syndrome or the

VACTERL complex. It may also occur in conjunction with genital anomalies, notably absence of the vas deferens in males and Müllerian anomalies in girls. **Bilateral renal agenesis** occurs in around 1 in 4000 pregnancies. Ultrasound features comprise absence of both kidneys (empty lumbar fossae) early anhydramnios, and lack of bladder filling. If the pregnancy proceeds to term, bilateral renal agenesis generally results in the early demise of the infant from pulmonary insufficiency and renal failure.

Cystic renal disease is reviewed in detail in Chapter 10. The form most commonly detected by prenatal ultrasonography is autosomal recessive polycystic kidney disease (ARPKD) which occurs in 1 in 20,000 live births. On ultrasound, the kidneys typically appear markedly enlarged and echogenic with poor or even reversed corticomedullary differentiation (Figure 4.5). However, the kidneys may appear normal up to the 20th week of gestation.

Unilateral multicystic dysplastic kidney (MCDK) is one of the commonest prenatally detected renal malformations (Figure 4.6). This partly because of its relative frequency (between 1:2500 and 1:4000 pregnancies) and partly

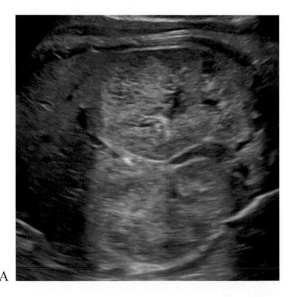
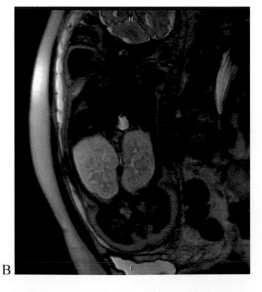

A   B

Figure 4.5 Prenatal imaging at 33/40 weeks showed markedly enlarged, bright kidneys consistent with infantile ARPKD. **(A)** Ultrasound shows echogenic kidneys. **(B)** MRI shows T2 hyperintense kidneys. The fetal bladder is empty, and there is severe oligohydramnios.

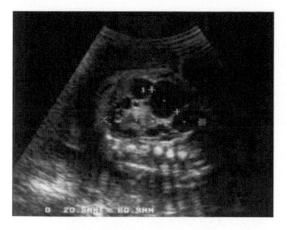

Figure 4.6 Multicystic dysplastic kidney at 22/40 weeks.

because of the ease with which the fluid-filled cysts can be visualized on ultrasound. Bilateral MCDK has an incidence of around 1:20,000 and is a lethal condition. The further investigation of MCDKs and the controversies surrounding their management are considered in Chapter 10.

Syndromes, Genital Anomalies

Many conditions involving the genitourinary system are routinely diagnosed prenatally. Among the commonest are myelomeningocele and sacral agenesis – which almost invariably give rise to neurogenic bladder dysfunction. Cloacal anomalies may be suspected in fetuses with a pelvic cystic structure (hydrocolpos), poorly visualized bladder, and bilateral hydronephrosis. Although bladder exstrophy is associated with a number of diagnostic features these are not always easy to detect with the result that only 50% of cases are diagnosed prenatally. Bowel distension may suggest an anorectal malformation, particularly if this is accompanied by other features of VACTERL (vertebral, anorectal, cardiac, esophageal fistula, renal, limb) anomalies. Isolated genital anomalies can also be detected prenatally – the most common being virilized genitalia in a female with 46 XX DSD due to congenital adrenal hyperplasia. Other forms of DSD may be identified because of discordance between genotype and prenatal ultrasonography.

Fetal intervention

Fetal diagnosis prompts the question of fetal intervention. Of the currently available fetal interventions, decompression of an obstructed fetal urinary tract and intrauterine closure of myelomeningocele are those of greatest relevance to pediatric urology. To date, the outcomes of both forms of intervention have been disappointing, with a significant incidence of perinatal complications and little evidence of benefit for bladder and renal function.

Vesicoamniotic shunting

The aims of this form of prenatal intervention for bladder outlet obstruction are:

1. To prevent pulmonary hypoplasia (the main cause of neonatal death)
2. To improve the outcome for renal function
3. To improve the outlook for bladder function

The commonest indication is to alleviate the effects of outflow obstruction due to posterior urethral valves. Although, fetal cystoscopic valve ablation and open vesicostomy have been reported the most commonly performed procedure consists of decompressing the obstructed urinary tract by use of a vesicoamniotic shunt. Under ultrasound guidance a trocar is inserted through the maternal abdominal wall and uterus into the bladder. A double-pigtail shunt is then introduced, with one end in the fetal bladder and the other in the amniotic cavity. If there is oligohydramnios it may be necessary to infuse fluid into the amniotic cavity to facilitate this maneuver (Figure 4.7).

Vesicoamniotic shunting is usually performed before 26 weeks. When performed after 26 weeks it is unlikely to lead to any improvement in pulmonary function. The selection criteria are quite complex and include; recent onset of oligohydramnios, functioning kidneys capable of urine output, normal karyotype and absence of co-existing congenital abnormalities. Serial fetal urine sampling is recommended to aid selection for intervention. High urinary levels of sodium, calcium, and β_2-microglobulin are predictors of poor renal function (Table 4.1). The combination of unfavorable fetal urine electrolyte markers

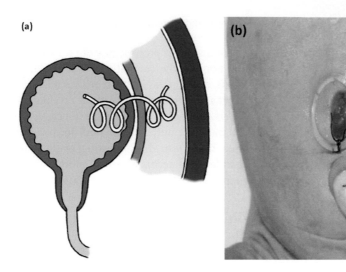

Figure 4.7 Vesicoamniotic shunt. (a) A double pigtail shunt diverts urine from the fetal bladder into the amniotic cavity. (b) Postnatal image showing the extra-abdominal portion of the shunt with associated prolapsed, hypertrophic bladder tissue.

Table 4.1 Threshold values of fetal urine parameters that predict good renal function

	Good prognosis
Sodium	<100 mEq/L
Chloride	<90 mEq/L
Calcium	<4 mEq/L
Osmolality	<210 mOsm/L
β_2-microglobulin	<10 mg/L
Total protein	<20 mg/dl

and/or echogenic kidneys with cortical cysts is a contraindication to shunting.

Although vesicoamniotic shunting appears to have the potential to improve pulmonary outcomes, the benefits (if any) for renal and bladder function remain unproven. The incidence of complications is high (45%) – including premature labor, shunt migration, shunt blockage, and chorioamnionitis. Further shunting procedures are often required, with an average of 2.5 shunt placements per pregnancy. The percutaneous shunting in lower urinary tract obstruction (PLUTO) trial was a randomized-controlled study to evaluate the efficacy and safety of vesicoamniotic shunting. Analysis of the initial results indicated that survival rates were improved by shunting but the prognosis for renal function remained poor. The

trial was terminated prematurely because of difficulties in recruiting sufficient patient numbers.

Myelomeningocele closure

The traditional surgical management of myelomeningocele consists of surgical closure in the early neonatal period. In utero surgical closure was proposed in the hope of improving neurologic outcomes. The first case was reported in 1997 and the results of an initial comparative outcome trial (management of myelomeningocele study [MOMS] were published in 2003. These demonstrated that in utero closure of the myelomeningocele was associated with a reduced requirement for ventriculoperitoneal shunting and improved early outcomes for cognitive and motor function. However, it did not lead to any improvement in bladder function. Complications of intrauterine closure of myelomeningocele include increased rates of premature birth and uterine dehiscence. Fetoscopic techniques have been developed as an alternative to open fetal surgery, with initial data suggesting they carry a lower risk of maternal complications.

Amnioinfusion

Amnioinfusion is a technique in which saline is infused into the amniotic cavity with the intention of alleviating the effects of oligohydramnios on pulmonary development. There have been recent case reports that the use of amnioinfusion in cases of bilateral renal agenesis permitted sufficient pulmonary development for postnatal survival followed by postnatal dialysis as a bridge to renal transplant. This is still considered an experimental intervention and should not be routinely offered.

Termination of pregnancy (therapeutic abortion)

Although this remains a controversial issue, termination of pregnancy for severe or lethal congenital abnormalities has long been legally permissible (subject to certain criteria) in many countries. The combination of prenatal diagnosis and termination of pregnancy may explain why the last two to three decades have seen declining numbers of referrals for severe but nonlethal urologic malformations such as prune-belly syndrome and cloacal and classic bladder exstrophy.

PRENATAL COUNSELING

When counseling expecting parents, clinicians should explain the differential diagnosis, the likely perinatal course (including required investigations,) and provide an overview of the longer term prognosis.

Counseling for the majority of cases of prenatally detected hydronephrosis should focus on reassuring parents. Mild hydronephrosis (SFU Grade I) is often a transient physiological phenomenon and even when it persists postnatally is unlikely to be clinically significant or require invasive investigation. More significant prenatally detected conditions such as ureteropelvic junction, vesico ureteral reflux, and unilateral multicystic dysplastic kidney may resolve without requiring operative intervention. Parents can also be reassured that even when operative intervention is required, the majority of children experience favorable outcomes.

When the prognosis is far less favorable (e.g. oligohydramnios, bilateral renal abnormalities,

and significant coexisting nonurologic condition) counseling will involve input from specialists in the relevant disciplines to ensure parents are fully informed on the implications for their child and the family. These discussions may include, for example the probable requirement for intermittent catheterization for children with neurogenic bladder and dialysis and future kidney transplant in urologic conditions posing a risk of renal insufficiency and chronic kidney disease. Broader issues relating to changes in lifestyle and financial implications of caring for a child with a long-term chronic condition will also need to be raised with the parents.

These are uncomfortable issues to discuss, but a full discussion is necessary to ensure that parents have all the information they need when making life-changing decisions.

Following the prenatal diagnosis of severe anomalies, parents must be reassured that whatever course of action they choose (aggressive medical intervention, limited medical intervention, comfort care, and termination of pregnancy) is valid, and that their medical team will support them in their decision.

KEY POINTS

- Most infants with prenatally detected hydronephrosis will require no intervention.
- Abnormalities of the renal parenchyma, ureter, and/or bladder suggest a clinically significant pathology.
- The urinary tract dilation (UTD) classification is the first system to unify descriptions of prenatal and postnatal hydronephrosis, and to provide guidance regarding initial management.
- Routine antibiotic prophylaxis, voiding cystourethrogram, and renography are unnecessary for the majority of patients diagnosed with prenatal hydronephrosis.
- The benefits of fetal intervention are uncertain, and fetal surgery should not be pursued outside of high volume centers.

FURTHER READING

Braga Luis H, Farrokhyar Forough, D'Cruz Jennifer, Pemberton Julia, Lorenzo Armando J. Risk Factors for Febrile Urinary Tract Infection in Children with Prenatal Hydronephrosis: A Prospective Study. J Urol. 2015;193(5S):1766–1771.

Capolicchio J-P, Braga LH, Szymanski KM. Canadian Urological Association/Pediatric Urologists of Canada guidelines on the investigation and management of antenatally detected hydronephrosis. CUAJ. 2017;12(4):85–92.

Morris RK, Malin GL, Quinlan-Jones E, Middleton LJ, Hemming K, Burke D, et al. Percutaneous vesicoamniotic shunting versus conservative management for fetal lower urinary tract obstruction (PLUTO): a randomised trial. Lancet. 2013;382(9903):1496–1506.

Nguyen HT, Benson CB, Bryann B, et al. Multidisciplinary consensus on the classification of prenatal and postnatal urinary tract dilation (UTD classification system). J Pediatr Urol. 2014;10:982–999.

Sairam S, Al-Habib A, Sasson S, Thilaganathan B. Natural history of fetal hydronephrosis diagnosed on mid-trimester ultrasound. Ultrasound Obstet Gynecol. 2001;17(3):191–196.

Urinary Tract Infection

STUART J O'TOOLE

Topics covered

Epidemiology of childhood urinary infection
Pathogenesis
Infecting organisms
Host factors
Diagnosis
Specimen collection, urine analysis
Clinical features

Age differences
Upper and lower tract infection
Investigation
NICE guidelines
International guidelines
Management

INTRODUCTION

Urinary tract infection (UTI) is one of the commonest disorders of childhood, affecting an estimated 82 000 children a year in the UK. A UTI may be the first indication of significant underlying pathology of the urinary tract which may require treatment to prevent ongoing or future renal damage. Diagnosing UTI in young infants can be problematic because the clinical features are often non-specific and reliable urine samples are difficult to obtain. Nevertheless, greater awareness of the importance and prevalence of UTI in children coupled with the availability of sensitive dipstick reagent strips has led to UTIs being detected on a far greater scale than in the past. In turn this has led to many more children with mild or asymptomatic lower tract urinary infections being referred for investigation. Standard protocols for the investigation and management of childhood UTI often dated from a time when children referred for investigation were those with more severe infection. As a consequence, many children with mild, lower tract UTIs have been subjected to unnecessary (and costly) invasive investigations. To address these concerns, healthcare organisations across the developed world have produced evidence-based guidelines on a selective approach to diagnostic imaging and recommendations on management. The published guidelines vary significantly – reflecting different healthcare philosophies. Those published in the UK place greater emphasis on the benefit to the population and costs to the healthcare system whereas guidelines published in North America place greater emphasis on the individual child.

Table 5.1 The age-related incidence of urinary tract infection in boys and girls

Age (years)	Boys (%)	Girls (%)
<1	1.0	0.8
<3	2.2	2.1
<7	2.8	8.2
<16	3.6	11.3
Lifetime	13.7	53.1

EPIDEMIOLOGY

The true incidence of UTI in children is far higher than was previously thought. In the 1960s, this was put at 0.02% for boys and 0.04% for girls, whereas current estimates have increased 20-fold (Table 5.1). In the first 12 months of life urinary infections occur more commonly in boys but thereafter (and particularly above 3 years of age) UTIs affect predominantly girls.

PATHOGENESIS OF URINARY TRACT INFECTION

UTIs occasionally result from haematogenous spread or the direct transmission of bacteria from other organs – e.g. vesico intestinal and genito-urinary fistulae. However, the overwhelming majority are "ascending infections" in which bacteria which have colonised the perineum or pre-putial sac gain access to the lower urinary tract via the urethra. Whether these bacteria go on to produce an established infection once they have entered the lower urinary tract is determined by the interplay of a number of factors set out in Figure 5.1. The concept of organisms multiplying within bladder urine is largely inaccurate and research has shown that bacterial replication occurs predominantly at an intracellular level, with organisms being shed into the urine from infected urothelial cells.

Organisms

Escherichia coli is responsible for around 85% of UTIs. The fimbriated forms of *E. coli* have the ability to adhere to receptors on the urothelial surface and are therefore particularly effective at colonising the urinary tract. P-fimbriated *E. coli* are particularly potent pathogens because of their adherence properties. Other common infecting organisms, in approximately descending order of frequency, are *Proteus vulgaris*, *Klebsiella*, *Enterobacter* and *Pseudomonas*.

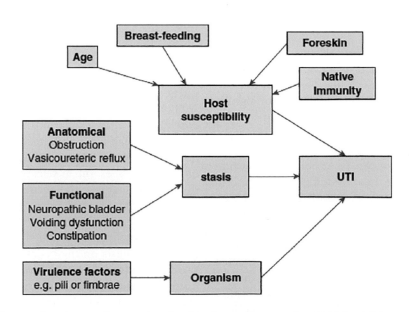

Figure 5.1 Host and pathogen factors involved in the pathogenesis of UTI in children.

Urinary Stasis

There is a substantial body of clinical experience which indicates that the risk of UTI is significantly increased by factors which impede the clearance of bacteria from the urinary tract. These include; urinary stasis due to obstruction, vesico ureteric reflux (VUR) and incomplete bladder emptying (due to outflow obstruction or dysfunctional voiding).

Anatomical Abnormalities

Because many more children with mild, lower tract infections are being referred for investigation than in the past, the relative proportion with significant underlying urological abnormalities has decreased from a historical figure of around 30% to closer to 10%. Even when anomalies are identified on investigation many are of limited clinical relevance. Examples include; minor grades of VUR, incomplete duplication anomalies and anomalies of renal ascent and fusion. Dysfunctional voiding characterised by infrequent toileting and impaired bladder emptying (particularly in girls) is a far more common predisposing cause of UTIs than anatomical abnormalities of the urinary tract.

Host Susceptibility

Many host factors can increase a child's susceptibility to urine infection. Premature infants are at greater risk (although breast-feeding appears to confer some protection). Other host factors linked to susceptibility or resistance to UTI include immunoglobulin A (IgA) secretion and blood group secretor status. The presence of a foreskin is an undoubted risk factor – particularly in the first year of life. The incidence of urinary infection is 10–20 times higher in uncircumcised boys than their circumcised peers. Although the increased risk of urinary infection in uncircumcised boys has been cited as one of the justifications for routine neonatal circumcision, the findings of large population-based studies indicate that over 100 boys would need to be circumcised in order to prevent one boy from developing urinary infection. Nevertheless, although routine neonatal circumcision is not a cost-effective measure for preventing UTIs in boys with normal urinary tracts there is growing evidence that circumcision reduces the risk of UTI in boys with underlying urological abnormalities such as posterior urethral valves and high grade VUR.

LABORATORY DIAGNOSIS OF URINARY TRACT INFECTION

Urine Collection

"Clean catch" midstream urine sample

A midstream urine (MSU) sample yields the most reliable results. Children who are toilet-trained can usually cooperate with this method of collection. For infants and children unable to provide a midstream specimen, the **non-invasive** alternatives include:

- **Adhesive collection bags** attached around the genitalia. This is the simplest and most commonly used method of collecting urine specimens in the very young. However, the results are only reliable if appropriate precautions have been taken to avoid contamination and if the voided specimen is sent promptly for culture.
- **Absorbent urine collection pads** placed inside the nappy. In this method, urine which has soaked into the pad is aspirated with a syringe and sent for microscopy and culture. Cotton wool balls may also be used but are less reliable. Contamination is common.

Invasive techniques

- **Suprapubic needle aspiration** is the ideal method of collection in sick infants in whom an urgent diagnosis is required. The procedure should be performed under ultrasound guidance, once it has been confirmed that there is urine in the bladder.

- **Urethral catheterisation** is distressing and is rarely appropriate for this purpose.

Although it is always preferable to obtain a urine sample before commencing treatment, there may be situations (e.g. a severely ill infant) when it is justifiable to commence antibiotic treatment even if a urine sample cannot be obtained.

Urine Storage and Transport

Once collected, the specimen should ideally be cultured within 4 hours to minimise the risk of contaminating organisms multiplying and yielding a false-positive result. If this is not feasible (e.g. in children presenting outside working hours), the sample can be refrigerated for up to 24 hours at +4.0°C or transferred to a vessel containing boric acid preservative.

Urine Dipsticks

The introduction of urine dipsticks with leucocyte esterase and nitrite reagents has been instrumental in facilitating the earlier diagnosis of UTI. Guidelines published by the UK's National Institute of Clinical Excellence make the following recommendations:

- **Leucocyte esterase and nitrite both positive** = definite evidence of UTI. Antibiotic treatment should be commenced.
- **Leucocyte esterase negative, nitrite positive** = presumptive evidence of UTI. Antibiotic treatment should be commenced and a urine sample sent for culture.
- **Leucocyte esterase positive, nitrite negative** – a urine sample should be sent for microscopy and culture but antibiotic treatment should not be commenced unless there is good clinical evidence of UTI.
- **Leucocyte esterase negative, nitrite negative** = negative result. Antibiotic treatment should not be started. Nor is it necessary for urine to be sent for microscopy and culture.

A positive result for protein does not denote infection. A trace of proteinuria is a common finding and is not a cause for concern. Heavier proteinuria may, however, signify renal disease and referral to a paediatric nephrologist should be considered if this is confirmed on a further test.

Urine Microscopy

When performed on a fresh uncentrifuged sample of urine, microscopy can be very useful in facilitating a prompt diagnosis and enabling treatment to be commenced without awaiting the results of culture. Results are generally expressed as absolute values or counts per high-powered field. Significant pyuria is defined as >10 WBC/mm^3. The concentration of motile bacteria can also be quantified, with 10^7 bacteria per ml being deemed significant. This figure corresponds to eight organisms per high-powered field. The interpretation of microscopy findings is summarised in Table 5.2.

Urine Culture

Provided the urine sample is uncontaminated, the criterion for the bacteriological diagnosis of urinary infection is a pure growth of >10^5 bacterial colony-forming units (CFUs) per ml. However, in a specimen which has been obtained by suprapubic aspiration, any growth of a Gram-negative organism is significant, as is a growth of greater than >500–1000 Gram-positive organisms. Following

Table 5.2 Interpretation of microscopy findings

Microscopy results	Pyuria positive	Pyuria negative
Bacteriuria positive	The infant or child should be regarded as having UTI	The infant or child should be regarded as having UTI
Bacteriuria negative	Antibiotic treatment should be started if clinically UTI	The infant or child should be regarded as not having UTI

the introduction of sensitive dipsticks, it has been questioned whether urine culture is still routinely necessary in all cases. However, at a time when multiple antibiotic resistance is increasing there remains a strong argument for sending a urine specimen for culture to identify the causative organism and establish its antibiotic sensitivities.

CLINICAL PRESENTATION AND DIAGNOSIS

History and Examination

It is important to enquire whether there is any family history of urological abnormalities, particularly VUR. The antenatal history is also important, specifically whether any abnormality was detected on antenatal ultrasound. In older, toilet-trained children, information should be routinely sought on:

- Voiding history (volume, frequency, stream, urgency)
- Fluid intake (volume, type)
- Bowel habits

Although **physical examination** is usually uninformative, it should nevertheless be performed routinely and should include the abdomen, genitalia, spine and lower limbs. Blood pressure should always be measured (although this can be difficult in small or fractious children). It is important that the appropriate equipment and paediatric blood pressure cuffs are always available in the outpatient clinic.

Clinical Features

The presentation of UTI can be non-specific and is influenced by the nature of the infection and the age of the child. Table 5.3 summarises the clinical features of UTI at different ages. It is important to maintain a high degree of suspicion and ensure that a urine sample is collected and tested for

Table 5.3 Presenting features of UTI in children at different ages

Frequency	Infant and toddler	Older child
Common	Fever irritability Vomiting Lethargy	Frequency dysuria
Less common	Offensive urine Poor feeding Failure to thrive	Offensive urine Incontinence Abdominal pain
Uncommon	Jaundice Failure to thrive Haematuria	Fever Vomiting Haematuria Loin tenderness

infection in any child with an unexplained fever exceeding 38.0°C. In addition to age-related differences, the clinical presentation is determined by whether the child is suffering from lower or upper UTI (Table 5.4).

Lower tract infection (cystitis)

Cystitis typically gives rise to bladder symptoms, with dysuria being almost universal. In addition, urinary frequency is common and often associated with secondary enuresis. However, suprapubic pain is comparatively rare. There is no fever or general malaise; indeed, many older children are able to continue attending school during the course of their illness.

Table 5.4 Symptoms of urinary tract infections

Lower urinary tract (cystitis)	Upper urinary tract (pyelonephritis)
Frequency/nocturia	Fever
Dysuria	Vomiting
Secondary enuresis	General malaise
Suprapubic pain	Loin pain
Hesitancy	Upper/central abdominal pain

Upper tract infection (pyelonephritis)

Fever is the most reliable clinical feature of upper tract UTI and, indeed, it is doubtful whether pyelonephritis ever occurs without a fever. Any temperature exceeding 38°C should be regarded as suspicious, although pyelonephritis is typically accompanied by a higher fever. Information on the presence or absence of fever is usually less reliable in children referred by general practitioners than those admitted directly to hospital from Emergency Departments.

The key diagnostic points can be summarised as follows:

- Infants and children who have bacteriuria and fever of 38°C or higher should be considered to have acute pyelonephritis.
- Infants and children presenting with fever lower than 38°C with loin pain/tenderness and bacteriuria should also be considered to have acute pyelonephritis.
- All other infants and children who have bacteriuria but no systemic symptoms or signs should be considered to have cystitis.

Other presenting features of UTI

The presence of haematuria is not in itself a guide to the severity or site of the infection. Haemorrhagic cystitis is the commonest cause. Urinary tract calculi should be suspected whenever the infecting agent is *Proteus* and it is important to be aware that stones may be present in the upper urinary tract without giving rise to any constitutional symptoms. Some boys referred with haematuria (with or without documented infection) may, in fact, have postmicturition bleeding due to urethritis rather than genuine haematuria. Epididymo-orchitis is an occasional presentation of urinary infection in boys of all ages and should arouse suspicion of some predisposing abnormality, such as urethral obstruction distal to the ejaculatory ducts or a duplication anomaly with the upper pole ureter draining ectopically into an ejaculatory duct (see Chapter 8).

Neonates and infants

UTI typically presents in this age group as a non-specific febrile illness, usually accompanied by vomiting (and quite often by diarrhoea). A dipstick urine test should always be performed in any infant with an otherwise unexplained febrile illness. Whenever possible a urine specimen should also be sent for microscopy and culture but this may not always be feasible because of difficulty obtaining a reliable urine sample in infants. Less common presentations of urinary infection in neonates and infants include failure to thrive (or frank weight loss) and prolonged jaundice in neonates. UTI may also occasionally present with haematuria (blood-stained nappy) or as epididymo-orchitis.

Children aged 2 years and older

Children as young as 2 years of age can usually give some account of their symptoms, and by 4 years, if not earlier, it should be possible to obtain a reasonably accurate history. The history and clinical features of the illness should provide a guide to whether the child is suffering from an upper or lower UTI. Pyelonephritis is sometimes accompanied by poorly localised upper abdominal pain but true loin pain is rare and, if prolonged, is more likely to signify obstruction than infection.

Potential pitfalls and sources of diagnostic confusion include:

- **Fever, abdominal/loin pain and dysuria in an older child**. This triad of symptoms associated with pyelonephritis can also be mimicked by acute inflammation of a retrocecal or pelvic appendix. In acute appendicitis, pain which occurs at the time of voiding is more likely to be localised to the abdomen rather than the urinary tract. In addition, the pain is more likely to be provoked or exacerbated by extension of the hip. The temperature is usually lower in appendicitis than in pyelonephritis.
- **Dysuria in the absence of other features of UTI.** Symptoms associated with vulvovaginitis in young girls are often, incorrectly

ascribed to UTI. Although the presence of white blood cells may be evident on urine microscopy, urine culture is either negative or may reveal a mixed growth. From the history it should be possible to distinguish between the features of dysuria associated with vulvovaginitis and dysuria due to a true UTI.

- Dysuria associated with **balanitis** may be confused with UTI in boys.

Classification of UTI

UTI can be classified according to whether it affects the **lower urinary tract (cystitis)**, **upper urinary tract UTI (pyelonephritis)**, whether it is **asymptomatic** or **symptomatic** and whether it is a single episode or recurrent. **Asymptomatic bacteriuria** (ABU) is predominantly a condition of school age girls who do not complain of symptoms of lower tract UTI despite having significant bacterial counts in their urine. There is some evidence that the bacterial strains found in the urine of girls with ABU are of lower virulence than the strains of bacteria responsible for causing symptomatic UTIs. Studies have demonstrated that ABU does not pose a risk of renal scarring in a child with an anatomically normal urinary tract. However, ABU is not an entirely innocent condition because there is considerable overlap between ABU and clinically significant infection. Not infrequently, girls with ABU subsequently experience (or have previously experienced) symptomatic UTIs.

INVESTIGATION: DIAGNOSTIC IMAGING

Established protocols and guidelines have been criticised for leading to over-investigation of children with lower tract infections and for not being cost-effective. Despite broad acceptance of new guidelines it seems likely that most paediatric clinicians will continue to recommend that all children presenting with proven urinary infection should undergo some form of investigation. However, a selective approach is required to ensure that normal children are not subjected to unnecessarily invasive investigations at the same time as ensuring that abnormalities which predispose to UTI (notably VUR) are not being missed.

The technical aspects of these investigations are considered in Chapter 3.

The different imaging modalities are summarized in Table 5.5.

Ultrasonography

Ultrasound is the ideal initial screening investigation because it is non-invasive, relatively inexpensive and does not entail exposure to radiation. European and North American guidelines recommend that all children presenting with a UTI should undergo an ultrasound scan. Somewhat controversially, however, the NICE (UK) guidelines state that an ultrasound scan is not routinely indicated in a child aged over 6 months who has experienced only a single uncomplicated UTI.

Ultrasonography is a reliable means of detecting obstructive and non-obstructive urinary tract dilatation, major degrees of renal scarring or dysplasia, most urinary calculi and almost all clinically significant duplication anomalies. It is also of value in demonstrating evidence of voiding dysfunction – which is apparent as a significant post void residual volume of urine and, in some cases, bladder wall thickening.

When an abnormality has been revealed by ultrasonography, the choice of further imaging is guided by factors which include the type of abnormality detected, the severity of infection (upper or lower tract) and the age of the child. The most widely used investigations are Tc-99m DMSA scintigraphy and either micturating cystourethrography (MCUG) or indirect radionuclide cystography (IRC). Suspected upper tract obstruction is investigated by dynamic renography using Tc-99m (MAG3).

One of the main limitations of ultrasonography is its poor sensitivity for detecting renal scarring and mild to moderate VUR. For example, ultrasonography has a false-negative rate of

Table 5.5 Strengths and weaknesses ("pros and cons") of the different imaging modalities available for the investigation of UTI in children

Investigation	Pros	Cons
Renal ultrasound with postvoid bladder views	Detects dilatation and allows measurement of renal size Detects major scarring Provides information on bladder dysfunction Visualises calculi and well tolerated	Poor at detecting scarring or reflux Operator dependent
DMSA	Most sensitive test for renal scarring and differential function	Relatively expensive and time consuming Requires IV cannulation
Indirect cystogram (MAG3)	Detects reflux during normal voiding Provides differential renal function Avoids the need for urethral catheterization	Child must be cooperative and toilet trained Poor sensitivity for detecting low-grade reflux Requires IV cannulation
Contrast micturating cystourethrogram (MCUG)	Most reliable test for detection of reflux Excludes urethral and other bladder pathology	Requires urethral catheterisation and incurs exposure to radiation

25–50% for the detection of grade III VUR and fails to identify renal scarring in 15–45% of cases.

The most controversial aspects of newer guidelines therefore relate to the role of further diagnostic imaging in children with normal ultrasound findings.

Indications for Further Imaging

Although, there are differences in the recommendations contained in current published guidelines they all advocate a far more limited use of DMSA and MCUG than in the past. Even in infants under 6 months of age these invasive investigations may not be routinely indicated following a single UTI which responds well to treatment within 48 hours. For children in the age range 6 months to 3 years with normal ultrasound findings the NICE guidelines recommend that DMSA should be reserved for those with recurrent UTIs or those with the type of clinical features listed in Table 5.6. However, this approach is arguable because, in practice, it is often difficult to establish retrospectively whether a UTI which was initially treated with

antibiotics in a community setting was accompanied by fever or not. Likewise, there may be insufficient information to determine whether a UTI responded well to treatment within 48 hours. The justification for DMSA as an early investigation is based on the argument that because ultrasonography is not a sensitive test for detecting renal scarring in young children, there is a significant risk that scarring and underlying VUR will be missed if it is not used fairly widely in this age group. There is broad agreement in the various guidelines that an MCUG may be indicated if there is upper tract dilatation on ultrasound. Where the guidelines differ is on the role of MCUG in children with normal ultrasound findings. Controversially, the NICE guidelines make no provision for MCUG in children aged 3 years and upwards (even those with recurrent or "atypical" UTIs) if the ultrasound findings are normal. It can be reasonably assumed that strict implementation of these guidelines would result in many cases of mild to moderate VUR in older children remaining undetected. It has been argued that this may not matter because the risk of new scarring is low after 3 years of age. However, the critics of the NICE guidelines point

Table 5.6 Clinical features which merit further investigation

- Severe infection with systemic symptoms indicating upper tract infection (pyelonephritis)
- Family history of VUR and/or renal scarring
- Poor urinary stream
- Palpable bladder or other abdominal mass (although these will generally be evident as abnormalities on ultrasound)
- Raised creatinine
- Failure to respond to treatment with suitable antibiotics within 48 hours
- Infection with organisms other than *E. coli*
- Age – although this is a weak discriminator, it is a factor when considering further investigation in view of the greater susceptibility of infants and young children to renal scarring. Most paediatric urologists continue to recommend further investigation in boys presenting with UTI in the first 6 months of life. However this is aimed more at detecting vesico ureteric reflux (VUR) than urethral obstruction, which usually gives rise to detectable abnormalities on ultrasound.
- Recurrent infection. This can be variously defined as:

  –two or more episodes of UTI with acute pyelonephritis/upper urinary tract infection, or

  –one episode of UTI with acute pyelonephritis plus one or more episodes of UTI with cystitis or

  –three or more episodes of UTI with cystitis

out that whilst new scarring may be uncommon it can undoubtedly occur after this age. Moreover, even if older children with VUR may be at a lower low risk of renal scarring they may still suffer from recurrent symptomatic UTIs and bouts of ill health which interfere with schooling and create considerable anxiety within the family. In such circumstances the results of a MCUG may be of considerable relevance to clinical management – for example by identifying those children who might benefit from endoscopic correction of their VUR. The relative merits of MCUG and IRC are considered in Chapter 3.

Some suggested imaging protocols are illustrated in Figures 5.2a, 5.2b and 5.2c. These are based on UK guidelines and can be compared with the imaging protocol recommended from the European Association of Urology (EAU) Guidelines (Figure 5.2d) and the American Academy of Pediatrics (AAP) guidelines (Figure 5.2e).

"Top-Down "versus "Bottom-Up" Approach to Imaging after a UTI

Normal ultrasound appearances of the urinary tract in a child with a history of presumed upper tract infection pose a potential dilemma

to the clinician. Is the urinary tract genuinely entirely normal or has the scan simply failed to identify VUR in a child who may be at risk of developing further UTI s and possible renal scarring? This question can be resolved by either a "top-down" or "bottom-up" approach. The "top-down" approach relies on a DMSA scan in the first instance. If this is normal it is assumed that even if the child does have VUR it is not clinically significant and a MCUG is not warranted. Alternatively, in the "bottom-up" approach a MCUG is performed as the first investigation. If this is negative (no evidence of VUR) no DMSA scan is performed. See also Chapter 6.

MANAGEMENT

Initial Management

Older children and those with mild to moderate UTI are usually treated in a community setting in the first instance and then referred for outpatient investigation. However, infants under 3 months and older children with clinical features of pyelonephritis should be referred promptly to

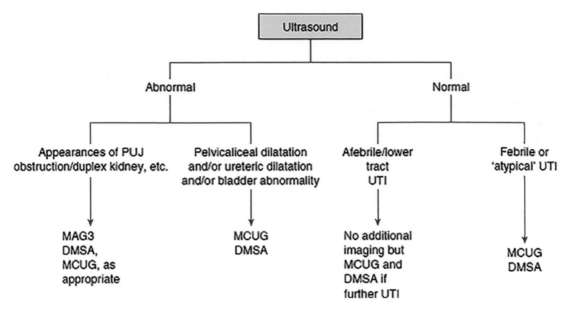

Figure 5.2 **(a)** Imaging protocol based on UK guidelines for infants aged 0–6 months.

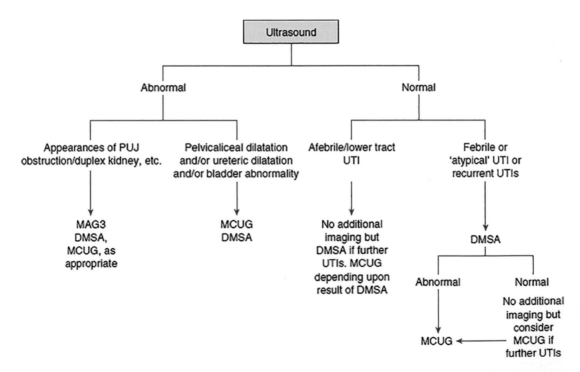

Figure 5.2 **(b)** Imaging protocol incorporating modified UK guidelines for young children aged 6 months to 3 years.

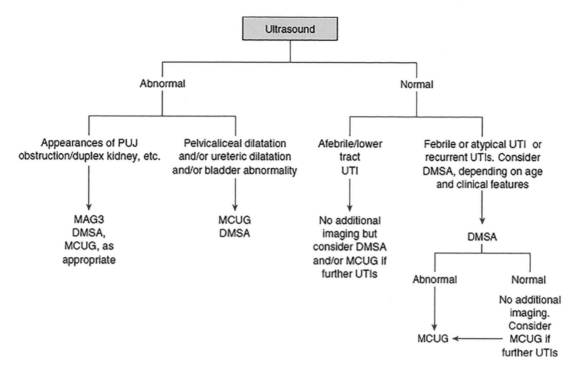

Figure 5.2 (c) Imaging protocol incorporating modified UK guidelines for children aged 3 years and upwards.

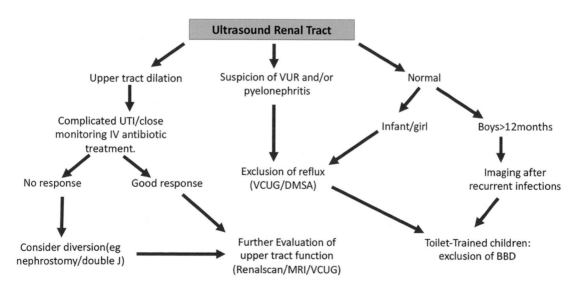

Figure 5.2 (d) European Association of Urology guidelines for assessment and treatment of febrile UTI. BBD, bladder bowel dysfunction.

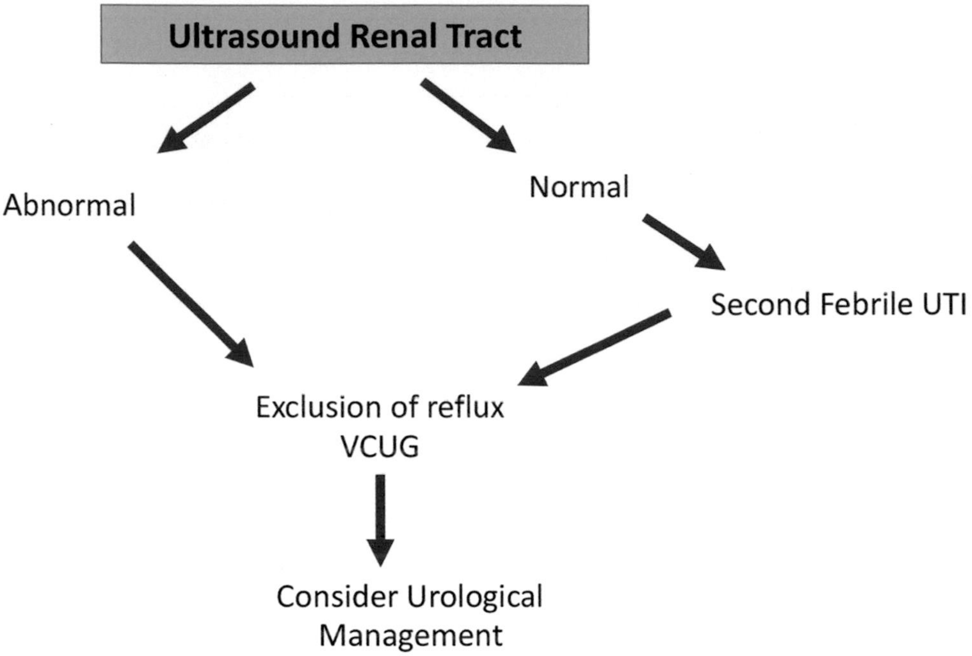

Figure 5.2 **(e)** Imaging recommendations taken from American Academy of Pediatrics guidelines for investigation and management of a child presenting with a UTI at 2–24 months of age.

a paediatric specialist at the outset. For infants under 3 months and for older children with presumed pyelonephritis (the groups at particular risk of renal scarring) treatment usually consists of an intravenous antibiotic such as cefotaxime or ceftriaxone. This typically comprises treatment with an intravenous antibiotic for 2–4 days followed by an oral antibiotic for a total duration of 10 days. If an aminoglycoside such as gentamicin is used, it is important to monitor blood levels. Depending upon the severity of the child's condition, oral rather than intravenous antibiotics may be considered (e.g. a 7–10 days course of cephalosporin or coamoxiclav). An ultrasound scan should be performed soon after admission in case there is a need for urgent intervention to bring the infection under control. Such interventions may include percutaneous nephrostomy in cases of upper tract obstruction complicated by infection (pyonephrosis) and percutaneous insertion of a suprapubic catheter in cases of bladder outflow obstruction.

Oral antibiotics are the first-line treatment for afebrile, lower UTI in children aged over 3 months. Although many clinicians now favour a short (3-day) course of treatment with an agent such as trimethoprim, cephalosporin, nitrofurantoin or amoxicillin there are others who still prefer to prescribe a longer course. The antibiotic should be switched to a more appropriate alternative if this is indicated by the results of sensitivities obtained from the MSU.

Longer-Term Management

Only a relatively small proportion of children require surgical intervention or ongoing management for abnormalities identified during the course of investigation. The majority of do not require urological intervention or follow-up. Nevertheless, some children, predominantly girls, suffer from recurrent UTIs despite having no underlying urological abnormality. In these children it is essential to identify and treat any predisposing factors – of which dysfunctional voiding is by far the most important. The role of constipation is more difficult to establish but there is a well-recognised association between these two "elimination disorders". Treatment is aimed at establishing a routine of regular and complete voiding coupled with measures designed to break the cycle of "holding back" – particularly in children who also experience habitual constipation. Even in the absence of VUR, a period of antibiotic prophylaxis may be helpful in some children by breaking the cycle of infection and allowing the bladder to settle down.

Other Conservative Measures

Cranberry juice has become increasingly popular as a prophylactic measure and although evidence of its effectiveness in children is lacking, some benefit has been shown in adult women. Probiotic yoghurts have also increased in popularity and, anecdotally, do seem to be beneficial in some children. However it is important that parents who do opt for alternative therapies should not disregard the three most important measures – increased fluid intake, treatment of constipation and, most importantly, treatment of voiding dysfunction to improve the frequency and effectiveness of bladder emptying.

KEY POINTS

- Urinary tract infection is one of the commonest disorders of childhood. Many more children with relatively asymptomatic lower tract urinary infections are being referred for investigation than in the past.
- Care is needed to obtain an uncontaminated urine sample for reagent dipstick testing and microscopy and culture whenever possible.
- It is important to confirm the diagnosis of urinary infection before submitting a child to any investigation which is more invasive than ultrasonography.
- Ultrasonography is the investigation of first choice but it is not a sensitive test for detecting vesicoureteric reflux and/or scarring.
- Further investigation is indicated if the initial ultrasound scan reveals an abnormality of the urinary tract. The

choice of further imaging is guided largely by the ultrasound findings.
- Further imaging (to look primarily for vesicoureteric reflux and/or renal scarring) may also be justified despite normal ultrasound findings. The indications for further investigation and the choice of imaging are determined by the age of the child, severity of infection and factors such as family history.
- Dysfunctional voiding is the most important factor predisposing to lower tract urinary infection in girls with normal urinary tracts. Management should be directed towards improving voiding function and treating constipation when present.

FURTHER READING

Christian MT, McColl JH, MacKenzie JR, Beattie TJ. Risk assessment of renal cortical scarring with urinary tract infection by clinical features and ultrasonography. Arch Dis Child. 2000;82(5):376–380.

National Institute for Health and Clinical Excellence. Guidelines on urinary tract infection in children. 2007. www.nice.org.uk/CG054

Newman TB. The new American Academy of Pediatrics urinary tract infection guideline. Paediatrics. 2011;128(3):572–575.

Singh-Grewal D, Macdessi J, Craig J. Circumcision for the prevention of urinary tract infection in boys: a systematic review of clinical trials and observation studies. Arch Dis Child. 2005;90(8):853–858.

Stein R, Dogan HS, Hoebeke P, Kocvara R, Nijman RJM, Radmayr C, et al. Urinary tract infections in children: EAU/ESPU Guidelines. Eur Urol. 2015;67(3):546–558.

Williams G, Craig JC. Long-term antibiotics for preventing recurrent urinary tract infection in children. Cochrane Database Syst Rev. 2019;4:CD001534.

Vesicoureteral Reflux

ROHIT TEJWANI and JONATHAN C ROUTH

Topics covered

INTRODUCTION

Vesicoureteral reflux (VUR) is defined as the retrograde flow of urine from the bladder into the upper urinary tract. It can be classified as primary or secondary. Primary VUR is due to an intrinsic failure of the valve mechanism at the ureterovesical junction whereas secondary VUR results from sustained exposure of the valve mechanism to the effects of elevated intravesical pressure. Secondary VUR is a feature of bladder outflow obstruction such as posterior urethral valves or functional abnormalities such as neurogenic bladder or severe dysfunctional voiding. This chapter is largely devoted to primary VUR because secondary VUR is covered in more detail in the other relevant chapters (9 and 13).

It has long been recognized that urinary tract infection (UTI) and pyelonephritis are important causes of morbidity in childhood. By the mid- to late-20th century, VUR was known to play a central role in linking UTI, pyelonephritis, renal parenchymal scarring, and end-stage renal disease (ESRD). As a result of better understanding of the natural history of VUR and the availability of safe and effective prophylactic antibiotics, continuous antibiotic prophylaxis (CAP) became adopted as the mainstay of the initial management of children with VUR in the 1970s. However, surgical management by ureteroneocystostomy (ureteric reimplantation) remained the treatment of choice for children experiencing recurrent/breakthrough UTIs or unresolved VUR. In the 1980s, endoscopic correction by injection of biocompatible materials (STING procedure) was introduced as a less invasive alternative to open surgery. More recently, robotic and laparoscopic ureteroneocystostomy have been added to the range of surgical options.

Numerous studies and controlled trials have been undertaken to compare the effectiveness of conservative and surgical management in preventing UTIs and renal scarring. However, these studies often yielded conflicting or inconclusive findings which failed to demonstrate any convincing advantage of one form of treatment over another. This probably reflects the difficulty in designing and conducting studies to take account of the many different variables in study populations. Meta-analyses have demonstrated a definite benefit from CAP in reducing the frequency of recurrent UTIs. However, the incidence of de novo renal scarring is relatively low in both medically and surgically treated patients and successful surgical correction of VUR has also been demonstrated to reduce the risk of recurrent UTIs.

Against this background of uncertainty, numerous professional organizations and national bodies have published guidelines for the diagnosis and management of UTI and VUR.

ETIOLOGY AND GENETIC BASIS OF VUR

The true incidence of VUR in children is difficult to ascertain with accuracy but the available evidence indicates that it can be found in 1–2% of younger children, decreasing in the older age groups. There is ample evidence that VUR has a strong genetic basis – with the incidence of VUR in infant siblings of affected children being approximately 30%, rising to 50% in the offspring of affected parents. Primary VUR is thought to represent the outcome of a developmental anomaly of the ureteral bud which typically results in a laterally placed ureteral orifice and defective valve mechanism caused by an abnormally short intramural/submucosal tunnel. Severe ureteral bud anomalies may be accompanied

by aberrant interaction with the metanephric mesenchyme leading to congenital renal dysplasia or hypoplasia. Attempts to identify a single "reflux gene" have been unrewarding and there have been very few studies with sufficient power to define the genetic basis of this condition. The available evidence indicates that nonsyndromic VUR has a polygenetic basis characterized by an autosomal dominant pattern of transmission with variable penetrance and expression. Amongst the genes expressed in the ureteric bud which have been have been implicated in VUR are *RET*, *PAX2*, *EYA1*, *SALL1*, *SIX1*, *SIX2*, *BMP4*, *TNXB*, and *GATA3*. Similarly, genes expressed in the metanephric tissue (*SLIT2*, *ROBO2*, and *SOX17*), have been linked to congenital renal malformations associated with VUR as have other genes expressed in the developing kidney such as *WNT4*, *FGF20*, *AGT*, *REN*, *ACE*, *AGTR1*, and *UMOD*.

It is hoped that ongoing and future genetic research may yield valuable insights into the genetic basis of VUR which could contribute to advances in diagnosis and management.

CAKUT (CONGENITAL ANOMALY OF THE KIDNEYS AND URINARY TRACT) AND REFLUX NEPHROPATHY

VUR is the commonest congenital anomaly of the kidneys and urinary tract (CAKUT). It is a major risk factor in the etiology of UTI and an important factor in bladder/bowel dysfunction (BBD). VUR is frequently identified as a causative or contributory factor in children with end-stage renal disease (ESRD). The presence of VUR is associated with a threefold increase in the incidence of acute pyelonephritis and pyelonephritic parenchymal scarring. However, the presence of VUR is not an essential prerequisite because both pyelonephritis and scarring can occur in the absence of VUR.

The term "reflux nephropathy" encompasses patterns of renal damage which may be the outcome of congenial dysplasia, acquired pyelonephritic scarring or, frequently, a combination of both mechanisms. However, the weight of experimental and clinical evidence indicates that the reflux of sterile urine at physiological voiding pressures does not cause renal scarring or impairment of renal growth. Reflux nephropathy accounts for more than 20% of children on end-stage renal failure programs and also poses a significant long-term risk of less severe forms of chronic kidney disease.

Severe congenital renal damage (renal dysplasia) is seen mainly in conjunction with high grade (IV–V) VUR (Figure 6.1). Histological studies of nephrectomy specimens in adults with severe reflux nephropathy have shown that whereas congenital renal damage is seen more commonly in males, pyelonephritic scarring is a far more important cause of long-term renal damage in females. Although, renal morphology is usually normal at the time of birth in children with low to moderate grades of VUR a small proportion may have renal hypoplasia a variant in which the normal renal outline is preserved but the kidney is reduced in size and contains fewer nephrons than a normal kidney. Pyelonephritic scarring can occur at any age but the kidneys of infants and young children

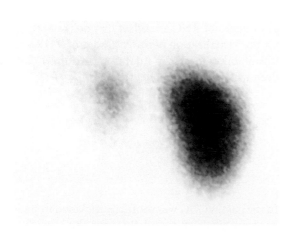

Figure 6.1 DMSA scan in a one month old infant with prenatally detected unilateral grade V VUR; 9% differential function in the affected kidney. No urinary tract infection prior to the DMSA. Findings demonstrate severe loss of function due to congenital dysplasia.

under the age of four are considerably more susceptible. In addition to gender-related differences there is considerable geographic, racial, and ethnic variation in rates of reflux nephropathy worldwide. Which of the different forms of medical and surgical management is most effective in protecting the kidney against acquired reflux nephropathy remains the subject of considerable controversy.

Presentation

Symptomatic presentation

Urinary tract infection (UTI) is the commonest form of clinical presentation. The incidence of VUR identified during the investigation of children with symptomatic UTIs has been historically quoted to be as high 30%. However, this figure is almost certainly lower in children with mild, predominantly lower tract UTIs. VUR is strongly associated with **Bladder and Bowel Dysfunction (BBD)** – a clinical syndrome defined by the coexistence of functional constipation and lower urinary tract symptoms (LUTS). Comorbid conditions associated with BBD include psychiatric/developmental disorders, and obesity.

Loin pain can occur as a symptom of **pyelonephritis** and pain may rarely denote the presence of **secondary pelvi-ureteric junction** obstruction. However, pain is not generally considered to be a feature of uncomplicated primary VUR. VUR sometimes comes to light for the first time in patients presenting with **renal insufficiency and/or hypertension** who may have little if any, history of documented symptomatic UTIs. In such cases the reflux nephropathy may be congenital in etiology or the late consequence of undiagnosed pyelonephritis in early childhood.

Asymptomatic Presentation

This includes VUR detected during screening of asymptomatic siblings and the offspring of parents with VUR and VUR identified during the investigation of infants with prenatally detected urinary tract dilatation (prenatal hydronephrosis [PNH]).

INVESTIGATION

Because the majority of children with VUR initially present with UTI, the diagnostic process usually commences with an ultrasound (US) scan of the urinary tract.

Ultrasound has the advantage of being a noninvasive investigation which does not entail any exposure to radiation. However, it is only capable of detecting those higher grades of VUR which give rise to detectable dilatation of the upper urinary tract. US is an unreliable routine screening test because of the high false negative rates in detecting lower nondilating grades of VUR. Nevertheless, US may still yield relevant information such as increased post void residual urine volume and bladder wall thickening in children whose VUR is linked to dysfunctional voiding. Renal scarring can also be visualized on US – although 99 m-Tc dimercaptosuccinic acid (DMSA) is the most sensitive imaging modality for this purpose. **Contrast-enhanced ultrasound (CEUS)** is a variant of ultrasonography which employs instillation into the bladder of a solution containing microbubbles which appear echogenic on US scanning. It has been advocated for the diagnosis of VUR but because it requires urethral catheterization and specialized equipment it has not found wide scale acceptance. (See Chapter 3.)

VOIDING CYSTOURETHROGRAPHY (VCUG)

Fluoroscopic voiding cystourethrography (VCUG) remains the definitive "gold standard" investigation for the diagnosis and evaluation of VUR. Following urethral catheterization, the bladder is filled with water soluble contrast and X-ray screening is performed during the filling and voiding phases. Various technical modifications have been introduced to reduce the exposure to radiation. Unlike other modalities VCUG not only permits grading of VUR but can also provide valuable additional anatomical information on the lower urinary tract which may be of considerable relevance in some cases. The most widely used grading system is the one originally devised by the International Reflux

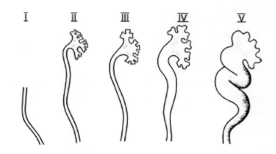

Figure 6.2 Grades of reflux (classification devised by international reflux study committee). Grade I: reflux into ureter only: Grade II reflux into non-dilated upper tract (pelvis and calyces); Grade III reflux accompanied by mild to moderate dilatation without "blunting" of calyces; Grade IV: moderate dilatation with some loss of normal calyceal appearances: Grade V gross dilatation and tortuosity with severe "blunting" of calyces.

Study in the 1970s (Figure 6.2). Nevertheless, the grading of VUR remains somewhat subjective – prompting some investigators to develop new diagnostic parameters such as the ureteral diameter ratio (UDR) or the VUR index (VURx).

Radionuclide cystography (RNC) was first introduced in the 1970s as an alternative to fluoroscopic VCUG, with the advantages that is does not require urethral catheterization and the radiation dose is lower (Figure 6.3). The technical details are described in Chapter 3. However, the advantages of RNC are offset by poor sensitivity for the visualization of lower grades of VUR and unsuitability for use in infants and younger children who are not yet toilet trained.

DIAGNOSTIC IMAGING FOR VUR AFTER URINARY TRACT INFECTION

In the past, VCUG was routinely included in standard protocols and guidelines for the investigation of children with UTIs. However, this resulted in many children (particularly those with lower tract UTIs) being over-investigated and subjected to unnecessary and invasive investigations which yielded negative results. There were also important cost implications. To address these concerns

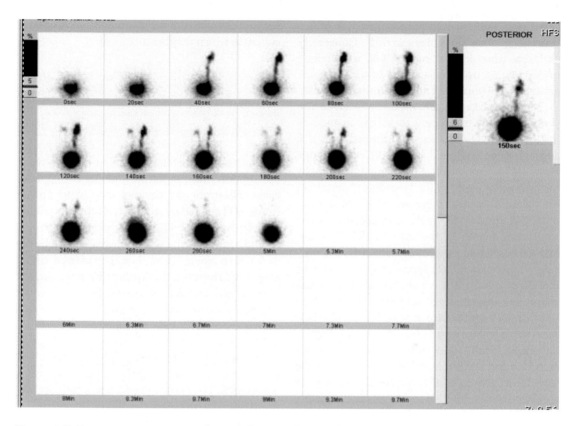

Figure 6.3 Representative images from indirect radionuclide cystogram.

evidence-based guidelines have been published by a number of professional organizations including the American Academy of Pediatrics (AAP), European Association of Urology and European Society for Paediatric Urology (EAU/ESPU), European Society of Paediatric Radiology (ESPR), and National Institute for Health and Clinical Excellence (NICE) in the United Kingdom. A more detailed review of these guidelines is contained in Chapter 5. The current AAP guidelines recommend that the use of renal and bladder ultrasound (RBUS) scan should initially be limited to children who have experienced a febrile UTI while the NICE guidelines state that RBUS is not necessary in a child aged over 6 months who has experienced a single "uncomplicated" lower tract UTI. There is considerable variation between guidelines with regard to the indications and timing of VCUG and DMSA in the diagnostic pathway. It should be noted, however, that relatively few studies have been undertaken to validate the different guidelines.

There is broad agreement in the guidelines that further investigations are indicated for those children who experience recurrent or febrile UTIs and those in whom the initial renal and bladder ultrasound scan demonstrated any abnormality (notably upper tract dilatation or evidence of renal damage). In addition, UTI caused by an "atypical" organism such as Pseudomonas or Proteus is generally regarded as an indication for further investigation.

In practice, however, many clinicians continue to routinely recommend a Renal and Bladder Ultrasound for any child who has experienced a documented or presumed UTI.

The principal dilemma lies in deciding on the extent of further investigation (notably VCUG and DMSA) in children with normal appearances of the urinary tract on ultrasound. Some of these children (mainly girls with nondilating VUR) would probably benefit from further investigation because the discovery of VUR might make them candidates for intervention, notably endoscopic correction, which could reduce their risk of further UTIs and possible scarring. Conversely, children who do not have VUR would have undergone an unnecessary and invasive investigation which would not alter their management.

The standard approach, which has been termed "bottom up", is to proceed to VCUG in the first instance with DMSA being performed later if it appears to be indicated by the VCUG findings. However, a fundamentally different philosophy (known colloquially as the "top-down" approach) has been advocated more recently which relies on RBUS and DMSA in the first instance. In the "top down approach" the use of a VCUG is limited to those children with evidence of renal scarring. Proponents of this approach argue that even if VUR is present if it is not accompanied by any changes in the renal parenchyma it is unlikely to be of clinical significance or pose a threat of future renal damage. Moreover, intervention is unlikely to be required if the kidneys appear entirely normal on RBUS and DMSA. If this argument is valid, the "top down" approach offers the advantages of fewer children being submitted to potentially distressing investigations and possible cost savings. However, the validity of this approach remains unproven and the findings of a recent meta-analysis have indicated that DMSA lacks the sensitivity and specificity to serve as a reliable screening for identifying children with high grade VUR. Criticism has been leveled at the NICE guidelines' highly selective indications for VCUG in the light of study findings which suggest that moderate or high grades of VUR are missed in a significant proportion of children when these guidelines are applied.

Faced with an abundance of (sometimes conflicting) guidelines how should the clinician decide how best to investigate a possible diagnosis of VUR in a child with UTI? Much will depend on factors such as the age and gender of the child, their medical history and clinical presentation, the diagnostic protocols employed by the institution's radiology department and possible cost implications. It is also essential that the parents are given all the information they need to make a fully informed contribution to the decision-making process. In consultation with the parents, however, it is ultimately for clinicians to decide on an evidence-based approach which is best suited to the needs of the individual child (and their parents) within the context of the institution and healthcare system in which they practice.

SCREENING FOR VUR IN SIBLINGS AND THE CHILDREN OF PARENTS WITH VUR

The rationale for sibling screening is based on an assumption that if VUR in a sibling is diagnosed early, measures can be implemented to prevent future UTI and renal scarring. Guidelines published by both the AAP and EAU recommend that parents should be informed about the increased genetic risk of VUR in siblings and should be offered sibling screening. However, the only feasible screening test is renal and bladder ultrasound (RBUS) – which has only a limited ability to detect VUR. Only if a sibling is found to have an abnormality on RBUS is VCUG recommended. If parents do not opt for screening, they (and the child's primary care physician) should be made aware that any documented or suspected UTIs should be treated promptly and any unexplained febrile episodes should be regarded as UTIs unless proven otherwise. The occurrence of UTI in a sibling of a child with VUR requires full evaluation, including VCUG.

The effectiveness of sibling screening in preventing UTIs and renal scarring has never been reliably established by randomized controlled studies – not least because of the difficulty in undertaking such studies. By one estimate, however, more than 30 asymptomatic siblings would need to be screened at a cost of US$56,000 in order to prevent a single febrile UTI. In summary, there is currently only very limited evidence to indicate that sibling screening is a worthwhile and cost effective measure. Screening is probably most useful in the first year or two of life but of very limited benefit in older siblings.

SCREENING FOR VUR IN CHILDREN WITH PRENATAL HYDRONEPHROSIS (PNH)

VUR may be manifest as dilatation of the fetal urinary tract – prenatal hydronephrosis (PNH) detected on prenatal ultrasonography. However, prenatal ultrasonography cannot reliably distinguish VUR from other causes of fetal urinary tract dilatation and a postnatal VCUG is required to confirm the diagnosis. Prenatally detected VUR is predominantly a condition of boys – in whom it is typically characterized by high grade VUR. By contrast, when VUR is diagnosed following clinical presentation with UTI, girls outnumber boys by a ratio of approximately five to one.

In the past, postnatal VCUG was performed routinely in all infants with PNH – including those with mild dilatation or "pelvi caliectasis" (corresponding to grades I and II in the Society for Fetal Urology [SFU]) classification. When performed routinely in infants with mild dilatation VCUG demonstrates an incidence of VUR of around 10%–15%. However, this VUR is usually low grade and of doubtful clinical significance. There is no convincing evidence that routine screening of all infants with prenatally detected hydronephrosis by VCUG is a worthwhile or cost effective means of preventing UTIs and renal scarring. For these reasons, American Urological Association and Society for Fetal Urology guidelines now advocate a more selective role for VCUG based on the following prenatal or early postnatal ultrasonographic criteria; ureteral dilatation (hydroureter), bladder abnormalities and moderate or severe grades of PNH, i.e. grades III–IV on the SFU scale. US appearances suggestive of duplex kidney should also be added to this list because of the high incidence of VUR into lower pole moieties.

TREATMENT OPTIONS FOR CHILDREN WITH VUR

Following the introduction of VCUG for the routine investigation of UTI in children in the 1960s and 1970s it became clear that VUR was far more common than had previously been recognized. This led to the introduction and wide scale use of surgical procedures for the correction of VUR. By the end of the 1970s, however, a more conservative approach had evolved which was underpinned by emerging evidence that VUR (particularly lower grades) has a strong tendency to resolve spontaneously during childhood (Table 6.1). In addition, the findings of clinical studies were being published which appeared to endorse the effectiveness of continuous antibiotic prophylaxis (CAP). In the mid-1980s the treatment options were further expanded by the introduction of a minimally invasive surgical intervention in the form of endoscopic correction.

The primary goal in the management of a child with VUR can be defined as the prevention of febrile UTIs and pyelonephritic scarring.

Table 6.1 Rates of spontaneous resolution and successful correction of vesicoureteral reflux pooled results of systematic reviews

	Spontaneous resolution at 1 year	Spontaneous resolution at 5 years	Open ureteroneocystostomy	Endoscopic injection dextranomer/ hyaluronic acid polymer
	Resolution Rate	Resolution Rate	% Successful correction VUR	% Successful correction VUR
Grade I	39%	92%	99%	89%
Grade II	28%	81%	99%	83%
Grade III	10%	42%	98%	71%
Grade IV	6%	16%	99%	59%
Grade V	-	-	81%	62%
Weighted average: all grades	17%	53%	97%	72%

However, another important goal is reducing the morbidity arising from recurrent lower tract UTIs which often impacts on general health and educational and social activities.

As far as possible, decisions on optimal management should be evidence based and individualized according to the child's gender, age, grade of VUR, clinical history (frequency and severity of UTIs), renal function, and any associated disturbance of bowel function. These decisions will also be strongly guided by parental preferences and the experience and clinical judgement of the clinician. The options currently available can be summarized as:

- Medical management with continuous antibiotic prophylaxis.
- Endoscopic correction by injection of bulking agents.
- Open or minimally invasive surgical correction by ureteroneocystostomy (ureteral reimplantation).

TREATMENT OF BLADDER/ BOWEL DYSFUNCTION

As already noted, there is a close relationship between bladder and bowel dysfunction and VUR and bladder symptomatology. When assessing a child with VUR it is essential to enquire about their bladder function. Ongoing dysfunctional voiding which is associated with infrequent or incomplete voiding is likely to increase susceptibility to ascending bacterial infection. In addition, elevated intravesical pressure secondary to detrusor instability associated with dysfunctional voiding may exacerbate the severity of any VUR which is present or prolong the duration of VUR which might otherwise have ceased spontaneously. Failure to address underlying bladder dysfunction will not only compromise the effectiveness of medical management but will reduce the chances of success following surgical management. The different types of functional voiding disorder and the various treatment options are considered in Chapter 12. It is also important to ensure that any associated bowel disorder, notably

habitual constipation, is recognized and actively treated. The success of medical management may be compromised if bowel function is not addressed because it is likely to exacerbate dysfunctional voiding and increase the risk of UTIs.

MEDICAL MANAGEMENT

This relies mainly on the use of continuous antibiotic prophylaxis (CAP) combined with other measures intended to reduce the risk of UTIs and normalize bladder function.

Since it was first described by Smellie and colleagues in the 1970s, CAP has been widely regarded as the standard approach for the initial management of VUR. In the majority of children with grades I to III VUR there is a high probability that it will resolve spontaneously during the course of childhood. The use of CAP in these children is intended to prevent UTIs and possible scarring while the VUR is in the process of resolving. Depending on their availability in different countries the most widely used prophylactic antibiotics are a trimethoprim-sulfamethoxazole combination, trimethoprim alone, nirofurantoin, and cephalexin. A major drawback of medical management by CAP is the extent to which its success is dependent on patient (and parental) compliance with long-term antibiotic usage. Some studies have suggested that compliance rates may be as low as 40%.

CAP has been the subject of several high-quality randomized trials, including the PRIVENT study, Swedish Reflux Trial, and RIVUR study. In addition, there have been a number of systematic reviews of the published data on CAP. A detailed review of the trial data is beyond the scope of this chapter but the key findings can be briefly summarized as follows: the weight of published data confirms that CAP significantly reduces the incidence of febrile and symptomatic UTIs in children with VUR. For example, in the Swedish Reflux Trial (in children with grades III–IV VUR) the incidence of febrile UTIs in the CAP arm of the study was 19% whereas the incidence of febrile UTIs in children allocated to the "surveillance" arm of the study was three times higher (57%). The evidence in relation to CAP and renal scarring is less clear cut. While some studies have identified an apparent reduction in new scar formation in children on CAP other studies have failed to find any statistically significant difference between children on CAP and controls. In part this probably reflects the fact that most scarring has already occurred by the time VUR is first diagnosed and the incidence of de novo scarring thereafter is relatively low, regardless of which type of management is adopted.

Some studies have reported that the benefit of CAP is independent of age, gender, and grade of VUR. However, the majority of studies have demonstrated that girls (particularly those with low to moderate grades of VUR) are considerably more likely to benefit from CAP than boys. Indeed, after the first year of life the overall incidence of UTIs in boys with primary VUR is low, regardless of how they are managed.

The results of the various reflux trials should be interpreted with some caution because only two (the PRIVENT and RIVUR trials) were judged by the authors of a recent metanalysis to be at low risk of bias. There is growing body of evidence that children on CAP are at increased risk of developing antibiotic resistant bacterial colonization and/or infection. This is likely to prove an increasingly relevant consideration for clinicians and parents when deciding on treatment.

SURGICAL MANAGEMENT

The options comprise endoscopic correction or ureteroneocystostomy (ureteral reimplantation) performed by either an open or minimally invasive technique.

Endoscopic Correction by Injection of Periureteral Bulking Agents

This approach was first described by Matouschek in 1981 and further developed and popularized by Puri and O'Donnell. Historically, various injectable materials were used for endoscopic correction including polytetrafluoroethylene (PTFE) – Teflon, collagen, polydimethylsiloxane (PDMS) – macroplastique and autologous chondrocytes. However, these were superseded by the introduction of dextranomer/hyaluronic acid (Dx/HA) copolymer "Deflux." In the United States, this continues to be the only injectable agent approved by the Food and Drug Administration (FDA).

TECHNICAL ASPECTS

Although various modifications have been described, the basic technique entails cystoscopic visualization of the ureteral orifice using an instrument with a "working channel" to accommodate a rigid or flexible needle. Under vision, the mucosa is punctured and the needle is advanced into a submucosal plane to facilitate injection of the implantable agent in the immediate vicinity of the ureteral orifice. In the standard technique, the injection is placed in a 6 o'clock position at the ureteral orifice but if the orifice is sufficiently wide to admit the tip of the cystoscope, an intra-ureteral injection is preferred. The implant is injected until a mound or "volcanic" bulge is formed and the ureteral orifice is elevated sufficiently to create a crescent shaped or slit-like orifice with a nipple-like appearance (Figure 6.4). After the injection has been completed the needle is left in position for 10–15 seconds to allow the gel to set and to minimize leakage.

Significantly, higher success rates (>93%) have been claimed for a technique termed the "double hydrodistention injection technique (HIT)".

Results of Endoscopic Correction

Caution is needed when interpreting the published success rates, not least because of differences in the definition of what constitutes a "successful" correction of VUR. Studies published from North American centers have typically defined success as the complete correction of VUR, i.e. no VUR visualized on follow up imaging. By contrast the authors of some European studies have extended their definition of "success" to include VUR which is still present but which has been downgraded to grades I–II from a higher grade. Reported success rates 3 months after treatment

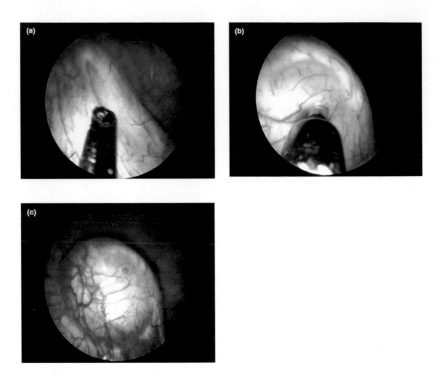

Figure 6.4 Correction of VUR by submucosal injection of dextran/hyaluronic acid polymer. See text for technical details.

are in the region of 75–80% (Table 6.1). However length of follow has a major impact on success rates, which typically decrease in relation to length of follow up. Moreover, more than one injection may be required to achieve correction of VUR. In the Swedish Reflux Trial, the initial success rate of endoscopic correction was 86% but 20% of treated children went on to develop recurrent VUR over the next 2 years.

The majority of published studies have focused on radiological outcomes, with little or no information on clinical outcomes with regard to UTI or renal scarring. The Swedish Reflux Study reported comparable rates of UTI in children managed by CAP or endoscopic correction (15% and 23%, respectively) but the incidence of new scarring was higher in those treated by endoscopic correction 12% vs. 6% p = 0.55.

Apart from failure to correct the VUR, complications are relatively rare – the most important being distal ureteral obstruction. Transient partial obstruction has been reported to occur in up to 5% of children but more severe or persistent obstruction requiring intervention is rare (<1% of cases). Some authors have claimed that even in cases where endoscopic injection does not achieve complete radiological correction of VUR, it may nevertheless contribute to a reduction in UTIs and clinical improvement in bladder function. In the United States, the uptake of endoscopic correction was not mirrored by any decrease in the number of ureteroneocystostomies. Moreover, in recent years the number of endoscopic corrections has plateaued. While, there is some evidence that initial enthusiasm for endoscopic correction may be waning, most pediatric urologists believe that it can be a useful intervention when used selectively. Examples include girls with VUR of moderate severity (grades II–IV) VUR and children with low to moderate grades of VUR who experience recurrent symptomatic breakthrough UTIs despite CAP. It is also the case that many parents may regard a simple surgical intervention to correct their child's VUR as a preferable alternative to prolonged antibiotic usage and the risks of antibiotic resistance.

Ureteroneocystostomy (Ureteral Reimplantation)

Open ureteroneocystostomy was widely adopted into pediatric urological practise in the 1950s and 1960s. Published success rates (defined by the complete correction of VUR) have been consistently reported to exceed 95% and ureteroneocystostomy has been shown to significantly reduce the risk of febrile UTI.

Despite technical differences in the various procedures the fundamental aim is similar: namely to replicate the normal one way valve mechanism at the uretrovesical junction by increasing the submucosal and/or intramural length of the distal ureteral segment as it enters the bladder.

The widely used Cohen technique is a cross-trigonal advancement procedure designed to elongate the submucosal course of the distal ureter within the bladder (Figure 6.5). Its appeal lies in its relative simplicity, high success rate in correcting VUR (97% or thereabouts) and low incidence of postoperative obstruction. Reflux into the lower pole ureter of a duplex kidney can also be reliably corrected using the Cohen technique. However, it is important that both duplex ureters are mobilized together within their common sheath and share the same submucosal tunnel in the bladder. Any attempt to re-implant the lower pole ureter on its own by separating the two ureters carries a risk of causing devascularization and/or damage to one or both ureters. In the Politano-Leadbetter technique, the ureter is initially mobilized intravesically. The ureter is then taken outside the bladder via the hiatus before being re-introduced into the bladder via a new hiatus created on the posterior bladder wall and drawn down to the trigone through a submucosal tunnel. Although largely superseded by the Cohen cross trigonal technique, the Politano-Leadbetter procedure retains a valuable role for grossly dilated refluxing ureters – particularly when it is combined with a Psoas Hitch procedure and reconstruction or ureteral tapering (Figure 6.6).

The extravesical technique originally described by Lich and Gregoir (Figure 6.7) has the advantage of causing less postoperative bladder discomfort. However, the extra vesical technique is less suited

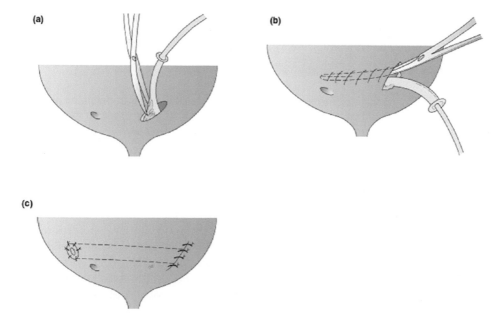

Figure 6.5 Ureteroneocystostomy by Cohen transtrigonal reimplantation technique. (a) Intravesical mobilization of ureter. (b) Creation of submucosal tunnel. (c) Ureter re implanted across the width of the trigone. The Cohen technique can be performed bilaterally and applied to duplex ureters and other variants.

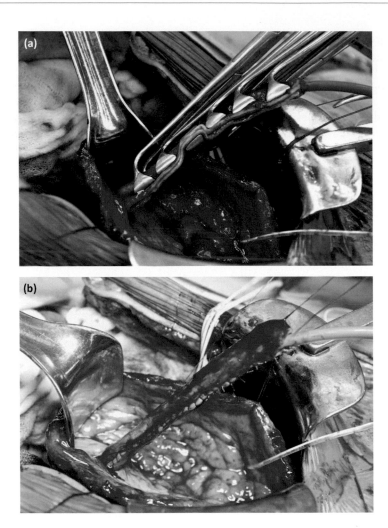

Figure 6.6 Tapering technique. (a) Forceps applied to dilated distal ureter to delineate portion of be excised during tapering. (b) After tapering, and prior to reimplantation of ureter in submucosal tunnel.

to dilated ureters and carries a well-documented risk of postoperative voiding dysfunction, which may occasionally amount to urinary retention. In summary, ureteroneocystostomy remains a highly effective option for children with high grade and/or symptomatic VUR (Table 6.1).

Minimally Invasive Ureteroneocystostomy

The role of minimally invasive techniques for the correction of VUR has been the subject of considerable controversy and there is considerable variation between different centers and pediatric urologists with regard to the indications, timing, and choice of technique. The technical aspects are considered in more detail in Chapter 23. Concerns have been raised regarding possible commercial influence, higher complication rates, and lack of evidence that minimally invasive procedures offer any significant advantages over current open surgical techniques. However, some of these concerns are being addressed as minimally invasive techniques evolve and become more widely adopted. This is clearly an area of ongoing technical research and development but for the time being many clinicians and parents will continue to favor open ureteroneocystostomy as opposed to a minimally invasive approach.

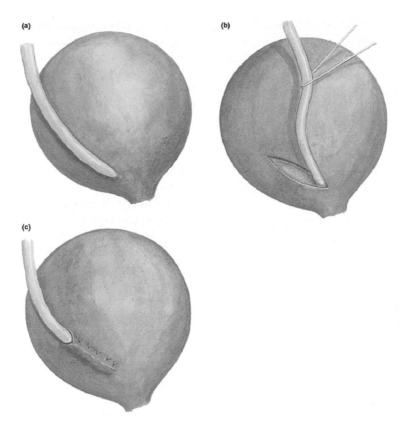

Figure 6.7 Extravesical (Lich-Gregoir) technique. Unsuitable for dilated ureters. (a) Ureter exposed and mobilized extravesically. (b) Detrusor muscle incised in the line of the ureter. Bladder mucosa exposed but not opened. (c) Detrusor closed around distal ureter to enclose it with submucosal tunnel.

Other Surgical Procedures

In some situations it may be necessary to consider other forms of surgical intervention.

For example, ureteroneocystostomy is probably best avoided in small infants with high grade VUR complicated by severe febrile UTIs because of the difficulty in creating an antireflux submucosal tunnel of adequate length in grossly dilated ureters. In addition, there are also concerns regarding long-term bladder dysfunction. In such cases a **cutaneous vesicostomy or refluxing ureterostomy** will provide effective temporary bladder decompression and drainage. Closure can either be performed as an isolated procedure or in combination with definitive correction of VUR during the second or third year of life.

There is growing evidence to support the use of **circumcision** boys with high grade VUR who are experiencing symptomatic breakthrough UTIs on CAP.

Nephroureterectomy may be a logical alternative to ureteroneocystostomy in children experiencing recurrent symptomatic UTIs who have high grade VUR associated with a poorly or non-functioning unilateral dysplastic and/or scarred kidney – particularly if this is thought to pose a potential long-term risk of hypertensive damage to the contralateral kidney. A minimally invasive approach is well suited for this purpose. The management of recurrent high grade VUR or obstruction following previous ureteroneocystostomy in a dilated ureter can be challenging. However, **Trans uretero ureterostomy (TUU)** can prove useful in these situations and may also be occasionally suitable as a primary procedure in cases of bilateral high grade VUR. TUU should only be considered if both ureters are dilated.

KEY POINTS

- VUR is an important cause of morbidity in children because of its role in urinary tract infection, pyelonephritis and renal scarring and its association with renal dysplasia.
- Reflux nephropathy may result from congenital or acquired renal damage - or a combination of both mechanisms.
- VUR is strongly associated with bladder and bowel dysfunction. Management of these conditions is an essential adjunct to management of the VUR itself.
- The role of different imaging techniques for the diagnosis of VUR remains controversial.
- Continuous antibiotic prophylaxis significantly reduces the incidence of symptomatic UTIs in children with VUR but carries a higher risk of inducing antibiotic resistant bacteria.
- Endoscopic correction and ureteroneocystostomy are effective ways of correcting VUR but may not always prevent the occurrence of further UTIs.

FURTHER READING

Holmdahl G, Brandstrom P, Lackgren G, Sillen U, Stokland E, Jodal U, et al. The Swedish reflux trial in children: II. Vesicoureteral reflux outcome. J Urol. 2010;184(1):280–285.

Peters CA, Skoog SJ, Arant BS, Jr., Copp HL, Elder JS, Hudson RG, et al. Summary of the AUA guideline on management of primary vesicoureteral reflux in children. J Urol. 2010;184(3):1134–1144.

Rivur Trial Investigators, Hoberman A, Greenfield SP, Mattoo TK, Keren R, Mathews R, et al. Antimicrobial prophylaxis for children with vesicoureteral reflux. N Engl J Med. 2014;370(25):2367–2376.

Routh JC, Bogaert GA, Kaefer M, Manzoni G, Park JM, Retik AB, et al. Vesicoureteral reflux: current trends in diagnosis, screening, and treatment. Eur Urol. 2012;61(4):773–782.

Shaikh N, Hoberman A, Keren R, Gotman N, Docimo SG, Mathews R, et al. Recurrent urinary tract infections in children with bladder and bowel dysfunction. Pediatrics. 2016;137(1).

Skoog SJ, Peters CA, Arant BS, Jr., Copp HL, Elder JS, Hudson RG, et al. Pediatric Vesicoureteral Reflux Guidelines Panel summary report: clinical practice guidelines for screening siblings of children with vesicoureteral reflux and neonates/infants with prenatal hydronephrosis. J Urol. 2010;184(3):1145–1151.

Wang HH, Gbadegesin RA, Foreman JW, Nagaraj SK, Wigfall DR, Wiener JS, et al. Efficacy of antibiotic prophylaxis in children with vesicoureteral reflux: systematic review and meta-analysis. J Urol. 2015;193(3):963–969.

Upper Tract Obstruction

KIM A R HUTTON and DAVID F M THOMAS

Topics covered

Acute and chronic upper tract obstruction
Diagnosis
Ultrasound
Isotope renography

Other imaging and diagnostic modalities
Pelviureteric junction obstruction
Vesicoureteric junction obstruction

INTRODUCTION

Upper urinary tract obstruction is an extremely important condition in children because it endangers renal function, poses a risk of potentially serious urosepsis and can cause distressing symptomatology. A high proportion of cases of possible upper tract obstruction are now identified prenatally following the discovery of fetal hydronephrosis or hydroureteronephrosis on maternal antenatal ultrasound scans. A substantial part of paediatric urological practice is now concerned with distinguishing between those infants who have significant obstruction demanding surgical intervention and those who can be safely managed conservatively.

The management of upper tract obstruction has been hindered by the indiscriminate use of terms such as 'idiopathic hydronephrosis' and 'pelviureteric junction (PUJ) obstruction' or 'vesicoureteric junction (VUJ) obstruction'

and 'primary megaureter' which are often used interchangeably. The use of other poorly defined terms such as 'physiological hydronephrosis' and 'transient hydronephrosis' further add to the confusion.

It is important to recognise that 'hydronephrosis' is not a pathological entity in its own right but simply a descriptive term denoting dilatation of the renal pelvis and calyces. Unfortunately, the term hydronephrosis is often used synonymously with PUJ obstruction. When this is accompanied by dilatation of the ureter the term 'hydroureteronephrosis' is used.

There are essentially four potential causes of upper tract dilatation:

- Urinary tract obstruction
- Vesicoureteric reflux (VUR)
- Developmental anomalies of the upper urinary tract
- Pathologically high rates of urine production ('flow uropathy')

In an attempt to achieve uniformity in the assessment of upper tract dilatation and obstruction a new classification was proposed following a multidisciplinary consensus conference held in the United States in 2014.

This classification (which is applicable to pre- and post-natal assessment) uses the following **criteria to evaluate the severity and clinical significance of upper urinary tract dilatation:**

1. Anterior-posterior renal pelvic diameter;
2. Calyceal dilatation;
3. Renal parenchymal thickness;
4. Renal parenchymal appearance;
5. Bladder abnormalities;
6. Ureteral abnormalities.

The findings of preliminary studies appear to validate the predictive value of this classification when applied to the clinical management of prenatally detected hydronephrosis. However, further studies are required to establish whether it offers any significant advantages over previously used scoring systems.

WHAT IS OBSTRUCTION AND HOW IS IT DIAGNOSED?

There is no universally accepted definition of obstruction nor is there a single investigation which is capable of providing an unequivocal diagnosis of obstruction in a dilated upper urinary tract. One widely used definition states that obstruction is any impairment to urine flow which, if left untreated will lead to progressive deterioration of function. However, this is not a very useful definition in clinical practice because it implies that the clinician should wait for evidence that the obstruction has caused renal damage before taking steps to prevent it. In clinical practice, decision-making is therefore guided by a combination of clinical factors and the evidence of imaging studies.

Acute Obstruction

The pathophysiology of acute obstruction has been studied in experimental animal models. In the first few hours, a sharp rise in intrarenal pressure is accompanied by a marked reduction in blood flow in the renal cortex. Some equilibration occurs after 24 hours but without prompt relief of the obstruction, rapid damage to the nephrons supervenes, with loss of approximately 50% of functioning nephrons after 6 days and irreversible loss of the entire function of the obstructed kidney within 6 weeks. However, acute obstruction is relatively rare in children. Possible causes include: impaction of a urinary calculus at the PUJ, acute PUJ obstruction or VUJ obstruction or early postoperative obstruction following a pyeloplasty or ureteric reimplantation which has not been protected by stenting.

Chronic Obstruction

This is encountered far more commonly in children but the pathophysiology is less well understood because of the difficulty in creating reliable experimental models.

Historically, it was far easier to justify a decision to intervene surgically because the majority of children with upper tract obstruction presented clinically with symptoms such as pain or urinary infection. Following the widespread introduction of antenatal ultrasound it became apparent, however, that the presence of mild to moderate upper tract dilatation is more prevalent in healthy, asymptomatic infants than was previously recognised. Indeed, some degree of dilatation of the fetal urinary tract is present in 1-2% of pregnancies. Even when obstruction has been demonstrated by the relevant investigations, the natural history is often characterised by progressive improvement and spontaneous resolution. The challenge is therefore to try to distinguish those infants in whom the dilatation/obstruction is destined to remain stable or resolve without affecting renal function from those with clinically significant obstruction which is likely to lead to loss of function unless intervention is undertaken to relieve it.

RADIOLOGICAL INVESTIGATION OF UPPER TRACT OBSTRUCTION

With the rare exception of acute obstruction by an impacted calculus, upper tract obstruction always gives rise to dilatation. However, the presence of dilatation does not always signify obstruction. Non-obstructive causes of dilatation include; VUR, developmental anomalies such as primary non-obstructive mega ureter and residual dilatation which may persist despite relief of obstruction in a previously obstructed system. Pathologically high urine flow, for example in diabetes insipidus, is a rare cause of dilatation.

Ultrasound

The diagnostic pathway usually starts with the ultrasound finding of dilatation (Figure 7.1).

The most valuable measurement derived from an ultrasound scan is the anteroposterior (AP) diameter of the renal pelvis at the renal hilum. In the neonate, this figure should not normally exceed 6 mm. However a diameter of 10 mm is usually taken as the upper limit of normal. Significant obstruction posing an active threat to renal function is most unlikely to be present if the AP diameter is less than 15 mm. Conversely, an AP diameter greater than 50 mm is almost invariably associated with impaired function, either at the time of initial assessment or during the course of follow up.

Additional parameters which may increase the sensitivity of ultrasound for the diagnosis of obstruction include calyceal dilatation (central or peripheral), thickness and ultrasound appearances of the renal parenchymal thickness and abnormal appearances of the ureters or bladder. The use of Doppler ultrasound has been described for the measurement of renal resistive index and assessment of jets of urine emerging from the ureteric orifices. However, this has not proved sufficiently sensitive to be of diagnostic value in a routine clinical practice.

The presence of ureteric dilatation is always an abnormal ultrasound finding because a ureter of normal calibre cannot be visualised on ultrasound.

Isotope Renography

The central role played by isotope renography in the diagnosis of upper tract obstruction is considered in detail in Chapter 3. In summary, dimercaptoacetyltriglycine (MAG3) labelled with metastable 99-Technetium (^{99m}Tc) is currently the radiopharmaceutical agent of choice.

In addition to quantifying differential function, dynamic renography provides serial gamma camera images of the kidneys and urinary tract and generates a graphic display of the uptake and clearance of the isotope from the kidneys over time. The use of dimercaptosuccinic acid (^{99m}Tc DMSA) is largely confined to assessing low levels of differential function when deciding between pyeloplasty and nephrectomy.

Diuresis renography provides a means of distinguishing between obstructed and non-obstructed dilatation.

The characteristics of the uptake and drainage curves, often referred to as the O'Reilly curves, fall into five well-recognised patterns (Figure 7.2):

- Type 1. Normal uptake with prompt washout
- Type 2. Rising uptake curve; no response to diuretic (obstruction)

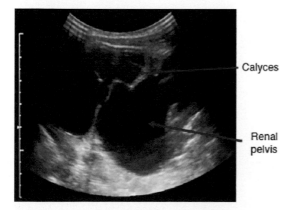

Figure 7.1 Postnatal ultrasound confirming antenatal ultrasound appearances of grossly hydronephrotic right kidney with marked dilatation of renal pelvis and calyces with thinned cortex.

Calyces

Renal pelvis

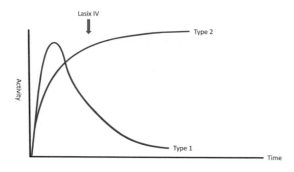

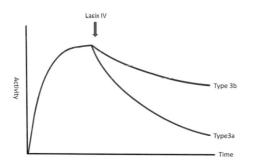

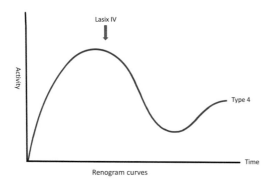

Renogram curves

Figure 7.2 Patterns of isotope renogram curves, as classified by O'Reilly and associates.

- Type 3a. Initially rising curve, which falls rapidly in response to diuretic (non-obstructive dilatation)
- Type 3b. Initially rising curve, which neither falls promptly nor continues to rise (equivocal)
- Type 4. There is a secondary peak suggesting obstruction precipitated by high urinary flow rates – the so-called Homsy's sign. Similar findings can be observed in patients with high grade VUR and no obstruction

Type 1 and type 3a curves are normal and non-obstructed. However, interpreting the clinical significance of type 2, type 3b and type 4 curves in children can often be more problematic.

Magnetic Resonance Imaging

Dynamic contrast-enhanced magnetic resonance imaging (MRI) can combine the anatomical information yielded by ultrasound with much of the functional information provided by renal scintigraphy. It has the advantage of providing anatomical and functional information in a single study without exposure to ionising radiation. The main drawback is the requirement for general anaesthesia or sedation in infants and younger children – although a 'feed and wrap' technique can be used in small infants.

The anatomical detail provided by dynamic contrast-enhanced MRI is excellent (Figure 7.3). In many centres dynamic contrast-enhanced MRI is replacing ultrasound and isotope as a 'one

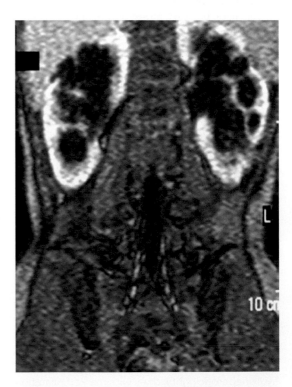

Figure 7.3 Contrast-enhanced MR scan demonstrating bilateral obstruction.

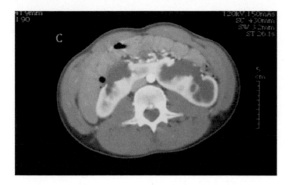

Figure 7.4 CT scan showing a horseshoe kidney with bilateral hydronephrosis due to bilateral PUJ obstruction. The isthmus can be seen crossing the abdominal aorta.

stop shop' imaging modality for the assessment of upper tract obstruction in children.

Computerised Tomography

Although not suitable for the routine assessment of upper tract obstruction in children, non-contrast and contrast-enhanced computerised tomography (CT) may be indicated in children presenting with obstruction due to calculi. CT may also be helpful delineating complex anatomy and aberrant renal vasculature – for example, horseshoe kidney (Figure 7.4). However, MRI has largely superseded CT in such cases.

Intravenous Urography

Intravenous urography (IVU), once the standard investigation for suspected upper tract obstruction, is now rarely used in children because the relevant functional and anatomical information can provided more accurately by other imaging modalities.

Retrograde Pyelography

This investigation entails cystoscopic catheterisation of the ipsilateral ureteric orifice and injection of X ray contrast to outline the upper urinary tract from below. It is not routinely performed prior to pyeloplasty by paediatric urologists in the United Kingdom but may still play a limited role – for example in identifying rare cases with obstruction at more than one level in the ureter.

Antegrade Pyelography

This contrast study, which is performed via ultrasound guided puncture of the kidney can be valuable for demonstrating obstruction distal to the PUJ and in cases of suspected recurrent PUJ obstruction following previous pyeloplasty.

Integrated Approach to Diagnostic Imaging

The aims of imaging are as follows:

- To determine whether the dilatation is genuinely due to obstruction.
- To establish the precise level of obstruction
- To measure differential renal function
- To assess the potential for recovery in poorly functioning kidneys
- To manage complications arising from infection in an obstructed system

Isotope renography is the principal investigation used to confirm or refute the diagnosis of obstruction but other imaging modalities may be needed to exclude reflux and non-obstructive dilatation. Renal ultrasound will usually provide adequate information on the level of obstruction. When this is unclear MRI is the investigation of choice, supplemented by antegrade or retrograde pyelography in difficult cases.

Differential renal function can usually be reliably assessed by MAG3 renography or dynamic contrast-enhanced MRI. However, in poorly functioning kidneys ^{99m}Tc DMSA isotope scintigraphy provides more accurate information and serves as a more reliable predictor of potential recovery of function. When percutaneous nephrostomy (PCN) has been performed to drain an infected/obstructed kidney, measurement of differential function (usually with ^{99m}Tc DMSA) should ideally be delayed until after 3–4 weeks of drainage.

PELVIURETERIC JUNCTION OBSTRUCTION

PUJ obstruction is characterised by impairment of urine transport across the pelviureteric junction leading to elevated renal pelvic pressures, dilatation of the proximal collecting system and the potential for nephron loss. It is a heterogeneous condition with a number of different causes and considerable variability in severity, clinical features, presentation and natural history. Estimates derived from antenatal screening place the incidence of PUJ obstruction in the range 1:750–1:1000. However, PUJ obstruction can also occur de novo as an acquired condition in older children.

The male to female ratio is approximately equal and the left kidney is more commonly affected than the right, by a ratio of approximately 2:1.

PUJ obstruction is associated with an increased incidence of other urinary tract anomalies such as:

- Multicystic dysplastic kidney (MCDK)
- Horseshoe kidney
- Ectopic kidney
- Duplex collecting systems (usually the lower moiety is affected)

Aetiology of PUJ Obstruction

Although the findings on diagnostic imaging, notably MRI, often provide a guide to the likely aetiology it is not usually until the time of operation that this can be established with certainty.

The causes of PUJ obstruction can be classified as follows:

Intrinsic obstruction (Figure 7.5a)

Typically, this comprises a short **stenotic segment** at the PUJ. However, in some cases, this may extend distally to involve a more extensive segment of proximal ureter. Although physical obstruction appears to play the most important role in children, functional obstruction due to an '**adynamic segment**' is very occasionally implicated as the likely cause. A number of histological abnormalities of smooth muscle and collagen have been reported and innervation abnormalities with reduced neural density and abnormalities of the interstitial cells of Cajal have also been described.

Extrinsic obstruction

Aberrant 'crossing' lower pole vessels are found in more than 30% of older children and adults undergoing pyeloplasty.

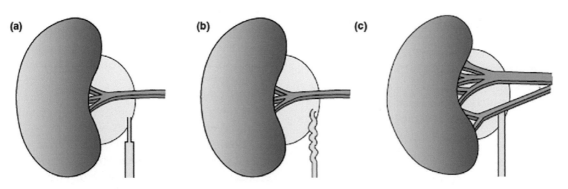

Figure 7.5 Aetiology of PUJ obstruction. (a) Intrinsic stenosis. Obstruction due to narrowing of a segment of ureter which is usually localised to the region of the pelviureteric junction but may extend over a length of several centimetres. (b) Ureteric folds. Tortuous segment of proximal ureter giving rise to varying degrees of obstruction. Straightening of this segment with growth may explain the spontaneous resolution of obstruction observed in a proportion of prenatally detected cases. (c) Extrinsic obstruction by crossing lower pole vessels.

In some cases, the presence of these vessels appears to be simply incidental to an intrinsic PUJ obstruction. However, in many cases, particularly older children presenting with intermittent loin pain, it is clear from the operative findings that the aberrant vessels are directly responsible for external compression and obstruction at the level of the pelviureteric junction. In suitably selected cases laparoscopic transposition of the lower pole vessels can successfully relieve the obstruction without the requirement for any surgical procedure on the pelviureteric junction itself.

In infants with prenatally detected PUJ obstruction, however, lower pole vessels account for less than 5% of cases requiring pyeloplasty.

In some cases the PUJ itself is normal in calibre but the proximal ureter is tortuous and obstructed by the presence of **kinks and folds** (Figure 7.5b). Overlying bands and adhesions may also be present. This variant of PUJ obstruction may have the potential to resolve spontaneously as the proximal ureter straightens with growth.

Intraluminal obstruction

A **urinary tract stone** which originated within the kidney may become impacted at the PUJ to cause acute or acute -on- chronic obstruction. Other causes include: **fibroepithelial polyps** arising from the renal pelvis (Figure 7.6), and **mycelial balls** resulting from fungal urinary tract infection – typically with *Candida albicans* (Figure 7.7).

High insertion of the pelviureteric junction

In cases where the PUJ is found to be high on the anterior wall of the dilated renal pelvis this is generally regarded as being a secondary phenomenon (upwards displacement of the PUJ due to progressive dilatation of the pelvis) – rather than the primary cause of obstruction.

Variants of PUJ Obstruction

Horseshoe kidney

The majority of horseshoe kidneys remain asymptomatic and do not cause urological problems.

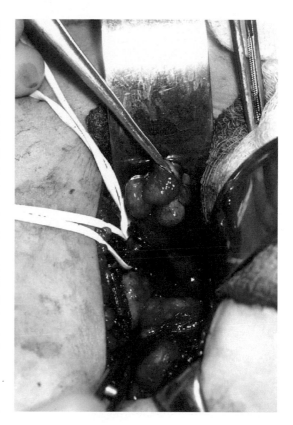

Figure 7.6 PUJ fibroepithelial polyps. Operative findings at open surgery in an 11-year-old boy presenting with loin pain. Preoperative imaging with ultrasound and isotope renography had shown hydronephrosis with obstruction at the PUJ. The intraluminal polyps, which resembled 'a bunch of grapes', were an unexpected finding on opening the 'bulky' upper ureter/PUJ region. Resection of all polyps together with an Anderson-Hynes dismembered pyeloplasty successfully relieved his symptoms and the obstruction. (Reprinted from paediatrics and child health, volume 18, edition 6, Kim A R Hutton and Ram Shrestha, surgical management of renal tract problems, page 260, Copyright 2008, with permission from Elsevier.)

The commonest complication is obstruction – which may be caused by the deviated course of the proximal ureter over the renal isthmus or, more commonly, by extrinsic compression by aberrant vasculature. On rare occasions a constellation of renal pathology can be encountered in the same patient – such as a horseshoe kidney,

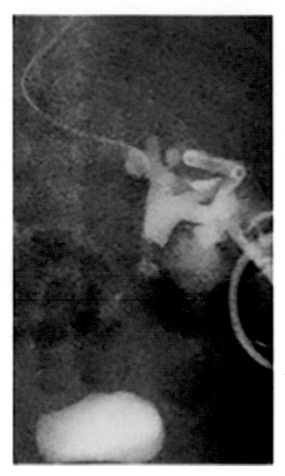

Figure 7.7 Renal fungal balls causing PUJ obstruction. A neonate born prematurely at 27 weeks gestation suddenly became completely anuric during the course of his intensive care treatment. A renal ultrasound showed marked bilateral hydronephrosis and echogenic material obstructing both PUJs. The patient required bilateral PCN insertion. In this right nephrostogram study a fungal ball can be seen obstructing the PUJ. The fungal balls and candida infection were successfully treated with the patient making a full recovery. (Reprinted from Paediatric Surgery International, Volume 20, Edition 10, R. Babu and K A R Hutton, Renal fungal balls and pelvi-ureteric junction obstruction in a very low birth weight infant: treatment with streptokinase, page 805, Copyright 2004, with permission from Springer Nature.)

renal duplication, and lower pole PUJ obstruction (Figure 7.8).

Retrocaval ureter

This rare anomaly, which more commonly affects the right ureter, originates from abnormal development of the posterior cardinal veins, the precursors of the inferior vena cava. Further investigation by MRI is indicated if this diagnosis is suggested by the ultrasound findings. A laparoscopic or robotic-assisted approach to treatment is preferable to open surgery.

Reflux in association with PUJ obstruction

Severe tortuosity and kinking of the proximal ureter associated with high grade VUR (e.g. grades IV and V) can sometimes give rise to fixed obstruction to the drainage of urine from the kidney. The diagnosis is confirmed by performing MAG3 renography with a catheter in the bladder to ensure that isotope does not reflux back to the kidney to interfere with interpretation of the findings. Antegrade pyelography may also be diagnostic. Depending on clinical factors the management options include conservative management, pyeloplasty (possibly combined with ureteric reimplantation), and ureteric reimplantation alone. It has been argued that pyeloplasty and ureteric reimplantation should not be performed simultaneously for fear of compromising the blood supply to the ureter. However, this appears to be a largely theoretical risk and in practice the two procedures can be safely combined if necessary.

Although primary ureteric reimplantation can be expected to correct the reflux it often fails to alleviate the secondary obstruction – thus necessitating a subsequent pyeloplasty.

Natural History of PUJ Obstruction

This is very variable, ranging from complete resolution to rapidly increasing obstruction causing deterioration in renal function. In a substantial proportion of cases the obstruction, whilst persisting, nevertheless remains stable for many years, with little or no impact on renal function. The later

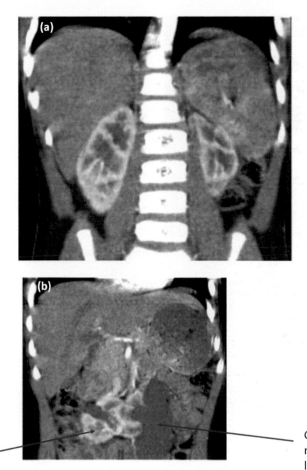

Functioning normal right lower moiety and isthmus

Grossly hydronephrotic, non-functioning left lower moiety of duplex horseshoe kidney

Figure 7.8 Bilateral renal duplication within a horseshoe kidney with left lower pole PUJ obstruction. This 5-year-old girl was referred with increasing left loin pain following conservative management of a prenatally detected uropathy. (a) Contrast CT image showing both upper poles. (b) Image showing the functioning right lower pole, 'chunky' isthmus and grossly hydronephrotic, non-functioning left lower pole. A left lower pole heminephrectomy with division of isthmus tissue overlying the aorta resulted in complete relief of her symptoms.

onset of PUJ obstruction in a previously normal kidney may be associated with aberrant lower pole vessels rather than intrinsic stenosis (Figure 7.9).

PRESENTATION

Prenatal detection: PUJ obstruction is the most common clinically significant uropathy detected during pregnancy. However, mild to moderate degrees of PUJ obstruction may not be present or may not yet have given rise to detectable dilatation at the time when routine fetal anomaly scans are performed in the second trimester. Such cases either remain undetected or are only detected if additional scans are performed later in pregnancy. The severity of dilatation (AP diameter of the renal pelvis) is a more accurate predictor of functional impairment than the gestational age at which dilatation was first detected.

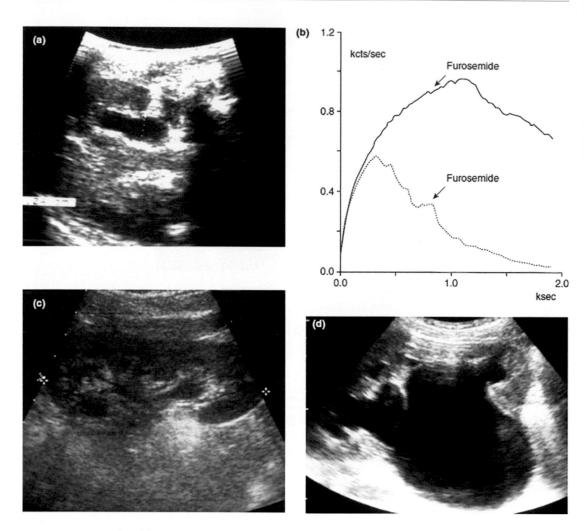

Figure 7.9 Unpredictable natural history of PUJ obstruction. (a) An ultrasound at 1 month of age. Appearances suggestive of PUJ obstruction, good renal cortex, AP diameter of renal pelvis (not shown) 18 mm. Conservative management was adopted. (b) Follow-up MAG study at 36 months showing type 3b O'Reilly curve (equivocal). Conservative management was maintained. (c) Ultrasound at 4 years of age. Complete resolution of dilatation, normal appearances of kidney. The child was discharged from further follow-up. (d) At 9 years of age he represented acutely with pain and infection. This ultrasound scan demonstrates severe dilatation due to recurrent PUJ obstruction. Pyeloplasty was curative.

Urinary tract infection used to be the commonest mode of presentation in infants and young children before the advent of prenatal ultrasound. In severe cases, infection within the obstructed system may progress to pyonephrosis – a serious condition characterised by high fever, systemic ill health, and ultrasound findings of debris within the collecting system.

Pain is typically encountered as a presenting feature of PUJ obstruction due to aberrant crossing vessels in older children. Although usually sited in the region of the loin, the pain may be more generalised within the abdomen, giving rise to possible diagnostic difficulties. Unlike non-specific abdominal pain, however, pain arising in the obstructed kidney usually persists for many hours or several days.

Haematuria may occur spontaneously, but is more commonly associated with minor trauma – to which obstructed kidneys are more susceptible. A grossly dilated kidney can sometimes present as an **abdominal mass** mimicking a Wilm's tumour. The distinction can be readily made with ultrasound, CT or MR imaging.

Occasionally, a dilated kidney comes to light as an **incidental finding** – for example, on an abdominal ultrasound performed for presumed non-specific abdominal pain, a CT scan performed for abdominal trauma or MR imaging for a spinal condition such as scoliosis.

Investigation

The diagnostic pathway has already been considered above. Typically, the sequence comprises ultrasound followed by ^{99m}Tc MAG3 dynamic renography. However, MRI is being increasingly used a the principal imaging modality. Other imaging modalities are only required in complicated cases: for example, to investigate secondary PUJ obstruction in the presence of gross reflux. DMSA scintigraphy is used to assess differential function in poorly functioning obstructed kidneys to guide the decision on whether to perform pyeloplasty or nephrectomy.

Management

Prenatally detected PUJ obstruction

The majority of infants are asymptomatic and would have remained undiagnosed (at least in infancy) if it had not been for the information yielded by the antenatal ultrasound scan.

The indications for pyeloplasty in children with prenatally detected PUJ obstruction remain controversial, although there is a broad consensus in favour of conservative management if differential function in the affected kidney is normal (defined as greater than 40%). The findings of early follow up studies reported from Great Ormond Street Hospital, UK indicated that when the initial AP diameter of the renal pelvis was less than 20 mm, 11% of patients eventually required a pyeloplasty for deterioration in function or symptoms. When the AP diameter

was 20–29 mm the pyeloplasty rate was 40% and when the AP diameter was 30–39 mm the pyeloplasty rate was 90%. Pyeloplasty (for reduced function or symptoms) was required in every child (100%) in those in whom the AP diameter exceeded 40 mm. Broadly comparable results for conservative management have been reported in other studies employing the system devised by the Society for Fetal Urology for grading the severity of prenatally detected hydronephrosis.

Fifteen to twenty percent of infants have bilateral dilatation. In these circumstances less reliance can be attached to the renographic assessment of differential function and greater weight must be attached to the severity of dilatation. In practice it is rare to encounter bilateral obstruction of equal severity, and if surgery is indicated it is usually reasonable to operate on the more severely dilated kidney and monitor the contralateral kidney. Only rarely is it necessary to operate on both kidneys simultaneously or in quick succession.

Conservative versus Surgical Management

The published outcome data have been derived almost entirely from observational studies and there have been very few randomised controlled trials of operative versus conservative management. The authors of a Cochrane review concluded (from the very limited trial data) that the majority of newborns and infants under 2-years of age who are managed conservatively do not experience significant deterioration in differential function, with only 20% coming to early pyeloplasty.

Incidentally detected PUJ obstruction

Conservative management can be adopted initially if the PUJ obstruction has been identified as an asymptomatic incidental finding and differential function is 40% or higher. Ultrasound follow up should be maintained until such time as the dilatation shows signs of resolving. Worsening hydronephrosis or the onset of symptoms are indications to proceed to surgery.

Infection (pyonephrosis)

Patients presenting with acute urosepsis are often very unwell with a high fever, tachycardia, a tender loin mass, and possible signs of haemodynamic instability. Initial management comprises resuscitation, urine culture, and intravenous antibiotics. Investigation comprises tests of renal function and septic markers and urgent ultrasound imaging of the urinary tract. The presence of debris in the collecting system is an indication to proceed to surgical intervention to decompress the obstructed kidney and drain the infected material. Ultrasound guided percutaneous nephrostomy is the preferred way of achieving this in children because it provides more rapid and effective drainage and is technically more straightforward than cystoscopic JJ stenting.

Once the condition has been stabilised, imaging is performed to confirm the diagnosis of obstruction (e.g. by antegrade pyelography via the nephrostomy catheter) and to assess differential function (e.g. by ^{99m}Tc DMSA scintigraphy). This information then permits a decision on whether to advise pyeloplasty or nephrectomy.

Symptoms (pain)

Children who present with classical episodic loin pain are almost invariably cured by surgical intervention. In the majority of cases, the obstruction is due to aberrant crossing vessels and the standard approach is to perform a pyeloplasty in which these vessels are transposed posteriorly to lie behind the anastomosis. However, an alternative approach (laparoscopic vascular hitch procedure) is being increasingly adopted. The PUJ is preserved intact and after the obstructing lower pole vessels have been mobilised from the PUJ they are anchored at a higher position on the anterior wall of the renal pelvis. The technical aspects are described in Chapter 23.

In summary, the indications for pyeloplasty are:

- Symptomatic PUJ obstruction, e.g. pain, infection, palpable renal mass
- Asymptomatic obstruction with reduced function (generally interpreted less than 40%) at the time of initial evaluation

- Asymptomatic obstruction and initial AP diameter of the renal pelvis equal to or greater than 30 mm
- Failure of conservative management, i.e. deteriorating function or increasing dilatation

Surgical Procedures

Although, the Anderson-Hynes dismembered pyeloplasty remains the most widely performed procedure for the correction of PUJ obstruction other options have also been described. These include balloon dilatation, endopyelotomy, and the vascular hitch procedure (in cases due to aberrant lower pole vessels). Primary ureterocalicostomy can yield good results in selected cases.

Anderson-Hynes dismembered pyeloplasty

Regardless of whether this is performed by an open or laparoscopic approach, the fundamentals of the technique are the same (Figure 7.10).

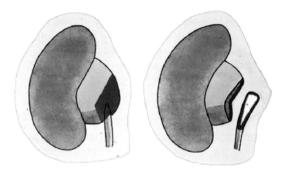

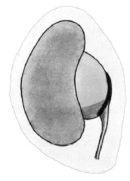

Figure 7.10 Anderson-Hynes dismembered pyeloplasty. The procedure of choice in children.

Gentle tissue handling, minimal mobilisation of the ureter, protection of the ureteric blood supply and creation of a widely patent, tension-free, watertight anastomosis all contribute to a successful outcome. Following excision of the PUJ, the proximal ureter is incised for a short length – 'spatulated'. Depending on surgical preference some of the redundant renal pelvis can be excised (reduction pyeloplasty) – although there is little evidence that this promotes more effective drainage postoperatively. Most paediatric urologists use interrupted sutures to begin the anastomosis between the spatulated ureter and renal pelvis. To minimise the risk of stenosis it is advisable to perform the anastomosis over a tube even if it is not intended to drain the kidney with an indwelling tube postoperatively.

Although many different methods of postoperative drainage have been described, published studies have mostly failed to demonstrate any statistically significant advantage of one over another.

Currently, the most widely used forms of postoperative drainage are either an indwelling JJ stent (with the drawback that this needs removing cystoscopically under a further general anaesthetic some 4–6 weeks postpyeloplasty) or an externalised pyeloureteral stent ('nephrostent'). This is, in effect, a JJ stent with an extension which crosses the renal pelvis, exits through the parenchyma or renal pelvis and emerges from the skin. Such stents can be easily removed without the need for a second anaesthetic, usually 1–2 weeks post-pyeloplasty. Some paediatric urologists prefer to avoid any form of transanastomotic stent, but rely instead on simple extrarenal drainage.

Open pyeloplasty

Despite the increasing number of pyeloplasties being performed by a laparoscopic or robotic-assisted laparoscopic technique there is still a very definite place for open surgery, particularly in the first few months of life. Depending on the age of the child and the surgeon's preference, open pyeloplasty can be performed via either an anterior, subcostal, extraperitoneal muscle splitting incision, or a muscle cutting loin incision.

The posterior lumbotomy approach provides more direct access to the kidney and is well tolerated postoperatively. However, the more limited access offered by this incision can create difficulties if the surgeon is forced to deal with unexpected anatomical findings or intraoperative problems.

The **minimally invasive open technique** is a modification of the open approach which utilises a smaller skin incision. In infants under 1 year of age an incision of 1–1.5 cm in length may be adequate. The incision is then deepened through underlying fascia and by manoeuvring the overlying skin incision the kidney can be exposed. If necessary, two narrow blade retractors can be used separate the edges of the skin incision. Decompression of the renal pelvis by needle aspiration allows the PUJ to be delivered out of the incision to enable the surgeon to perform the anastomosis. When used selectively this technique can offer a high success rate with a very short (<24 hours) hospital stay.

Laparoscopic and robotic-assisted laparoscopic pyeloplasty

The technical aspects of minimally invasive procedures and their relative advantages and drawbacks are considered in detail in Chapter 23. In a recent survey, 50% of paediatric urologists stated their preference for a minimally invasive approach in children aged 2 years and upwards.

Robotic-assisted laparoscopically pyeloplasty (RALP) offers a number of advantages over conventional laparoscopic pyeloplasty (LP) and has shorter learning curve. However, costs are higher for RALP.

Other Surgical Procedures

Laparoscopic transposition of crossing lower pole vessels

The technical aspects of the vascular hitch procedure are described in Chapter 23.

Endourological interventions

The use of balloon dilatation and endopyelotomy have both been reported children but the results are inferior to pyeloplasty. Nevertheless, there may be a very occasional role for antegrade or retrograde endopyelotomy in cases of failed pyeloplasty in older children due to a short (<10 mm) stricture at the PUJ.

Ureterocalicostomy (Figure 7.11)

In this procedure, the ureter is detached from the renal pelvis and anastomosed directly to the most dependent lower pole calyx. Ureterocalicostomy is only appropriate in cases with severe caliceal dilatation and cortical thinning. Although rarely indicated as a primary procedure, ureterocalicostomy may provide more effective drainage than pyeloplasty in cases of recurrent PUJ obstruction or PUJ obstruction occurring in a horseshoe kidney.

Pyeloplasty in duplex kidney

PUJ obstruction in a duplex kidney almost invariably affects the lower pole. It is usually caused by stenosis at the point where the lower pole pelvis

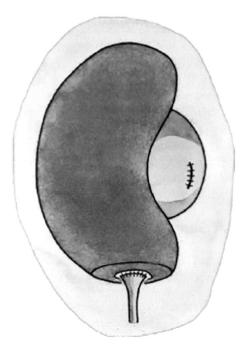

Figure 7.11 Ureterocalicostomy. The ureter is disconnected from the renal pelvis and the pelviureteric junction closed. The ureter is then anastomosed directly to the lower pole calyx.

joins the ureter descending from the upper pole. The anastomosis is performed using a modified 'fish mouth' technique to minimise the risk of obstruction to drainage from the upper pole. When the obstruction is caused by aberrant crossing vessels the surgical technique is determined by the individual operative findings.

Nephrectomy

When deciding whether to advise pyeloplasty or nephrectomy, most paediatric urologists apply an arbitrary 'cut off' value for differential function in the range of 10–15%. ^{99m}Tc DMSA scintigraphy is the most reliable method for obtaining an accurate measure of differential function in these circumstances. To assess the potential for recovery of function a period of temporary percutaneous nephrostomy drainage or JJ stent insertion may be helpful in borderline cases.

Complications of Dismembered Pyeloplasty

- Wound infection
- Urinary infection
- Haematoma
- Stent related problems
- Urine leak
- Urinoma formation
- Recurrent obstruction

The majority of paediatric urologists in the United Kingdom employ some form of intrarenal postoperative drainage in the belief that it reduces the risk of complications. Nevertheless, early postoperative complications of some type occur in 5%-10% of cases.

Follow-Up and Surgical Outcomes

Postoperative follow up relies mainly on ultrasound. If this clearly demonstrates that the dilatation is resolving (or reduced in severity) it can be reasonably assumed that the operation has successfully relieved the PUJ obstruction and it is not necessary to confirm this with a ^{99m}Tc MAG3 renogram. However, this investigation is advisable if ultrasound demonstrates persisting dilatation with no discernable reduction in its severity. Nevertheless, it may be a considerable time before renogram drainage curves revert to normal in kidneys which were grossly dilated before pyeloplasty. Dismembered pyeloplasty is a good operation, with a long-term success rate of >95%. Most failed procedures are diagnosed within 3 years of surgery and redo pyeloplasty, open or minimally invasive, has a high success rate (80–100%).

VESICOURETERIC JUNCTION OBSTRUCTION

Ureteric dilatation (megaureter) is classified as follows:

- **Obstructed megaureter**: The obstruction is usually intrinsic with either stenosis or an adynamic segment of distal ureter at the VUJ (Figure 7.12). Secondary causes include: tumour, scarring and fibrosis, neuropathic bladder, or bladder outflow obstruction. Most cases are due to primary obstruction at the VUJ, and hence the synonym '**VUJ obstruction**'.
- **Non-refluxing, non-obstructed megaureter**: The aetiology of such cases is often unclear

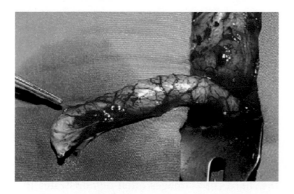

Figure 7.12 Obstructed megaureter. The ureter has been mobilised and divided at the level of the bladder. Dilatation of the ureter proximal to a short stenotic segment at the vesicoureteric junction.

but it is thought that many represent the legacy of 'burnt-out' VUJ obstruction, in which the original obstruction has resolved, leaving residual dilatation.
- **Refluxing megaureter**: Occasionally obstruction and reflux co-exist simultaneously within the same ureter.

Aetiology of Primary VUJ Obstruction

This is characterised by a marked discrepancy between the diameter of the terminal segment of the distal ureter and the dilated, often tortuous, length of ureter above it. Although a narrowed stenotic segment can be identified in some cases, in others the distal ureter is relatively normal in calibre and only appears narrow by comparison with the dilated ureter. In such cases the obstruction is thought to be functional in aetiology, with failure of normal coordinated urine transport across the distal ureter and vesico ureteric junction. Histological studies have demonstrated a range of abnormalities including a reduction in interstitial cells of Cajal (thought to be important for normal ureteric peristalsis), smooth muscle hypertrophy, and collagen deposition.

Clinical Presentation

Most cases of primary obstructed megaureter are now detected prenatally. Data derived from routine prenatal ultrasound screening point to an incidence of 1:1500–1:2000. Megaureter occurs more frequently in males, the left side is more commonly affected than the right and 25% of cases have bilateral involvement. Infants with prenatally detected primary megaureter are almost invariably asymptomatic. However, the condition is not always detected prenatally and some children still present clinically with symptoms of urinary infection, loin pain, haematuria, failure to thrive, an abdominal mass, or associated urolithiasis. VUJ obstruction can also present occasionally with intermittent loin pain, in a manner similar to intermittent PUJ obstruction (Figure 7.13).

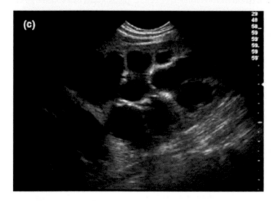

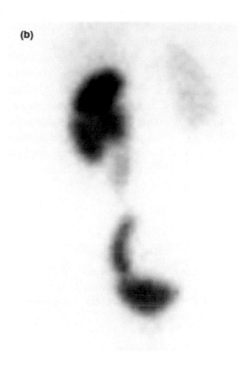

Figure 7.13 (a) Intravenous urogram in a 12-year-old girl with a long history of intermittent abdominal pain diagnosed as 'abdominal migraine'. Ultrasound (not shown) and IVU performed between episodes of pain were consistent with non-obstructive dilatation. (b) MAG3 renogram shows good preservation of function. The findings were interpreted as non-obstructive dilatation consistent with 'burnt out' obstructed megaureter. (c) However, an ultrasound scan performed acutely during an episode of pain demonstrated a dramatic increase in the severity of caliceal dilatation. Diagnosis: intermittent VUJ obstruction. Her symptoms resolved completely following surgery.

Investigation

Ultrasound cannot distinguish between dilatation due to obstruction and dilatation associated with the higher grades of VUR. For this reason an MCUG is an essential investigation in the assessment of children with megaureter.

Once reflux has been excluded an isotope renogram is then required to quantify differential function and to assess drainage. However, it is important to be aware that drainage curves may be difficult to interpret because clearance of isotope from a capacious, grossly dilated upper tract is often delayed even in the absence of obstruction. Moreover, closer scrutiny of the 'hard copy' images often demonstrates that although isotope has drained from the kidney (interpreted as non-obstruction) it has simply emptied into the capacious ureter rather than draining into the bladder. In clinical practice, the diagnosis of significant obstruction often has to rely on information on differential function and ultrasound assessment of changes in the severity of dilatation- in addition to drainage curve data.

Management of Prenatally Detected Obstructed Megaureter

The majority of infants with prenatally detected VUJ obstruction are healthy and asymptomatic at birth. Early surgical intervention (because of reduced differential function) is required in around 10% of cases and a further 10–20% of children will eventually require surgery for the indications outlined below. Conservative management has a long-term success rate of 70–80%.

Indications for surgical intervention:

- Impaired differential function (<40%) on initial assessment
- Increasing dilatation and/or deterioration of differential function on follow up
- Occurrence of symptoms (typically febrile urinary infection)

The severity of dilatation on initial assessment is a reasonable predictor of the likely success or failure of conservative management with a ureteric diameter ≥14 mm indicating an increased risk of surgery being required during the course of follow up.

Urinary infection of mild to moderate severity is not an automatic indication for surgery if other parameters (differential function, ureteric diameter 1 cm or less) are favourable. A period of antibiotic prophylaxis and trial of conservative treatment are appropriate in such cases, but surgery is indicated in the event of recurrent or severe infection.

Stone formation associated with stasis in a dilated but non obstructed ureter has been reported to occur as late complication of otherwise – successful conservative management.

Surgical Procedures

The definitive treatment of VUJ obstruction consists of excising the distal ureteric segment and reimplanting the ureter into the bladder. JJ stenting and endoscopic balloon dilatation have also been reported as temporising (or even definitive) alternatives to reimplantation.

Most paediatric urologists prefer to avoid reimplantation of megaureters in the first year of life because of the disparity in size of the dilated ureter and the small capacity bladder. Moreover, there is strong anecdotal evidence that this type of surgery in small infants carries some risk of later neurogenic bladder dysfunction due to damage to pelvic innervation sustained during dissection in the vicinity of the bladder. Despite these reservations, however, some paediatric urologists have claimed good results and low complication rates following reimplantation of megaureters in the first year of life.

Endourological interventions

The use of a JJ stents was initially described as a temporising manoeuvre but it has since been reported that a prolonged period (>6 months) of indwelling stent drainage may be curative in its own right. Success rates ranging from 26% to 66% have been reported. However, stent insertion by a purely endoscopic technique may not be technically possible in a small infant and open cystotomy may be required. A complication rate of up to 70% has been reported, including; urinary infection, stent migration, and deterioration in function – leading in some cases to nephrectomy. Higher success rates of 70–100% have been claimed when JJ stenting is combined with high pressure balloon dilatation or use of ureteroscopic endoureterotomy.

Temporary urinary tract diversion

Historically, severe forms of obstructed megaureter in small infants were sometimes managed by temporary cutaneous ureterostomy pending definitive surgery at a later age. A novel alternative has recently been described, which consists of a temporary internal diversion in which the dilated ureter is divided proximal to the obstructing segment and an end to side anastomosis is performed with the bladder – thus converting the obstructed megaureter into a refluxing megaureter. Definitive reconstruction is then performed at around 1 year of age.

Excision of obstructing segment and ureteric reimplantation

The standard open surgical technique consists of excision of the obstructing ureteric segment and intravesical reimplantation of the ureter into the bladder in a way that ensures good upper tract drainage without introducing VUR. Where the dilatation is of mild to moderate severity this may be achievable with a conventional Cohen cross-trigonal tunnel technique. For more severely dilated ureters, however, a Politano-Leadbetter reimplantation is usually indicated. This can be combined with reducing the diameter of the distal ureter using one of the techniques described below. A psoas hitch procedure is advisable to prevent kinking and obstruction at the entry point of the ureter into the bladder (Figure 7.14). More recently, a combination of excision of the obstructing segment, remodelling

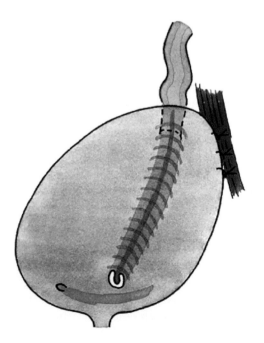

Figure 7.14 The politano-leadbetter reimplantation procedure combined with psoas hitch, which is often better suited to megaureters than the Cohen cross-trigonal reimplantation technique.

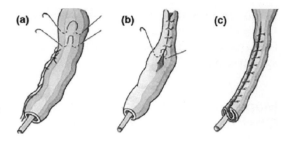

Figure 7.15 Method of ureteric plication using the Starr technique.

and an extravesical antireflux procedure has been reported to yield excellent results.

Ureteric tailoring

This may be required to achieve an antireflux reimplantation in grossly dilated ureters. The available techniques include:

- Hendren excisional tapering
- Kalicinski plication and folding
- Starr ureteral imbrication (Figure 7.15)

Laparoscopic and robotic surgery

A number of different approaches are being developed for the minimally invasive management of obstructed megaureter – including tailoring and different reimplantation techniques. Satisfactory early results have been reported in small series of patients but medium and long-term results are still awaited. As with other forms of innovative minimally invasive urological surgery in children, a high level of expertise is required.

Surgical Complications

These comprise:

- Wound infection
- Urinary infection
- Haemorrhage
- Stent related problems
- Recurrent VUJ obstruction
- VUR

Follow-Up and Surgical Outcomes

This typically consists of a postoperative ultrasound scan 4–6 weeks after surgery (or JJ stent removal) followed by an ultrasound and isotope renogram at around 6–12 months. Excision of the obstructing segment combined with ureteric reimplantation usually results in reduction in the severity of dilatation and good preservation of differential function. Any postoperative VUR tends to be low grade and can be managed conservatively. The outcomes of surgical management of obstructed megaureter are generally very good with reported overall success rates in the region of 90–95%.

KEY POINTS

- PUJ obstruction is a heterogeneous condition with a number of different causes and a variable natural history.
- Hydronephrosis due to PUJ obstruction accounts for 30–50% of clinically significant prenatally detected uropathies. A renal pelvic AP diameter exceeding 30 mm is associated with a significant likelihood of functional impairment. Conversely, an AP diameter of less than 15 mm is most unlikely to denote significant obstruction.
- Magnetic resonance imaging can combine anatomical and functional information in a single investigation and may in time become the investigation of choice. Drawbacks are the additional cost and requirement for anaesthesia in younger children.
- Laparoscopic and robotic-assisted pyeloplasty are being increasingly used for reconstruction particularly in children who are no longer infants. Advantages are improved cosmesis,

reduced postoperative pain and a shorter hospital stay.
- Primary obstructed megaureter can be managed conservatively in the majority of cases with surgery being limited to specific indications. Controversy continues to surround some aspects of the surgical management in the first year of life.

FURTHER READING

Chacko JK, Koyle MA, Mingin GC, et al. The minimally invasive open pyeloplasty. J Pediatr Urol. 2006;2(4):368–372.

Dekirmendjian A, Braga LH. Primary non-refluxing megaureter: analysis of risk factors for spontaneous resolution and surgical intervention. Front Pediatr. 2019;7:126.

Jude E, Deshpande A, Barker A, et al. Intravesical ureteric reimplantation for primary obstructed megaureter in infants under 1 year of age. J Pediatr Urol. 2017;13(1):47.e1–47.e7.

Nguyen HT, Benson CB, Bromley B, et al. Multidisciplinary consensus on the classification of prenatal and postnatal urinary tract dilation (UTD classification system). J Pediatr Urol. 2014;10(6):982–998.

Varda BK, Wang Y, Chung BI, et al. Has the robot caught up? National trends in utilization, perioperative outcomes, and cost for open, laparoscopic, and robotic pediatric pyeloplasty in the United States from 2003 to 2015. J Pediatr Urol. 2018;14(4):336. e1–336.e8.

Weitz M, Portz S, Laube GF, et al. Surgery versus non-surgical management for unilateral ureteric-pelvic junction obstruction in newborns and infants less than two years of age. Cochrane Database Syst Rev. 2016;7:CD010716.

Duplication Anomalies, Ureteroceles and Ectopic Ureters

PARVIZ HAJIYEV and BERK BURGU

Topics covered

Classification
Embryology
Pathology and definitions

Investigations
Management

Complete or partial duplication of the upper urinary tract is a relatively common congenital anomaly with autopsy and radiological data indicating an overall incidence of the order of 1–3%. The most common form is partial (incomplete) duplication, in which two ureters emerge separately from the kidney but then converge to form a single ureter draining via a single ureteric orifice. Partial forms of duplication rarely give rise to clinical problems and may be picked up as an incidental finding during urological investigation for unrelated symptoms.

Complete forms of duplication are characterized by two separate collecting systems in the duplex kidney with ureters which remain separate throughout their length, entering the lower urinary tract via two separate ureteric openings.

Complete duplication is much rarer, occurring in less than 1% of individuals, mainly females. Unlike partial duplication, complete duplication anomalies are often of clinical significance. They may be associated with a range of symptoms and complications including urinary tract infection, urinary incontinence, bladder outflow obstruction and functional renal damage. Duplication occurs bilaterally in 40% of cases but the anatomical pattern is often different between the two upper tracts.

Complete duplication is frequently detected on routine prenatal ultrasound screening but further evaluation with diagnostic imaging is required postnatally. Clinical presentations include urinary tract infection, urinary incontinence, obstructed voiding, pain and urolithiasis.

Upper tract duplication has a familial tendency and there is an incidence of 8% in close relatives.

EMBRYOLOGY

This is considered in Chapter 1 but can be briefly summarized as follows:

During the fourth week of gestation the ureteral bud branches off from the mesonephric duct and advances toward the metanephric blastema to initiate development of the embryonic kidney from around 32 days. A single ureteral bud will usually induce normal nephrogenesis and give rise to a single renal pelvis and normal calyces. Division (bifurcation) of the ureteral bud before it enters the metanephros results in partial duplication – with the ureteral anatomy being determined by the level of bifurcation. Complete duplication occurs when the mesonephric duct gives rise to two separate ureteral buds which each make contact with the metanephric blastema (Figure 8.1). A ureteral bud derived from an aberrant (ectopic) position on the mesonephric duct is more likely to penetrate and abnormal part of the metanephric blastema – resulting in defective nephrogenesis and renal dysplasia.

In complete forms of duplication the more caudal of the two ureteral buds (draining the lower pole of the kidney) has a tendency to open in a superior and lateral position in relation to the trigone. This may result in a shorter intramural course of the distal ureter in the bladder predisposing to reflux into the lower pole moiety of the duplex kidney.

Paradoxically, the ureter draining the upper pole moiety invariably drains in a more distal (caudal) position in the urinary tract than the lower pole ureter. This characteristic feature of the ureteral anatomy in upper tract duplication is described as the Meyer-Weigart law. In females, an ectopic upper pole ureter may enter the lower urinary tract at the bladder neck or more distally at a level below the bladder neck and striated sphincter muscles. In the most severe forms of ectopia, the ureter opens at the introitus or drains into the vagina. In males, however, an ectopic upper pole ureter always drains at a supra sphincteric level, typically connecting with the vas, seminal vesicle or ejaculatory duct. The embryological origin of ureteroceles remains poorly understood.

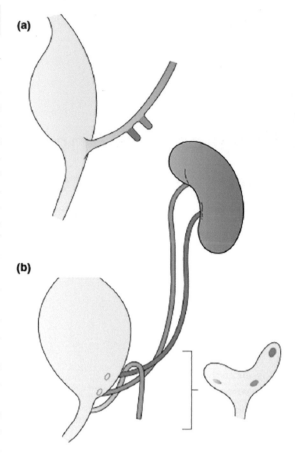

Figure 8.1 Embryological origins of complete duplication. (a) Accessory ureteral bud (blue) arising in an abnormally cephalad position on the mesonephric duct (green). (b) By 12 weeks the upper pole ureter has been carried with the mesonephric duct to an abnormally distal ectopic location. The more caudal ureteral bud (red) may become incorporated into a superolateral position on the trigone, with a short submucosal tunnel predisposing to reflux. The relative positions of the ureteral orifices on the trigone are also illustrated. The characteristic anatomical patter of duplex ureters is defined by the Meyer-Weigart law.

CLASSIFICATION

Upper tract duplication is subdivided into

- Complete duplication
- Partial duplication

The anomalies associated with complete duplication include

- Upper pole: ureterocele, ectopic ureter, upper pole renal dysplasia
- Lower pole: vesicoureteral reflux

The anomalies associated with partial duplication include

- Pelvi ureteric junction obstruction (lower pole)
- "Yo yo" reflux between the two ureters above their point of convergence. However, this is a doubtful clinical entity in children of unknown clinical significance

Ureteroceles (Figure 8.2)

These are classified as

- Intravesical (entirely within the bladder)
- Extravesical or ectopic (ie, a portion extends beyond and below the bladder neck into the urethra)

A ureterocele is defined as a cystic dilation of the intravesical segment of the distal ureter. The overall incidence of duplex system ureteroceles is 0.02% – with the majority (80%) occurring in females. The renal cortex drained by a ureter

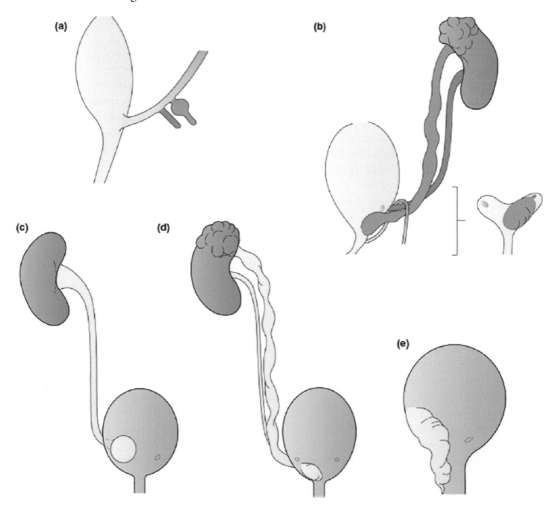

Figure 8.2 Ureteroceles. (a) Cystic dilatation of upper ureteral bud with aberrant interaction with the metanephric blastema leading to (b) duplex ureterocele and dysplastic upper pole moiety. (c) Single system orthotopic ureterocele. (d) Duplex ectopic ureterocele. (e) Large prolapsing caecouretrocele extending down between the deficient trigone and urethra anteriorly and vagina posteriorly.

terminating in a ureterocele is often dysplastic and the ureter and upper pole collecting system are dilated (hydronephrotic). A ureterocele may lie entirely within the bladder, in which case it is unlikely to interfere with voiding and urinary continence. However, up to 50% of duplex ureteroceles are termed "ectopic" because they extend extravesically and encroach upon the bladder outlet and proximal urethra. The largest variety is the caeco ureterocele, which extends further down into the urethra and may appear as a cystic mass in perineum by the external urethral meatus. Ectopic ureteroceles can cause bladder outflow obstruction giving rise to voiding dysfunction and elevated intravesical pressure – which may have the potential to cause obstructive damage to the contralateral kidney. Elevated intravesical pressure caused by a prolapsed ectopic ureterocele may also exacerbate any existing vesicoureteral reflux (VUR) into the ipsilateral lower pole.

The majority of infants with duplex system ureteroceles are now identified by prenatal ultrasonography. In infants in whom the abnormality has not been identified prenatally, the most common clinical presentation is with urinary tract infection in the early months of life.

Less frequently, the condition presents with symptoms of voiding dysfunction and outflow obstruction. Although rare, prolapsed ectopic ureterocele is nevertheless the most frequent cause of urethral obstruction in girls and may occasionally be accompanied a visible cystic swelling.

In addition to symptoms caused by outflow obstruction, other symptomatic presentations in older infants and children include febrile or non-febrile urinary infections, failure to thrive and recurrent abdominal/pelvic pain. Duplication may rarely present with urolithiasis secondary to infection and obstruction.

Whereas the majority of ureteroceles occur in duplex systems, approximately 10% of ureteroceles are associated with a single (non-duplex) upper urinary tract. These ureteroceles (termed "orthotopic" or "single system") are almost always intravesical and do not interfere with voiding. Dilatation of the ipsilateral ureter and upper tract is only of mild or moderate severity and function in the ipsilateral kidney is usually either normal or only mildly impaired.

ECTOPIC URETER

This is defined as ureter which enters the urinary tract in a more caudal position than the normal point of entry on the trigone. The estimated incidence is 0.01% and it occurs mostly in females – in whom the ectopic ureter may open into the urethra, vagina or, very rarely, the cervix or uterus. In males, an ectopic duplex ureter may drain into the proximal urethra, ejaculatory duct or seminal vesicles.

Depending on the level at which the ectopic enters the lower urinary (or genital) tract in relation to the sphincter complex it is defined as being either supra sphincteric or infra sphincteric.

Supra Sphincteric Ectopic Ureter

Because affected children are continent the diagnosis is usually made following the finding of dilatation of the upper pole ureter and/or collecting system on routine prenatal screening or during the investigation of urinary tract infection.

Infra Sphincteric Ectopic Ureter (Figure 8.3)

As with supra sphincteric forms of ectopic ureter, this anomaly may be identified following the discovery of dilatation on prenatal ultrasound screening. Alternatively, it may come to light during investigation of urinary tract infection or symptoms. The classic symptomatic presentation is with constant dribbling of urine which is superimposed upon an otherwise normal pattern of voiding and urinary continence. In theory, this characteristic pattern should serve to distinguish ectopic ureter from other causes of urinary incontinence but in practice the clinical picture may be less diagnostic. For example, some girls remain dry overnight when lying horizontally and others may experience pooling of urine in the vagina which may enable them to remain relatively dry for variable periods during the daytime. The picture may also be complicated if the girl also suffers from wetting due to dysfunctional voiding – as well as experiencing urinary leakage

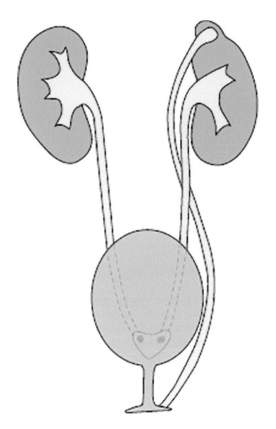

Figure 8.3 Diagrammatic representation of infra sphincteric ectopic ureter.

from the ectopic ureter. Finally, small volumes of urine collecting in the vagina may become infected and present as a vaginal discharge – a relatively common symptom in girls which does not usually merit imaging of the urinary tract.

Physical examination is rarely confirmatory and the diagnosis is based on the characteristic pattern of the incontinence and the findings of imaging studies. Because duplication is commonly bilateral the presence of a complete or partial duplex system on one side should always raise suspicion of a contralateral duplex system with an occult upper pole and ectopic ureter.

VESICOURETERAL REFLUX

Complete duplication is accompanied by VUR into the ipsilateral lower pole ureter in approximately 50% of cases. This is usually identified during postnatal evaluation of prenatally detected cases or during the investigation of urinary tract infection.

COMPLICATIONS OF PARTIAL DUPLICATION

The term "Yo Yo" reflux is applied to the possible crossflow of urine between the two ureters of a partial duplication (limbs of a Y) above their convergence to form a single ureter. Although, postulated as a possible cause of loin pain in adults there is no evidence that it causes any symptoms in children. Pelvi ureteric junction obstruction in duplex systems almost invariably occurs in the lower pole of a partial duplex kidney (bifid pelvis).

INVESTIGATION

During the physical examination the external genitalia and urethral orifice should be inspected, looking for dampness in the region of the introitus. Very occasionally a bulging ureterocele can be observed (Figure 8.4).

ULTRASONOGRAPHY

Using ultrasound, it is possible to assess the distribution and severity of dilatation (hydro ureter

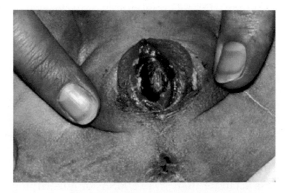

Figure 8.4 Prolapsed ureterocele emerging at the introitus of a neonate.

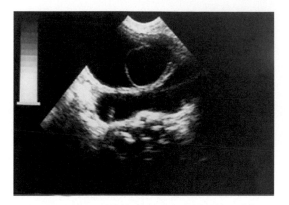

Figure 8.5 Bladder ultrasonography demonstrating large ureterocele and dilated upper pole ureter behind the bladder.

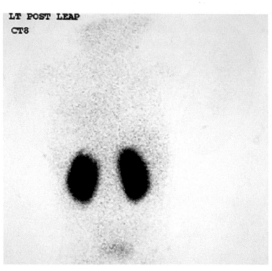

Figure 8.6 DMSA scintigraphy in a child with bilateral duplex system ureteroceles. Left upper moiety non-functioning, minimal function in thin rim of renal parenchyma in hydronephrotic right upper moiety. Normal function in both lower moieties.

and hydronephrosis) and the appearances of the renal parenchyma in the upper and lower poles of both kidneys. A ureterocele can almost always be visualized on ultrasound, providing the bladder is full (Figure 8.5). Likewise, an ectopic ureter which is dilated can be visualized lying behind the bladder. However, cases of "cryptic duplication" may be missed on ultrasound because the upper pole is small and dysplastic and the ectopic ureter is not dilated and not readily detectable on ultrasound.

RADIONUCLIDE SCAN

Functional imaging with ^{99m}Tc dimercaptosuccinic acid (DMSA) scintigraphy is performed to assess the distribution of function between the two kidneys and between the upper and lower pole moieties of a duplex kidney (Figure 8.6). ^{99m}Tc DMSA can also help to identify an occult duplex system by demonstrating poorly functioning dysplastic upper pole parenchyma associated with an infra sphincteric ectopic ureter. Dynamic renography with ^{99m}Tc MAG3 has the advantage of providing information on drainage as well as differential function but is less accurate than ^{99m}Tc DMSA for quantifying differential function in the two moieties of a duplex kidney.

VOIDING CYSTOURETHROGRAPHY (VCUG)

The VCUG plays an important role when planning management of duplication anomalies. It is an essential investigation if there is any suggestion of lower pole VUR (which is present in approximately 50% of cases) and also provides dynamic anatomical information on the ureters, bladder and urethra. This may be particularly helpful in demonstrating partial obstruction of the bladder neck and proximal urethra by a prolapsing ureterocele.

Reflux into the lower pole of a complete duplex kidney has a characteristic appearance which is likened to a "drooping flower" (Figure 8.7). Reflux into the upper pole of a complete duplex system is rare. When a VCUG demonstrates reflux into both poles this is usually indicative of a partial duplication. The finding of contralateral VUR may be an important factor when devising an overall plan of management.

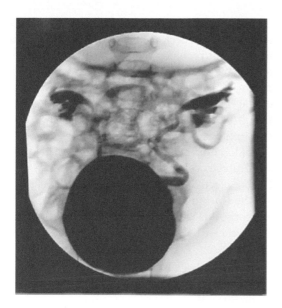

Figure 8.7 VCUG demonstrating bilateral lower pole VUR with characteristic "drooping flower" appearances. Displacement of left lower pole ureter by grossly dilated upper pole ureter.

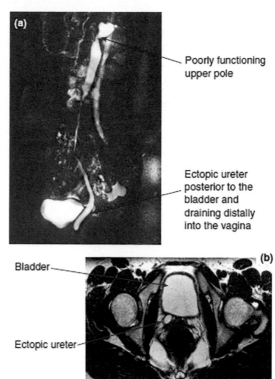

Figure 8.8 MR Urogram demonstrating an "occult" duplex ectopic ureter which could not be visualized by other imaging techniques.

MAGNETIC RESONANCE UROGRAPHY

Magnetic resonance (MR) urography has been used on a selective basis for investigating complex patterns of duplication and detecting a poorly functioning dysplastic upper pole associated with infra sphincteric ectopic ureter. However, it is rapidly becoming the first line investigation of choice in girls whose urinary incontinence is suspected to be related to a possible ectopic ureter (Figure 8.8). MR urography can yield information on function as well as providing an accurate delineation of anatomy and vasculature. It does not entail any exposure to radiation but is relatively costly and requires the use of sedation or general anesthesia to ensure the child remains still for the duration of the scan.

CYSTOSCOPY

Although not routinely indicated, cystoscopy can nevertheless make an important contribution to diagnosis and management in selected cases. For example, visual assessment by cystoscopy (and vaginoscopy) may provide valuable additional information on ureteroceles which was not forthcoming from diagnostic imaging and it may also occasionally identify an occult ectopic ureteral orifice. Endoscopic techniques are widely used for the surgical management of ureteroceles and may also be used for endoscopic correction of VUR.

MANAGEMENT

Upper tract duplication is characterized by considerable diversity of anatomy and function. In addition, it may either be detected prenatally or present clinically with differing symptoms, notably urinary tract infection or urinary incontinence. Accordingly, there is no single approach to management – which must be adapted to account of the anatomy, function and presenting features of each individual case.

Prenatally Detected Duplication

The majority of infants with prenatally detected upper tract duplication are asymptomatic at the time of birth and have no abnormal clinical findings on examination.

The aims of management of infants with prenatally detected duplex kidneys can be summarized as:

- Prevention of febrile urinary tract infections which might pose threat of new pyelonephritic scarring or progression of existing renal damage.
- Relief of obstruction.
- Correction of anatomical abnormalities which would otherwise be destined to cause symptoms, notably urinary incontinence, in later childhood.

However, the long-term natural history of asymptomatic infants who have been born with less severe forms of duplication is not well documented. For this reason, it is important to avoid submitting healthy infants to surgical intervention which is not justified or which is needlessly invasive.

A number of studies have reported the successful conservative management of some forms of prenatally detected duplication such as intravesical ureteroceles associated with non-functioning/cystic dysplastic upper pole tissue or upper pole moieties which appear non-obstructed on dynamic renography. However, the duration of follow up in such studies has been relatively short (<10 years) and the longer term outcomes of conservative management are not yet known.

Endoscopic Incision

This is the least invasive form of intervention and is used mainly to decompress an intravesical ureterocele and facilitate drainage in an obstructed

upper pole system. In infants with prenatally detected ureteroceles, it is performed with the intention of reducing the risk of infection in the obstructed system and protecting the upper pole parenchyma from infective and/or obstructive damage. It can also be used as temporizing measure in children who present with severe infection in the upper pole system.

Endoscopic puncture of a small or medium sized ureterocele can be performed with a 3 Fr Bugbee electrode or with holmium laser inserted via the working channel of a 7.5–10 Fr pediatric cystoscope (Figure 8.9). Alternatively, the ureterocele can be incised with an electrical hook

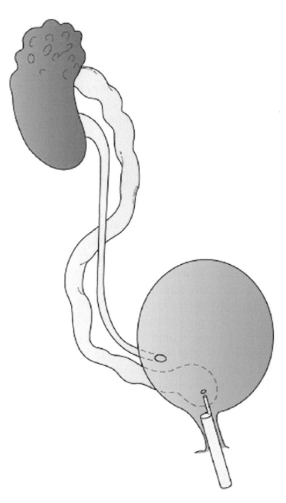

Figure 8.9 Diagrammatic representation of simplest intervention-endoscopic puncture. The ureterocele can also be incised more extensively by cold knife or laser.

or cold knife. The horizontal incision should be sited close to the junction between the uretero-cele and bladder wall to prevent the creation of a potentially obstructive flap and to reduce the risk of inducing reflux.

The main drawback of endoscopic incision is that it can cause the onset of reflux in a previously non-refluxing system. This occurs in approximately 50% of cases and is associated with a significant incidence of urinary infection. For this reason, endoscopic incision results in a requirement for subsequent secondary surgical intervention in at least 20% of cases.

Endoscopic incision can also be applied to the management of extravesical ureteroceles. However, an additional incision distal to the bladder neck at the lowest part of the uretero-cele is advisable to prevent the decompressed ureterocele from filling with urine and causing bladder neck obstruction at the time of voiding. Although, endoscopic incision of an extravesi-cal ureterocele may be a worthwhile short-term measure is rarely curative and additional surgical intervention is required in the majority of cases.

Depending on its size and degree of dilatation of the upper tract dilatation, a single system, orthotopic ureterocele can also be managed by endoscopic incision. However, because this carries a significant risk of inducing reflux some pediatric urologists favor surgical excision of the ureterocele combined with ureteral reimplantation. This is a relatively straightforward procedure with a high success rate.

Upper Pole Heminephrectomy or Heminephroureterectomy (Figure 8.10)

Although now being performed less frequently, this procedure retains a valuable role when the upper moiety is non-functioning or poorly functioning and the collecting system and ureter are grossly dilated. The definitive surgical management of a large and/or ectopic ureterocele consists of removing the upper pole moiety and as much of the ureter as can be accessed through a flank incision. A second (groin) incision is then used to remove the remaining (distal) section

of ureter. A suprapubic incision and transvesi-cal approach are required to provide adequate access to the region of the bladder neck for excision of a prolapsing ectopic ureterocele (caecoureterocele). This is a technically challenging operation because the bladder neck is often deficient in the vicinity of the ureterocele and bladder neck reconstruction may be required. The parents should be advised of the possible risk of sphincter weakness incontinence. In this context, however, there is good published evidence that bladder neck/sphincter weakness in such cases is more likely to be related to a preexisting congenital anatomical deficiency than a complication of the surgery.

Intravesical ureteroceles and some extravesi-cal ureteroceles can be managed by upper pole heminephrectomy and excision of an accessible length of ureter performed through a single loin incision. Once the ureter has been transected, urine is aspirated from the ureterocele and residual length of distal ureter – leaving the decompressed ureterocele and "ureteral stump" in situ. When used selectively this "simplified approach" constitutes definitive treatment in the majority of patients, with only 10–20% requiring subsequent excision of the ureteral stump and ureterocele and reimplantation of the lower pole ureter.

The various procedures described above are being increasingly performed by a minimally invasive (laparoscopic or robotic assisted) rather than open surgery.

Ectopic Ureter

Supra-sphincteric

In most cases, the ipsilateral upper pole is non-functioning and heminephrectomy (open or laparoscopic) is sufficient. However, this type of ectopic ureter is occasionally associated with reflux into the upper pole moiety – for which it is also necessary to remove the ureter. In the rare cases in which there is a worthwhile degree of function in the upper pole the ectopic upper pole ureter and the lower pole ureter can be reimplanted together "en-bloc" into the bladder.

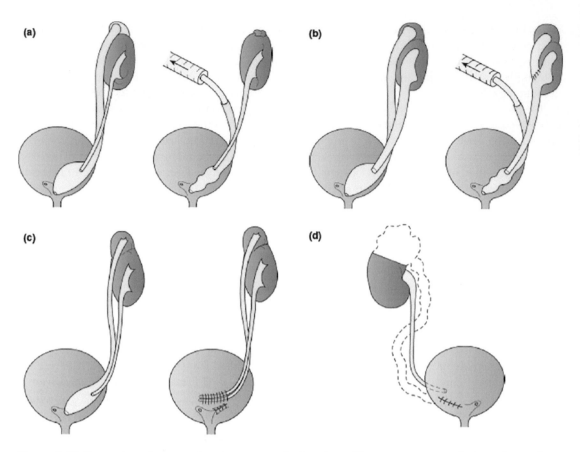

Figure 8.10 Examples of conventional open surgical options. There are many variations depending on the anatomy and function in the individual case. (a) "Simplified Approach" normal lower moiety, non-functioning upper moiety. Upper pole heminephrectomy combined with excision of ureter accessible through the same incision. Aspiration of residual upper pole ureteral stump. (b) Pyelopyelostomy. Ureters anastomosed at the level of the kidney. Upper pole ureteral stump aspirated and left in situ. Alternatively, both ureters can be anastomosed in the pelvis adjacent to the bladder – ureteroureterostomy (see text). (c) Excision of ureterocele and reimplantation of both duplex ureters in their common sheath. (d) Heminephroureterectomy with excision of ureterocele. Definitive surgical treatment but a major operation requiring two incisions or a laparoscopicallly assisted procedure.

Infrasphincteric

An upper pole heminephrectomy is sufficient in such cases because it removes the renal parenchyma responsible for excreting the small amount of urine which eventually emerges from the opening of the ectopic ureter to cause incontinence. It is not necessary to remove the ectopic ureter – although it may be reasonable to do so if the heminephrectomy is performed laparoscopically since this does not require any additional incisions.

Ureteroureterostomy

Ureteroureterostomy or pyelo pyelostomy used to be limited to the small proportion of cases in which there was sufficient function in the upper pole to justify its conservation. However, these techniques are being increasingly applied to cases with a poorly functioning upper pole moiety.

In the technique of distal ureteroureterostomy the upper pole ureter is anastomosed to the lower pole ureter in the pelvis. Before performing this procedure, however, it is important to confirm that there is no reflux into the lower pole ureter. If the VCUG demonstrates that reflux is present the alternative options are to perform ureteroureterostomy in conjunction with an antireflux procedure or, alternatively to reimplant both ureters together in their common sheath.

Ureteral Clipping

This novel technique has been reported for the management of symptomatic ectopic ureters associated with a non-functioning upper moiety. Using a laparoscopic approach the ectopic ureter is visualized and then clipped (ligated) – thus preventing the passage the urine responsible for causing incontinence. Initial results in small numbers of patients have been promising but follow up has been relatively short and there are uncertainties regarding the long-term outcome of the hydronephrosis which develops in the upper pole following occlusion of the ectopic (upper pole) ureter.

The management of VUR in duplex systems is mainly concerned with lower pole VUR in complete duplication and follows a very similar approach to the management of VUR in single systems – as described in Chapter 6. However, the rate of spontaneous resolution is lower than in single systems. For this reason, greater consideration should be given to surgical intervention if the child is experiencing symptomatic urinary tract infections.

Endoscopic correction is a reasonable option for low grades of VUR (particularly in partial duplication) but success rates are lower than for comparable grades in single systems. For moderate or high grade VUR ureteral reimplantation is usually required. When performing ureteral reimplantation, both ureters should be mobilized and reimplanted together in their common sheath to avoid jeopardizing the vascularity of both ureters. However, this may not always be feasible if one of the two ureters is dilated and it is necessary to perform ureteral tapering.

Extensive loss of function in the ipsilateral lower moiety is usually due to congenital dysplasia rather than pyelonephritic scarring. The management consists of removing the poorly functioning lower pole together with as much of the refluxing lower pole ureter as possible without compromising the adjoining upper pole ureter.

BILATERAL SINGLE ECTOPIC URETERS (FIGURE 8.11)

This is an extremely rare abnormality which occurs mainly in females. A single ureter on each side drains in an ectopic location in the proximal urethra. The ureteral ectopia is accompanied by congenital weakness of the bladder neck and striated sphincter and greatly reduced functional capacity of the bladder. Both ureters are usually

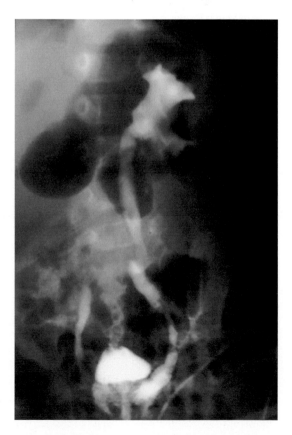

Figure 8.11 Intravenous urogram demonstrating bilateral single ectopic ureters. Both ureters drain extravesically and the bladder is of small capacity.

dilated and there are varying degrees of renal dysplasia. This anomaly typically presents with continuous dribbling urinary incontinence in childhood or, more rarely, with features of renal impairment in infancy.

The primary treatment consists of reimplantation of the ectopic ureters into the bladder. However, further procedures such as bladder augmentation and sphincter enhancing surgery are often required. As a last resort to achieve continence it may be necessary to perform surgical closure of the bladder neck closure combined with a Mitrofanoff procedure.

Treatment should be individualized according to the anatomy, function and presentation of each case.
- Ureteroceles can be treated by endoscopic incision but there is a relatively high requirement for secondary surgery.
- A range of open surgical options are available. Uretero-ureterostomy is being increasingly performed as an alternative to heminephrectomy.

KEY POINTS

- The anatomy of complete ureteral duplication is described by the Meyer-Weigart Law.
- Partial duplication is relatively common and is not usually of clinical significance. Complete duplication is rarer and more frequently gives rise to clinical symptoms and morbidity.
- The upper pole moiety of a complete duplex system which is associated with a ureterocele or ectopic ureter is often poorly functioning or dysplastic.
- MR urography is a valuable investigation for demonstrating an "occult" duplex system suspected of causing urinary incontinence in a girl.
- Vesicoureteral reflux is the commonest complication affecting a lower pole moiety.
- There is no single approach to the management of upper tract duplication.

FURTHER READING

Fufezan O, Tatar S, Dee AM, Cramariuc R, Asavoaie C, Cosarca M. Large spectrum of complete urinary collecting system duplication exemplified by cases. Pictorial essay. Med Ultrason. 2013;15:315–320.

HK Le, G Chiang. Current urology reports, 2018 - Springer long-term management of ureterocele in duplex collecting systems: reconstruction implications

JR Dillman, AT Trout, EA Smith. Abdominal Radiology, 2016 – Springer MR urography in children and adolescents: techniques and clinical applications.

Malik RD, Pariser JJ, Gundeti MS. Outcomes in pediatric robot-assisted laparoscopic hemi-nephrectomy compared with contemporary open and laparoscopic series. J Endourol. 2015;29:1346–1352.

Sander JC, Bilgutay AN, Stanasel I, Koh CJ, Janzen N, Gonzales ET, et al. Outcomes of endoscopic incision for the treatment of ureterocele in children at a single institution. J Urol. 2015;193:662–666.

Posterior Urethral Valves and Other Urethral Abnormalities

DIVYESH Y DESAI and PATRICK G DUFFY

Topics covered

Posterior urethral valves
Anatomy/pathophysiology
Presentation/investigation
Treatment
Prognosis

Long-term management
Anterior urethral diverticulum
Urethral duplication
Other urethral pathology

POSTERIOR URETHRAL VALVES

Introduction

Urethral obstruction in children is usually congenital in origin – with posterior urethral valves (PUV) being by far the commonest cause. Posterior urethral valves give rise to changes in the upper urinary tract which reflect the severity and duration of bladder outflow obstruction in fetal life. Severe obstruction which has been present from early gestation is associated with varying degrees of congenital renal dysplasia, which is the principal cause of renal insufficiency and chronic kidney disease (CKD) in PUV patients. Long-term morbidity also includes symptomatic bladder dysfunction which often persists despite successful treatment of the valves themselves.

Posterior urethral valves carried a mortality rate of almost 100% during the early years of the 20th century and remained as high as 50% until the 1950s. By contrast, the mortality reported in one recent series was only 0.3%. However, this reduction in early mortality has come at the expense of a greater proportion of the surviving children suffering from chronic renal failure. Posterior urethral valves are confined to males, in whom the incidence is of the order 1 in 4000–6000 live births. Although some familial cases have been reported, including in siblings, no established genetic predisposition has been identified and PUV generally behaves as a sporadic anomaly.

Anatomy

Hugh Hampton Young in 1919 described the first classification of posterior urethral valves based on postmortem dissection studies. He described three types, Type I being the commonest (95%) which consisted of co-apting leaflets with a proximal attachment to the distal verumontanum extending through the region of the external urethral sphincter to attach to the anterior urethral wall. Type III valves are uncommon (5%) and are best described as a transverse perforated membrane in the bulbar urethra with no attachment to the verumontanum. Type II valves, are described as leaflets that extend upwards from the verumontanum to the anterior aspect of the posterior urethra. It is unlikely that Type II valves constitute a genuine pathological entity and they are generally regarded as being non-obstructive mucosal folds of no clinical significance.

Some authors have challenged Young's classification which identified three distinct patterns of valvular obstruction. Dewan and Ransley's anatomical and endoscopic studies point to a single configuration comprising an obliquely orientated congenital obstructive posterior urethral membrane (COPUM) with a variably sized eccentric aperture located within it which arises from the verumontanum and extends through the region of the external urethral sphincter to attach to the anterior urethral wall (Figure 9.1). It has been argued that urethral instrumentation, including catheterisation, disrupts the valve membrane in the midline to create the appearance of two separate, side-by-side valve leaflets described as the classical Type I valves by Young.

Pathophysiology

Posterior urethral valves are thought to originate from abnormal interaction between the mesonephric ducts and the urogenital sinus around the seventh week of gestation. Dilatation of the fetal urinary tract secondary to obstruction caused by PUV can detected on ultrasonography as early as 14 weeks gestation.

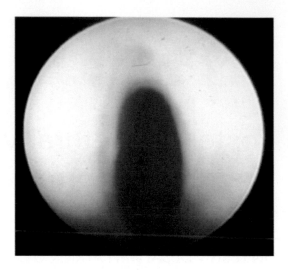

Figure 9.1 Endoscopic appearance of intact valve membrane prior to endoscopic ablation.

Studies of experimentally induced fetal bladder outflow obstruction in various animal models have established the following:

- Early outflow obstruction leads to abnormalities in bladder wall components with an increase in the collagen element, aberrant innervation and renal dysplasia. The characteristic histological features of renal dysplasia include the persistence of primitive tubules and the presence of abnormal mesenchymal derivatives such as cartilage interspersed between normal renal tissue.
- Obstruction in later gestation results in the typical features of chronic bladder outflow obstruction and raised intravesical pressure, without the occurrence of renal dysplasia.
- Intrauterine intervention to relieve experimentally induced obstruction in fetal animal has been shown to result in resolution of hydro-ureteronephrosis. This is accompanied by reversal of the detrusor hypertrophy and more normal innervation of bladder wall muscle.

In man, the clinical features of PUV may be at any point on a wide spectrum of pathology ranging from relatively mild obstructive changes to gross changes in the bladder and upper tracts accompanied by severe renal dysplasia.

Thus, the long-term prognosis in an individual with posterior urethral valves is determined by a combination of abnormal development of the urethra, bladder, kidneys and the ureters, and secondary consequences of congenital outflow obstruction on the development and function of bladder and the upper urinary tract.

The relative contribution made by these different factors to the long-term outcome for bladder and renal function is often difficult to determine, and therefore predicting long-term outcomes can be difficult. The urinary tracts of boys with posterior urethral valves must therefore be monitored through childhood, adolescence and early adulthood.

Presentation

The fetus

More than 80% of cases are detected on prenatal ultrasound. Although the underlying urethral anomaly dates from the seventh to the ninth week of gestation, dilatation of the urinary tract may not develop until later in pregnancy. In 55% of prenatally detected cases of PUV abnormal ultrasound findings are visualised on routine maternal ultrasound scans performed between 16 and 20 weeks. In the remaining cases, the appearances of the fetal urinary tract are normal in the second trimester, and the condition only becomes apparent on scans performed in later pregnancy – mainly for obstetric indications.

Functional outcome is closely linked to the gestational age at which dilatation becomes apparent, and studies have shown that when the condition is detected at 16–20 weeks the prognosis is more likely to be poor, especially if oligohydramnios is present. Oligohydramnios is a manifestation of fetal oliguria or anuria. In pregnancies which proceed to term, a severely affected newborn infant may demonstrate features of Potter's syndrome (characteristic Potter's facies and skeletal "moulding" deformities) with death supervening in the early neonatal period due to pulmonary hypoplasia. Biochemical constituents of fetal urine such as sodium, calcium and

Table 9.1 Ultrasound features of posterior urethral valves in the fetus

| **Male fetus** |
| Bilateral upper tract dilatation |
| Persistently distended full bladder |
| **Predictors of poor functional outcome and early-onset renal failure** |
| Detection before 24 weeks' gestation |
| Bladder wall thickening |
| Echo-bright kidneys (renal dysplasia) |
| Oligohydramnios |

b_2-microglobulin have been studied as possible predictive markers of renal function. However, there is considerable overlap with normal values and their prognostic sensitivity is less reliable than information yielded by detailed evaluation of the ultrasound appearances. In addition to dilatation and renal dysplasia (bright kidneys), predictive findings may include pulmonary hypoplasia, urinary ascites and perinephric urinomas (Table 9.1). In cases where dilatation does not develop until later in gestation, the prognosis is generally good.

The neonate

When symptoms are present these usually relate to bladder outflow obstruction or, less commonly, to clinical manifestations of impaired renal function. Clinical features of listlessness, poor feeding, irritability and failure to thrive are common. The urinary stream, if witnessed, is usually poor. The bladder is palpable in most instances; the kidneys may also be palpated. Urinary ascites is occasionally present and does not necessarily denote a poor prognosis.

The infant

Presentation in infancy is generally with urinary infection and in the majority of cases there are no immediately obvious signs of PUV. Gram-negative sepsis and renal failure with gross electrolyte disturbance were common forms of presentation but with increasing detection by prenatal ultrasound and greater awareness of the features of urinary infection in infants it has become much less common for PUV to present with sepsis than in the past. Chronically impaired renal function is usually manifest as poor growth and general failure to thrive.

The older child

Presentation may include manifestations of renal failure such as growth retardation, urinary infections, haematuria or voiding symptoms (typically prolonged voiding, rather than a poor urinary stream). However, "late presenting" cases of PUVs are often at the milder end of the spectrum of severity and may occasionally be diagnosed during the investigation of diurnal or nocturnal enuresis.

Investigations

Prenatal

The presence of posterior urethral valves can only be inferred from the ultrasound appearances of a distended fetal bladder and dilated upper tracts (Figure 9.2). Alternative diagnoses include urethral atresia (which is always lethal), prune-belly syndrome, megacystis–microcolon intestinal hypoperistalsis syndrome and high grade primary vesicoureteric reflux. However, the diagnosis of PUV

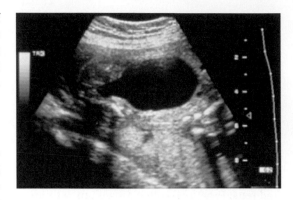

Figure 9.3 Ultrasound illustrating the diagnostic "keyhole sign." Dilated (thick-walled) bladder and dilated posterior urethra.

can be made with more certainty if these findings are also accompanied by dilatation of the posterior urethra – the so-called "keyhole sign" (Figure 9.3).

Postnatal

Ultrasonography is the initial investigation. Relevant findings in the upper tracts may include; dilatation (which is sometimes unilateral), perinephric urinoma (a rare occurrence) and changes in the renal cortex denoting dysplasia (e.g. "echo bright" parenchyma and cysts). Ultrasound appearances of the bladder include; bladder wall thickening, trabeculation and sacculation. There may or may not be residual urine retained in the bladder. If voiding views can be obtained, ultrasound may demonstrate dilatation of the posterior urethra.

Micturating cystourethrography (MCUG) provides the definitive diagnosis, with a range of findings, as illustrated in Figures 9.4–9.6. Vesicoureteric reflux is present in 40–60% of cases at the time of initial evaluation and is unilateral in approximately two-thirds of cases.

Initial assessment also includes measurement of electrolyte balance and renal function. It should be noted, however, that serum creatinine levels in the first 48 hours of life are a reflection of maternal renal function and it is not until the infant is a few days of age that the plasma creatinine becomes a reliable measure of his own renal function.

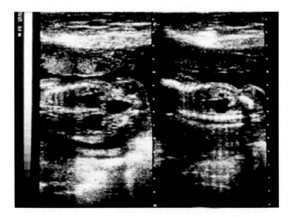

Figure 9.2 Prenatal ultrasound demonstrating marked dilatation of both fetal kidneys and the fetal bladder. The fetal spine and thorax are clearly visible in both these longitudinal images.

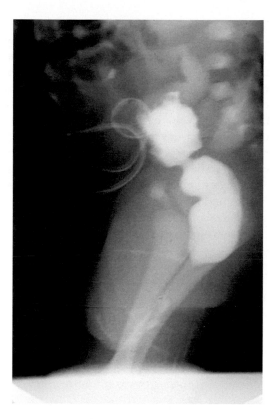

Figure 9.4 Newborn infant: micturating cysto-urethrogram (MCU). Grossly dilated posterior urethra, indentation by prominent bladder neck, small trabeculated bladder.

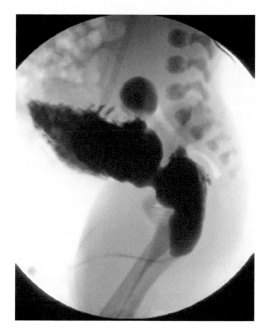

Figure 9.5 Newborn preterm infant, prenatal diagnosis. Heavily trabeculated bladder with diverticulum, prominent bladder neck and demarcation between dilated posterior urethra and non-dilated distal urethra at the site of the valve membrane.

Treatment

The fetus

The rationale for fetal intervention is based on the findings of studies in experimental animals which indicated that obstructive renal damage could be ameliorated by intrauterine decompression of the obstructed fetal bladder. However, the extent to which these experimental findings can be applied to the clinical setting in humans is debatable. Initially, fetal intervention in humans took the form of hysterotomy and open fetal surgery but this was soon superseded by ultrasound guided insertion of a shunt between the obstructed fetal bladder and amniotic cavity. (See Chapter 4) One metanalysis of 10 published studies identified a higher survival rate in shunted fetuses and a higher percentage

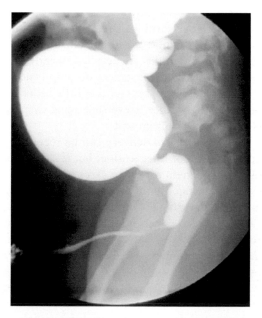

Figure 9.6 MCU in a boy presenting in the first year of life with urinary infection. Smooth-walled non-trabeculated bladder, unilateral grade IV reflux.

of infants with normal renal function at 6 months to 2 years of age. However, the results of comparative studies are difficult to critically assess because of differences in selection criteria and other weakness of methodology. In the United Kingdom the multicentre percutaneous shunting in lower urinary tract obstruction (PLUTO) trial was established with the aim of evaluating and comparing survival rates and outcomes for renal and bladder function following vesicoamniotic shunting. Although the trial was discontinued because of inability to recruit sufficient numbers of subjects, preliminary data did not appear to identify any significant benefit for renal function.

Fetal cystoscopy and intrauterine valve ablation has been reported as an alternative to vesico amniotic shunting and there is limited evidence to suggest that this approach might that have a higher early survival rate. However, it has only been used on a very limited scale and no long-term results are available.

In summary, although the published results of fetal intervention have generally been disappointing, vesico amniotic shunting may have a limited role to play when used on a selective basis.

Termination of pregnancy is probably the most common form of prenatal intervention, particularly when severe dilatation and associated oligohydramnios are detected in early pregnancy. In these circumstances decompression of the obstructed urinary tract is of little benefit for renal function, since irreversible renal dysplasia is almost invariably present.

Elective preterm delivery can be regarded as another form of intervention, but it is probably of limited benefit except in cases where there is evidence of rapidly progressing late-onset dilatation. In deciding the optimum timing for elective early delivery the predicted benefit for renal function must be carefully balanced against the risk of pulmonary immaturity in preterm infants.

Regardless of the controversies surrounding fetal intervention, there is a universal consensus that prenatal diagnosis has proved beneficial by facilitating prompt postnatal treatment of PUVs and a corresponding reduction in the risk of severe sepsis and pyelonephritic renal damage.

The neonate

To minimise risks of metabolic disturbance and urinary tract infection (UTI), the obstructed urinary tract should be decompressed promptly by either urethral or suprapubic bladder catheter drainage. Once this has been achieved, there is no compelling urgency to proceed to definitive treatment of the posterior urethral valves. Plasma biochemistry should be monitored during the first 7–21 days to obtain a measurement of baseline renal function (nadir creatinine) which serves as a reasonably reliable predictor of the later functional outcome.

Endoscopic valve ablation

The definitive management of posterior urethral valves consists of surgical resection or ablation of the obstructing valve membrane. For this purpose, modern miniaturised endoscopes (Figure 9.7)

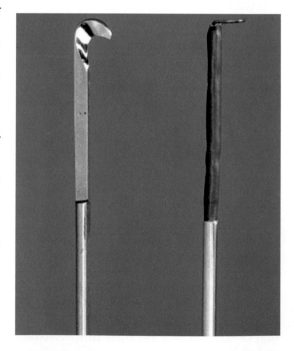

Figure 9.7 Cold knife and cutting resectoscope loop for use with neonatal resectoscope. The availability of instruments designed for neonatal use including lasers has simplified management and greatly reduced the incidence of instrumentation-induced urethral trauma.

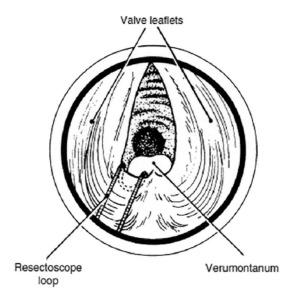

Valve leaflets

Resectoscope
loop

Verumontanum

Figure 9.8 Position of the cutting loop prior to ablation of the valve membrane.

can be used safely even in small premature neonates. The valve leaflets are incised from margin to base (rather than fully resected). These incisions are conventionally performed in the 5 and 7 o'clock positions (Figure 9.8) – with a further incision at the 12 o'clock position if required. To minimise the risk of any damage to surrounding tissues we prefer to incise the valve membrane with a cold knife blade rather than a cutting diathermy loop. Incision of the valve membrane at two or three sites is sufficient to relieve the obstruction. It is not necessary to attempt complete removal of the valve tissue and, indeed this carries some risk of damage to adjoining tissues. Practice varies with regard to catheter drainage following the procedure but this is advisable if significant intraoperative bleeding has been encountered. We favour a follow-up cystoscopy 6–12 weeks later to ensure completeness of valve ablation. Some paediatric urologists combine this procedure with a circumcision performed under the same anaesthetic.

The majority of boys can be effectively and safely managed by definitive primary surgical treatment of their posterior urethral valves. Urinary tract diversion is performed less

frequently than in the past and there is no convincing evidence that it leads to any improvement in the prognosis for renal function. Nevertheless, there are still indications for urinary diversion in individual cases.

Vesicostomy

Primary cutaneous vesicostomy drainage is used for the management of boys with markedly impaired renal function and/or gross vesicoureteric reflux. In our centre its use for this purpose has been largely superseded by refluxing ureterostomy. However, primary cutaneous vesicostomy remains a useful option in situations when miniaturised instruments are unavailable.

The stoma is created at the apex of the bladder to minimise the risk of prolapse. Closure is undertaken after subsequent valve ablation at around 6–18 months of age depending on the initial indication for selecting vesicostomy and the child's level of renal function (Figure 9.9).

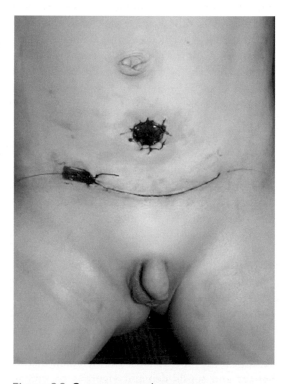

Figure 9.9 Cutaneous vesicostomy.

Supravesical diversion

Bilateral end ureterostomies or pyelostomies are rarely performed because:

- Defunctioning the bladder may adversely affect its development and later function.
- Vesicostomy usually provides equally effective drainage and is easier to manage by parents.

Refluxing ureterostomy

This is an elegant way of overcoming the high storage and voiding pressures in the bladder which may persist in infancy despite successful valve ablation. A low lying loop of dilated ureter is exteriorised in a configuration which permits external drainage of urine into a nappy whilst retaining continuity of drainage between the kidney and bladder. Refluxing ureterostomy has a number of advantages including; maximising drainage from the ipsilateral kidney, serving as a "safety valve" to protect both kidneys from elevated bladder pressure during storage and voiding, maintaining a pattern of bladder emptying and filling (termed "cycling") and retaining the potential for normal bladder emptying in the future. The urinary tract is usually reconstituted between 2 and 3 years of age in preparation for toilet training.

Urinary leaks

Urinary ascites and perinephric collections or "urinomas" respond to a short period of bladder drainage. Large or persistent perirenal collections may occasionally require ultrasound-guided percutaneous aspiration or open drainage.

The infant

Urinary infection in infants with previously undiagnosed PUVs is often complicated by septicaemia and gross disturbances of electrolyte and acid–base balance – of which hyperkalaemic acidosis is the most serious. The metabolic disturbances and sepsis demand vigorous treatment, which should be undertaken in cooperation with a paediatric nephrologist. The urological priority is to ensure prompt and effective drainage of the obstructed urinary tract. Definitive treatment of the posterior urethral valves should be delayed until the infant's general condition has been stabilised and the infection has been effectively treated – usually after 2–7 days. Vesicostomy or refluxing ureterostomy may sometimes be the most appropriate primary intervention, with treatment of the valves being deferred until closure of the vesicostomy or ureterostomy around the time of toilet training.

The older child

With few exceptions, endoscopic ablation of the valves is the initial treatment.

Prognosis

Approximately one-third of individuals have significantly impaired renal function and approximately 20% develop stage 5 CKD (end-stage renal failure). However, the full extent of renal insufficiency associated with PUV in the long-term does not become fully apparent until adolescence or early adulthood. Factors implicated in the aetiology of chronic renal failure include:

- Primary renal dysplasia.
- Secondary damage from bladder outflow obstruction. This occurs principally in utero, but may also occur in the postnatal period if undiagnosed obstruction persists after birth.
- Urinary infection and pyelonephritis – mainly in association with vesicoureteric reflux.
- Secondary damage from ongoing high pressure bladder dysfunction which persists despite successful valve ablation.

The incidence of CKD in the first decade of life is not reduced by prenatal diagnosis because this is largely determined before birth by the severity of congenital renal dysplasia. However, prenatal diagnosis may nevertheless be of some benefit in those boys who do not have renal dysplasia by reducing the obstructive and/or infective damage to their kidneys which might otherwise have occurred if the diagnosis of PUV had been delayed until later in infancy or childhood.

The importance of ongoing bladder dysfunction, which is manifest clinically as impaired continence, has received greater recognition in recent years. Published evidence of urodynamic studies has demonstrated that patterns of bladder dysfunction tend to change over time, with detrusor overactivity being superseded by a pattern of detrusor decompensation, sometimes termed "myogenic" failure. This is accompanied by weakening detrusor contractility and progressive increase in bladder capacity. Obligatory polyuria in the early stages of chronic renal insufficiency results in large residual volumes of poorly concentrated urine being retained within the bladder.

Urodynamic studies undertaken in the authors' unit have shown a uniform pattern of bladder dysfunction 1 year after successful relief of outflow obstruction by valve ablation. During the filling phase, the functional capacity of the bladder is reduced but bladder compliance is unimpaired despite the detrusor overactivity. The voiding phase is characterised by a distinctive biphasic or polyphasic detrusor pressure profile coupled with high voiding detrusor pressures and incomplete bladder emptying.

By the age of 5 years, however, bladder function has changed and falls into three distinct patterns based on voiding dynamics. A proportion of boys have proceeded to develop a largely normal voiding pattern on urodynamic evaluation. A second group continue to exhibit a biphasic or polyphasic detrusor pressure profile with high detrusor pressures on voiding and incomplete bladder emptying. Finally, a small proportion of boys are already showing evidence of bladder decompensation ("myogenic failure").

Predictors of a poor renal function

PRENATAL

- Maternal oligohydramnios, regardless of the gestational age
- Early detection (<20 weeks) on prenatal ultrasound of echogenic "bright" renal cortex and pelvicaliceal dilatation

POSTNATAL

- Presentation in the first 12 months of life (if not already detected prenatally)
- Persistently elevated plasma creatinine level at 6 months of age
- Proteinuria
- Bilateral vesicoureteric reflux
- Impaired continence at 5 years of age upwards

INDICATORS OF GOOD RENAL FUNCTION

- Presentation in later childhood
- Protection of the upper tracts by a "pop-off" phenomenon

The most common **"pop-off" mechanism** is unilateral high-grade vesicoureteric reflux. The combination of unilateral high grade VUR and a non-functioning or poorly functioning ipsilateral dysplastic kidney is termed the "VURD" (VU reflux dysplasia) syndrome. This is believed to act as a "safety valve" which confers some degree of protection to the developing contralateral kidney by reducing its exposure to the high intravesical pressure in the obstructed bladder. However, the importance of the "pop-off" phenomenon as a protective mechanism has probably been overstated. Although it may impart some medium-term benefit, a proportion of boys nevertheless progress into renal failure regardless of the VURD syndrome. Other less common forms of "pop-off" mechanisms include urinary ascites, perinephric urinoma and a large bladder diverticulum.

Follow-Up and Long-Term Management

All boys with PUVs require long-term follow-up. A suggested protocol is illustrated in Table 9.2. Once overall function has stabilised, differential renal function is monitored by MAG3 (mercaptoacetyltriglycine) renography or by dimercaptosuccinic acid (DMSA) scintigraphy. Successful relief of the outflow obstruction by valve ablation generally results in some reduction of the severity of upper tract dilatation. However, some degree of dilatation tends to persist during childhood.

Table 9.2 Follow-up protocol for patients with posterior urethral valves

Routine at every visit
Height and weight
Blood pressure
Urinary tract ultrasonography
Urine dipstick, serum creatinine and electrolytes
As indicated
Isotope renography (MAG3 or DMSA) – baseline at age 3 months and at age 5 years
Flow rate – after successful toilet training and annually
Video urodynamics – age 5 years and repeated if any change in symptoms or increasing PVR
Formal estimation of GFR – age 1 and 5 years, pre- and post-pubertal growth

This may be unilateral but is more commonly bilateral. Possible explanations include:

- Incomplete relief of bladder outflow obstruction.
- Persisting vesicoureteric reflux.
- Ureterovesical obstruction secondary to occlusion of the ureterovesical junction by a thick-walled bladder (rare).
- Exposure of the upper tracts to high pressures generated by bladder dysfunction (reduced compliance, detrusor instability).
- Ureteric decompensation, particularly in conjunction with polyuria.

Dilatation which shows no sign of improvement in the first few months after valve ablation is an indication for endoscopic re-evaluation to exclude the possibility of residual valvular obstruction or stricture formation.

Persistent or increasing dilatation in mid to late childhood may occur in response to the high obligatory output of dilute urine which occurs when the concentrating ability of the kidneys declines with the onset of early chronic renal failure (tubular defect). Investigation should therefore be aimed at reassessing glomerular and tubular renal function.

Vesicoureteric reflux resolves in 30–60% of cases following valve ablation. However, this is less likely in the presence of bladder dysfunction or when the ipsilateral kidney is poorly functioning.

Neonatal circumcision is performed routinely by some surgeons to minimise the risk of UTI. Although this was previously performed on a largely anecdotal basis it is now supported by a body of stronger evidence. Even if circumcision has not been performed as a prophylactic measure it should be actively considered in any boy with PUV who experiences breakthrough urinary infections despite antibiotic prophylaxis. Other forms of surgical intervention, such as open or endoscopic correction of VUR or nephroureterectomy are rarely indicated

Bladder dysfunction

Around two thirds of boys experience some degree of lower urinary tract symptoms and 15–30% suffer from varying degrees of urinary incontinence. As already noted, urodynamic studies typically demonstrate detrusor overactivity and hypercontractility between 1 and 3 years of age. As this pattern gradually resolves, bladder capacity increases and voiding pressures reduce to more normal levels between the ages of 4 and 7 years. By adolescence and early adulthood this pattern of bladder dysfunction has often been superseded by hypocontractility and large post void residual volumes. Although most boys have become dry by the end of adolescence, men with a history of PUV continue to have a higher incidence of lower urinary tract symptoms.

Because of the potentially harmful behaviour of the bladder despite valve ablation, some paediatric urologists advocate the routine use anticholinergics – which, in some cases may be accompanied by clean intermittent catheterisation. However, there is no agreement on the duration of this form of management and, as yet, no convincing evidence that it leads to improved outcomes for renal or bladder function in the longer term.

Diurnal enuresis secondary to bladder dysfunction and detrusor overactivity often responds to detrusor antispasmodics such as oxybutynin or alternative anticholinergics.

Intermittent catheterisation should be considered when detrusor decompensation is associated with large volumes of residual urine. In practice, urethral self-catheterisation rarely proves acceptable to boys with posterior urethral valves because, in contrast to patients with neuropathic bladder, they have a normally sensate urethra and experience urethral discomfort during catheterisation. In addition, secondary bladder neck hypertrophy often makes it difficult to negotiate the catheter into the bladder. For these reasons, effective long-term intermittent catheterisation is usually dependent on the creation of a continent catheterisable (Mitrofanoff) channel. When used selectively, the combination of Mitrofanoff procedure and CIC has been reported to result in a marked improvement in quality of life for boys and adolescents with severe urinary incontinence. However, whilst this approach is also associated with a reduction in the severity of upper tract dilatation it does not appear to avert or delay the onset of end-stage renal failure because this is largely determined by preexisting renal damage and congenital dysplasia.

Augmentation cystoplasty

The role of augmentation cystoplasty is controversial because it inevitably introduces a requirement for CIC (usually by a Mitrofannoff channel) and, as yet, has not been demonstrated to contribute to any long-term preservation of renal function. At the present time, bladder augmentation is probably best considered for boys under 3–4 years of age with severe renal impairment for whom renal transplantation is on the horizon. As previously described, the storage and voiding characteristics of the "valves bladder" are still potentially hostile and it may not be possible to await spontaneous improvements in bladder function before proceeding to renal transplantation. In this situation, bladder augmentation is preferable to urinary diversion as a means of ensuring that the lower urinary tract is safe for transplantation. The long-term complications of enterocystoplasty (mucus stone formation, metabolic disturbance, etc) can be avoided by augmenting the

bladder with a vascularised segment of dilated ureter (ureterocystoplasty) rather than bowel. Ureterocystoplasty is often more applicable to boys with PUVs as they are more likely to have a dilated ureter associated with a non-functioning ipsilateral kidney than children undergoing augmentation for neuropathic bladder.

OTHER URETHRAL ABNORMALITIES

Anterior Urethral Valves, Diverticula and Megalourethra

These anomalies, which are also confined to males, are much less common than posterior urethral valves. Although distinct entities in their own are right, these anomalies can also be regarded as constituting a continuum of urethral pathology. For example, it is difficult to define the point at which the urethral dilatation proximal to anterior urethral valves can be regarded as a diverticulum, and similarly the point at which an extensive diverticulum becomes a megalourethra.

Anterior urethral valves

As classically described, these take the form of either a fenestrated diaphragmatic membrane or a mucosal cusp arising from the ventral wall of the urethra. In 40% of cases the valve is sited at the bulbar urethra, whereas in 30% it is at the penoscrotal junction and in 30% in the penile urethra. The presentation is with obstructive symptoms, such as a poor urinary stream, hesitancy or urinary retention. Secondary changes in the upper urinary tracts are rare. MCUG demonstrates the obstruction, and treatment is by endoscopic incision.

Urethral diverticulum

In the more common wide-mouthed form, the diverticulum is usually located in the region of the penoscrotal junction. The distal lip may give rise to a form of valvular obstruction as the diverticulum becomes progressively distended. The presentation is either with obstructive symptoms or with postmicturition dribbling. The rarer saccular lesions have a narrow neck and may occur anywhere along the length of the penile urethra, including in the fossa navicularis. This form of diverticulum tends to present with urinary infection and may very occasionally be associated with stone formation within the diverticulum. Treatment is by endoscopic incision or resection of the obstructing lip. If the diverticulum is large it may be necessary to perform open excision by a perineal approach.

Megalourethra

This rare condition is characterised by marked dilatation of the penile urethra in the absence of any evident obstruction. Megalourethra may be associated with lack of corpus spongiosum or, in the extreme form, with complete absence of the corpora cavernosa. In such cases the penis amounts to little more than a floppy sac comprised of skin externally and urethral mucosa internally. Megalourethra often occurs in conjunction with other congenital abnormalities, particularly prune-belly syndrome.

Cowper's Gland Cysts (Syringocoele)

These paired structures, located on either side of the urethra at the level of the urogenital diaphragm, are each drained by a duct which runs distally through the corpus spongiosum to enter the bulbar urethra. Distension of the ducts, or of the glands themselves, may cause urethral compression or, if the anterior wall of the cyst ruptures into the urethra, may result in the formation of an obstructive membrane. The management is the same as for anterior diverticulum.

Urethral Duplications

These rare anomalies may be sagittal or collateral. Of these, the sagittal pattern is more common and takes the form of two channels running one above the other in the sagittal plane whereas in the collateral form the duplicate urethras run side by side. The most common sagittal configuration is represented by an orthotopic principal urethral channel with an epispadiac accessory urethra lying dorsal to it. In some cases both urethras leave the bladder separately and remain separate throughout their length, whereas in other cases the two urethras unite distally to form a single channel. In the so-called "spindle" variety the urethra separates into two components before reuniting again more distally. In "Y" patterns of duplications, an accessory urethra diverges from the main channel to emerge in the perianal region or the perineum. Reconstruction is dependent upon individual anatomy but nearly always entails excision of the narrower accessory urethra.

Posterior Urethral Polyps

These fibroendothelial lesions arise from the verumontanum. Small polyps are usually discovered incidentally during the course of endoscopy for some unrelated indication. Larger lesions comprising a polypoid head floating freely on an extended stalk have a tendency to extend upwards through the bladder neck to give rise to acute, transient episodes of urinary retention. Haematuria or frank urethral bleeding may also occur. Diagnosis is by cystourethroscopy or MCUG (Figure 9.10). Most polyps can be excised endoscopically, although an open transvesical approach may be required for complete excision of large polyps.

Urethral Strictures

The aetiology, investigation and management of post-traumatic strictures are considered in Chapter 22. Occasionally a urethral stricture is discovered in a boy who has no previous history of external injury, urethral instrumentation or catheterisation. In very young boys the aetiology can be assumed to be congenital, but in the older age group the possibility of previously unrecognised trauma is an alternative explanation. Whether congenital or acquired, such strictures are generally mild and respond well to endoscopic urethrotomy. Formal urethroplasty is rarely required.

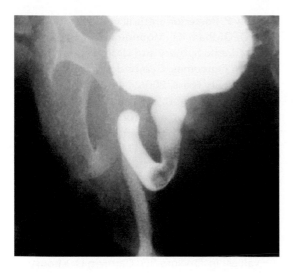

Figure 9.10 MCUG outlining a posterior urethral polyp prolapsing from its point of origin into the membranous and bulbar urethra.

Cobb's Collar

The clinical status of this anomaly is arguable. Its principal significance is as an occasional radiological finding on MCUG which appears as a short, narrowed segment of urethra immediately distal to the urogenital membrane. On endoscopy, the findings consist of little more than a soft, non-obstructing concentric ring. Cobb's collar has sometimes been implicated as a possible cause of voiding disorders, notably enuresis. However, it is more generally believed that in children it is essentially an incidental radiological or endoscopic finding without any clinical significance.

Urethritis

Although well recognised by paediatric urologists, the occurrence of urethritis in boys and adolescents is poorly documented in the literature. The clinical features of this uncommon condition are non-specific and its aetiology is poorly understood. Urethritis occurs mainly in boys aged 6 years and upward. The presenting features include dysuria, penile discomfort and urethral discharge or urethral bleeding – usually consisting of no more than spotting on the underclothes. Attempts to culture a specific organism are unrewarding. In the absence of other features, cystourethroscopy is not indicated, as it rarely makes a practical contribution to clinical management. However, when urethroscopy is performed, the findings are characterised by erythema of the anterior and bulbar urethra, with a granular appearance and strands of fibrinous exudate. There is no specific treatment other than, perhaps, a 6 weeks course of analgesic anti-inflammatory medication such as Ibuprofen. Other suggested treatments for urethritis have included steroids and a period of indwelling catheter drainage. However, there is no reliable evidence that the duration or severity of the urethritis is reduced by either approach. The condition is self-limiting, although it sometimes runs a protracted course.

KEY POINTS

- The original classification of PUV devised by Young is outdated. Congenital urethral obstruction generally conforms to a uniform anatomical pattern, although there is considerable variability in the severity of obstruction and the degree of congenital damage to the upper tracts.
- The majority of cases are detected prenatally. The gestational age at diagnosis and the characteristics of the prenatal ultrasound findings provide a guide to prognosis. Prenatal intervention improves the outcome of lung function in the presence of severe oligohydramnios but there is little if any evidence that prenatal intervention benefits renal function.
- Despite relief of the urethral obstruction in early postnatal life, bladder function is abnormal in up to 70% of boys. The pattern evolves during childhood and if unaddressed may contribute to deteriorating upper tract function and the onset of renal failure in late childhood or early adult life.

- Approximately one-third of individuals with posterior urethral valves are destined to develop chronic renal failure (as a consequence of dysplasia, obstruction, infection and bladder dysfunction). Careful follow-up should be maintained into adulthood.

FURTHER READING

Nassr AA, Shazly SAM, Abdelmagied AM, Araujo Ju'nior E, Tonni G, Kilby MD, Ruano R. Effectiveness of vesicoamniotic shunt in fetuses with congenital lower urinary tract obstruction: an updated systematic review and meta-analysis. Ultrasound Obstet Gynecol. 2017;49:696–703.

Cuckow P. Posterior urethral valves. In: Stringer MD, Oldham KT, Mouriquand PDE (eds), Paediatric Surgery and Urology: Long-Term Outcomes. Cambridge: Cambridge University Press, 2006: 540–554.

Holmdahl G, Sillen U. Boys with posterior urethral valves: outcome concerning renal function, bladder function and paternity at ages 31 to 44. J Urol. 2005;174:1031–1034.

Glick Philip L, Harrison Michael R, Noall Rhoda A, Villa Robin L. Correction of congenital hydronephrosis in utero III. Early mid-trimester ureteral obstruction produces renal dysplasia. J Paediatric Surg. 1983;18(6):681–687.

Zderic SA, Canning DA. Posterior urethral valves. In: Docimo SG, Canning D, Khoury A, Pippi Salle JL (eds), Textbook of Clinical Pediatric Urology, 6th Edition. London: Taylor & Francis, 2019: 1087–1107.

Cystic Renal Disease

DAVID F M THOMAS

Topics covered

Autosomal recessive polycystic kidney disease (ARPKD)

Autosomal dominant polycystic kidney disease (ADPKD)

Multicystic dysplastic kidney (MCDK)

Multilocular renal cyst

Simple renal cyst

INTRODUCTION

Cystic renal pathology is relatively common across all ages from birth into late adulthood. Multicystic dysplastic kidney (MCDK) and autosomal recessive polycystic kidney disease (ARPKD) are the main forms recognised in childhood whereas autosomal dominant polycystic kidney disease (ADPKD) is the commonest form in adults.

POLYCYSTIC RENAL DISEASE

This group of disorders is characterised by the presence of microscopic and/or macroscopic cystic tissue distributed diffusely throughout the parenchyma of both kidneys.

There are two major forms: autosomal recessive polycystic kidney disease (ARPKD) and autosomal dominant polycystic kidney disease (ADPKD).

Recent research suggests that although ARPKD and ADPKD result from different mutations, both conditions exhibit similar defects in signalling pathways of the cilia lining the tubules.

AUTOSOMAL RECESSIVE POLYCYSTIC KIDNEY DISEASE (ARPKD) (FIGURE 10.1)

Incidence

ARPKD is the form of polycystic renal disease most commonly encountered in children, with a reported incidence of between 1:10 000 and 1:40 000. It is caused by mutations of the PKHD1 gene located on chromosome 6. As an autosomal recessive condition, it is associated with a 25% risk in siblings.

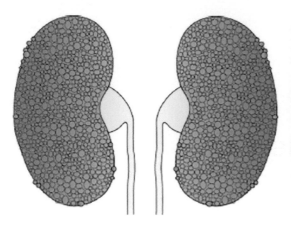

Figure 10.1 Autosomal recessive polycystic renal disease (ARPKD). Diffuse bilateral renal enlargement.

Pathology

The kidneys are considerably enlarged with loss of normal corticomedullary differentiation but typically retain a normal renal outline. The renal parenchyma is extensively replaced by cylindrical, radially orientated cysts which are usually less than 2 mm in diameter (Figure 10.2). ARPKD is also accompanied by varying degrees of liver involvement which is characterised by bile duct abnormalities termed "biliary dysgenesis".

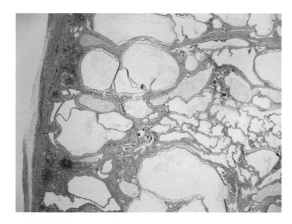

Figure 10.2 Histological appearances of ARPKD. Diffuse distribution of small cysts throughout the renal parenchyma.

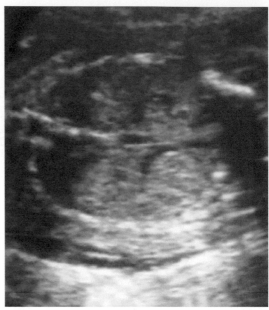

Figure 10.3 Prenatal ultrasound appearances of autosomal recessive polycystic kidney disease.

Presentation

Autosomal recessive polycystic kidney disease is accompanied by characteristic appearances of the kidneys on ultrasonography (Figure 10.3). When visualised prenatally, the additional ultrasonographic findings of oligohydramnios or reduced bladder volume are predictors of severe impairment of renal function. Fetal magnetic resonance imaging (MRI) has also been used to enhance the sensitivity of prenatal diagnosis with a view to possible termination of pregnancy. Nevertheless, the accuracy of prenatal counselling remains somewhat limited despite advances in imaging and genetic sampling.

Clinical Features and Diagnosis

Enlargement of the kidneys causes abdominal distension which is usually readily apparent at birth. The "mass effect" created by the presence of grossly enlarged kidneys may be sufficient to cause respiratory distress due to splinting of the diaphragm. Pulmonary hypoplasia secondary to oligohydramnios may be an additional factor.

Neonates may be initially anuric and can develop acute renal injury. Milder forms of ARPKD may occasionally remain undetected until later childhood when they present with hypertension or manifestations of liver involvement.

The diagnosis of ARPKD is established by a combination of clinical features in conjunction with ultrasonographic imaging of the kidneys and liver.

Treatment

Initial ventilatory support may be required in severely affected infants and unilateral nephrectomy may be considered to alleviate diaphragmatic splinting due to the presence of particularly large kidneys.

Medical management is directed at the treatment of hypertension, prevention of malnutrition, and measures designed to minimise anaemia and bone disease associated with chronic kidney disease. Children progressing to end-stage renal disease may require unilateral or bilateral nephrectomy to control hypertension or to create space to facilitate peritoneal dialysis or accommodate a transplanted kidney. Specific treatment may be required for the complications of hepatic disease such as portal hypertension and a small number of children will require a combined liver-kidney transplant.

Prognosis

The mortality rate is highest in the first month of life. For children who survive the neonatal period the reported 5 years survival rate is 87%, with a 67% survival rate at 15 years.

AUTOSOMAL DOMINANT POLYCYSTIC KIDNEY DISEASE (ADPKD) (FIGURE 10.4)

Incidence

This is the commonest form of inherited renal disease with a reported incidence of between 1:200 and 1:1000. Approximately 10% of adults on end-stage renal replacement programmes have

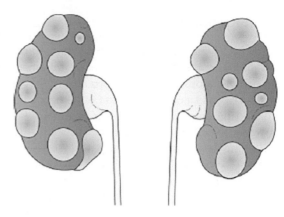

Figure 10.4 Autosomal dominant polycystic kidney disease. Discrete cysts of varying size interspersed between areas of normal renal parenchyma.

ADPKD. Mutations of the PKD1 gene located on chromosome 16, account for 85% of cases whereas most of the remaining cases are due to mutations of the PKD2 gene on chromosome 4.

Pathology

On histological examination the cysts are lined by tubular epithelium and the intervening renal parenchyma may be normal or show evidence of glomerulosclerosis. Extrarenal manifestations include hepatic cysts and cerebral aneurysms.

Presentation

ADPKD is occasionally detected antenatally on fetal ultrasonography but in most affected individuals, cysts do not develop or become apparent until later in life. ADPKD also may come to light as an incidental finding of bilateral renal cysts in asymptomatic children undergoing ultrasonography for other indications or during family screening for the condition. Even when cysts are present, ADPKD usually remains asymptomatic in this age group. However, ADPKD may occasionally give rise to haematuria, hypertension or loin pain in older children or adolescents. In the majority of affected individuals the clinical manifestation do not supervene until adulthood – typically with hypertension, abdominal pain, palpable renal masses, haematuria or other urinary symptoms.

Management

ADPKD is managed expectantly, with follow-up aimed at the detection and early treatment of complications, notably hypertension. This is primarily managed with the use of angiotensin-converting enzyme inhibitors or angiotensin 2 receptor blockers. Flank pain associated with enlarging cysts can be treated with cyst aspiration or sclerosis. Nephrectomy is occasionally indicated for the management of severe hypertension. Following clinical trials, Tolvaptan, a competitive vasopressin receptor 2 antagonist has recently been introduced to delay the rate of cyst development and the decline in renal function in adults with ADPKD with mild to moderate chronic kidney disease.

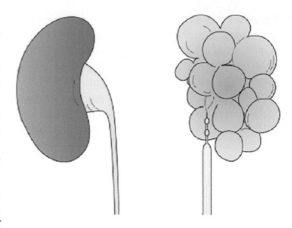

Figure 10.5 Multicystic dysplastic kidney (MCDK). Kidney replaced by collection of cysts of varying size. Ureteric atresia.

Prognosis

When ADPKD is diagnosed incidentally or as a result of family screening, normal renal function is usually maintained until early adulthood. Thereafter, there is considerable individual variability in the natural course of the condition and the rate of progression to end-stage renal disease. Adults with the PKD1 mutation develop end-stage renal disease at a younger age than those with the PKD2 mutation.

Incidence

Published studies put the prevalence of unilateral MCDK between 1:2500 and 1:4300 live births. Bilateral MCDK (which is invariably lethal) is estimated to occur in 1:20 000 pregnancies.

MULTICYSTIC DYSPLASTIC KIDNEY (MCDK) (FIGURES 10.5, 10.6)

MCDK was historically regarded as a relatively rare congenital abnormality which usually presented as an abdominal mass in the neonatal period. Nephrectomy was the standard management. Following the introduction of routine prenatal ultrasonography, however, it soon became apparent that the true prevalence of MCDK is far higher than was previously suspected. But in the majority of cases the MCDK is clinically undetectable and the infant is entirely asymptomatic and outwardly normal.

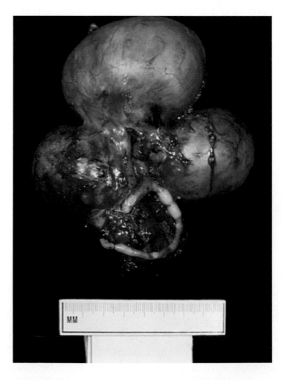

Figure 10.6 Nephrectomy specimen MCDK. (Courtesy of Mr P G Ransley.)

Aetiology/Embryology

MCDK is typically associated with the presence of an occluded atretic segment in the proximal ureter but it is sometimes seen in conjunction with distal ureteric obstruction. Although MCDK is usually a sporadic anomaly, examples of familial occurrence have also been reported in which MCDK is inherited as an autosomal dominant trait with variable penetrance.

Pathology

The histological appearances consist of irregular collections of non-communicating cysts of varying size lined by cuboidal or flattened tubular epithelium. Renal parenchyma, where present, is dysplastic and consists of small islands or flattened plates of abnormal tissue interposed between cysts.

Presentation

Clinical presentation. This is typically as a visible/palpable abdominal mass which is detected in the neonatal period. On palpation, the surface of a MCDK is "knobbly" and irregular in contour – in contrast to other neonatal renal masses such as hydronephrosis or polycystic kidney which typically have a smoother surface.

Incidental postnatal ultrasound finding. A MCDK which has not already been detected prenatally may occasionally be identified on ultrasonography during the evaluation of an infant with coexisting congenital anomalies such as oesophageal atresia.

Prenatal ultrasonography. This is now by far the commonest presentation. The majority of prenatally diagnosed MCDKs (>90%) are small and are not clinically apparent at birth.

Diagnosis

Apart from occasional similarities with severe hydronephrosis the diagnosis of MCDK does not usually present problems. The distinctive ultrasonographic features include:

- Multiple non-communicating round or oval cysts.

- Presence of interfaces between the cysts.
- Absent renal sinus.
- Non-medial location of largest cyst
- Absence of solid parenchymal renal tissue.

A kidney which contains solid renal tissue is, by definition, not a MCDK. The failure to recognise this important diagnostic criterion has led the authors of some case reports to wrongly attribute hypertension to abnormal kidneys which were not, in fact, MCDKs. Genuine MCDKs are characterised by a complete absence of uptake of radionuclide tracer (0% differential function) on a DMSA scan. However, many paediatric urologists no longer perform confirmatory functional imaging with DMSA or MAG3 if the ultrasonographic appearances fulfil all the diagnostic criteria of MCDK. Any uptake of radionuclide (even a small percentage) denotes the presence of some functioning tissue and effectively excludes the diagnosis of MCDK. Kidneys which contain solid tissue or demonstrate radionuclide uptake on functional imaging represent an intermediate form of dysplastic kidney which probably poses a greater risk of potential complications than a genuine MCDK. Contralateral or ipsilateral vesicoureteric reflux (VUR) can be demonstrated on routine micturating cystourethrography in around 20% of cases. However such VUR is usually low-grade, has a high tendency for spontaneous resolution and usually poses a low risk of symptomatic urinary tract infection (UTI). For this reason many paediatric urologists no longer routinely perform a micturating cystourethrogram (MCUG) but limit its use to infants with ipsilateral or contralateral upper tract dilatation on ultrasonography. If a MCUG is not performed it is nevertheless important to advise parents and general practitioners (GPs) of the importance of ensuring that the urine is tested for possible infection in the event of urinary symptoms or an unexplained febrile illness. A documented urinary tract infection in a child with MCDK is an indication for a MCUG.

Natural History

Numerous studies have shown that prenatally detected MCDKs have a strong tendency to involute, i.e. shrink in size and disappear on ultrasound. Approximately 30% of MCDKs are no longer detectable on ultrasonography by 1 year and 50% by 5 years. After 10 years 60–70% of prenatally detected MCDKs can no longer be visualised on ultrasound. It seems highly likely that a significant proportion of individuals diagnosed with unilateral "renal agenesis" as adults may, in fact, have been born with MCDKs which then underwent spontaneous involution.

Hypertension

Hypertension has been ascribed to MCDKs in a number of case reports. However, the validity of at least some of these reports is questionable since they appear to relate to other forms of dysplastic kidney (containing significant elements of solid renal tissue) rather than genuine MCDKs.

A literature review of 29 published studies totalling 1115 MCDKs identified an incidence of hypertension of 0.5%. However, a large prospective study found no instances of hypertension in 202 children with MCDKs followed for a median of 8.1 years. A series of 454 children with hypertension reported from a major UK children's hospital did not contain a single case of MCDK. Only 1 MCDK was encountered in a series of 21 children undergoing nephrectomy for hypertension reported from the same institution. In summary, the weight of reliable evidence points to a very low risk of hypertension (probably of the order 0.5%) which does not justify performing "prophylactic" nephrectomy in asymptomatic infants and children.

It is also important to note that removing the MCDK does not necessarily abolish the risk of hypertension because of well documented instances of hypertension arising from pathology in the contralateral kidney.

Malignancy

As with case reports of hypertension, the credibility of the diagnosis of MCDK in some reported cases of malignancy is questionable. A review of 105 published series of prenatally detected MCDKs coupled with registry data on 900 MCDKs identified a total of 3 cases of Wilms tumour. However, no Wilms tumours were encountered in two prospective long-term studies in the UK totalling more than 600 prenatally detected MCDKs. Wilms tumour Registry data in the United Kingdom and United States point to a similar picture. In summary, the published data suggest that the risk of developing malignancy (notably Wilms tumour) in a MCDK very low – and probably no higher than 1:5000.

Other Complications

These are rare. Urinary tract infections are far more likely to be associated with concurrent VUR or some other coexistent anomaly rather than the MCDK itself. Symptomatic VUR is usually low grade and can be managed conservatively or by endoscopic correction. Varying degrees of contralateral pelviureteric junction obstruction are present in 5–10% of cases and are managed conservatively or surgically according to their severity.

Surgical Management

The last two decades have witnessed a marked shift away from nephrectomy in favour of conservative management.

Nevertheless, the following are generally recognised as valid indications for nephrectomy:

a. A clinically apparent renal mass – particularly when this appears to be giving rise to discomfort or other symptoms associated with a large MCDK.
b. Uncertainty surrounding the diagnosis and/or the presence of a solid component or functioning tissue.

Paediatric urologists who advocate the practice of "prophylactic" nephrectomy often cite parental preference to justify surgical intervention ("the parents were counselled and chose nephrectomy"). With rare exceptions this cannot be regarded as a legitimate indication because parents are strongly influenced by the inherent bias of the surgeon and the manner in which information is presented to them (particularly if this includes any mention of malignancy).

Technical Aspects of Nephrectomy

MCDKs can be removed by either an open or laparoscopic approach. The traditional approach entails the use of either a short incision anterior to the tip of the 12th rib or a posterior lumbotomy incision. Aspiration of cyst fluid facilitates removal through a small incision. Laparoscopic nephrectomy can be performed by either a retroperitoneal or transperitoneal approach – the latter being more appropriate if the MCDK is in an ectopic location. Any benefits of laparoscopic nephrectomy are marginal in view of the simplicity and low morbidity with which a MCDK can be removed through a limited incision which leaves a small cosmetic scar.

Conservative Management

Some paediatric urologists prefer to maintain ultrasound surveillance (typically on an annual or biannual basis) until the MCDK has undergone complete involution and is no longer visible on ultrasonography. However, other paediatric urologists discontinue regular surveillance after the age of 5–6 years (the age at which any theoretical risk of Wilms tumour has passed). Ninety percent of children with MCDK demonstrate compensatory hypertrophy in their contralateral kidney. It would seem logical to pay particular attention to following up the 10% of children who do not develop compensatory hypertrophy since this may be indicative of a greater long-term risk of hyperfiltration damage in the solitary contralateral kidney.

Regardless of the age at which a child is discharged from urological follow-up it is prudent to arrange for their blood pressure to be checked by a paediatrician or GP on an annual basis, continuing into adult life.

MULTILOCULAR RENAL CYST (FIGURE 10.7)

This rare renal abnormality (which is also termed cystic nephroma, benign multilocular cystic nephroma etc.) can create diagnostic difficulty

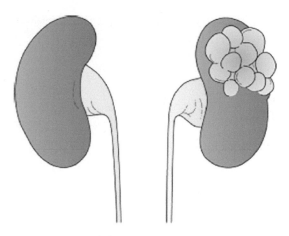

Figure 10.7 Multilocular renal cyst.

because of similarities with cystic forms of Wilms tumour.

Aetiology

It is unclear whether multilocular renal cyst should be regarded as a neoplasm or a developmental anomaly. Although, malignancy associated with multilocular renal cyst has been reported in adult life, it is not generally regarded as a premalignant lesion in children. Multilocular renal cyst usually occurs sporadically with no evidence of an inherited basis. A very rare association has been reported with pleuropulmonary blastoma – premalignant lung cysts.

Incidence

There are no reliable data but the incidence is probably in the range 1:200 000–1:250 000. Multilocular renal cyst has a bimodal age distribution, with one peak in infancy and a second peak in early adult life. Children account for 30–50% of cases.

Presentation

Multilocular renal cyst usually presents with haematuria, loin pain or an abdominal mass. Very rarely it comes to light as an incidental finding on ultrasound during the investigation of unrelated symptoms.Diagnosis is by ultrasound

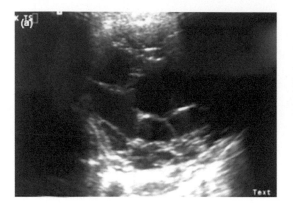

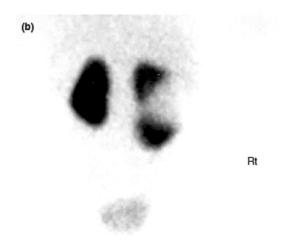

Rt

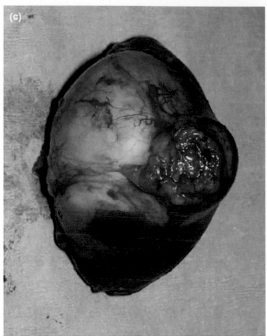

Figure 10.8 (a) Ultrasound scan demonstrating multilocular cystic lesion. (b) Non-functioning cystic lesion in the midzone of the right kidney demonstrated on DMSA. (c) Nephrectomy specimen. Distortion of the renal outline by the tense intrarenal lesion. Histology confirmed benign multilocular cyst.

complemented by CT (Figure 10.8a, b, c) and/or MRI. A DMSA radionuclide scan is also helpful to delineate functioning renal parenchyma if nephron sparing surgery is being considered. Typically the multilocular cystic lesion is localised within the renal parenchyma, but it may extend into the collecting system or distort the renal capsule. An experienced paediatric radiologist should be able to differentiate multilocular renal cyst from other forms of renal pathology, but even with sophisticated imaging it may sometimes be difficult to distinguish it from a cystic variant of Wilms' tumour.

Management

The use of nephron-sparing surgery, i.e. partial nephrectomy has been reported. This may be appropriate in certain circumstances, such as a multilocular renal cyst arising in a solitary kidney but nephrectomy nevertheless remains the generally accepted form of management – particularly if there is the slightest degree of diagnostic uncertainty.

SIMPLE RENAL CYST (FIGURE 10.9)

The rarity of unilateral simple cysts in children compared with adults has been interpreted as evidence that they are acquired rather than congenital in aetiology.

Simple cysts are usually asymptomatic in children and tend to be discovered as incidental findings on ultrasound scans performed for unrelated indications. In the assessment

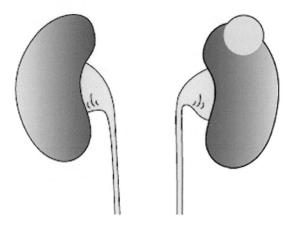

Figure 10.9 Simple renal cyst.

of a child presenting with a solitary cyst it is important to enquire about the family history because the presence of a single cyst may very occasionally represent an early manifestation of ADPKD. The presence of bilateral cysts points to a diagnosis of ADPKD. Not all simple cysts are asymptomatic and some give rise to pain which usually responds to surgical removal or de roofing of the cyst. Asymptomatic cysts can be safely managed conservatively, with ultrasound follow up being discontinued after 2–3 years if the cyst remains asymptomatic and unchanged in size (Figure 10.10). When intervention is indicated, the surgical options are similar to those used for symptomatic renal cysts in adults. Percutaneous aspiration of the

cyst carries a high risk of recurrence. However, this can be reduced by injecting a sclerosing agent such as alcohol into the cyst after aspiration. Surgical options include deroofing and subtotal excision (or marsupialisation) of the cyst wall by either an open or laparoscopic approach. Recurrence is uncommon.

KEY POINTS

- A clear understanding of the different types of cystic renal disease is essential in order to be able to recognise the important differences in their clinical significance and prognosis.
- Autosomal recessive polycystic kidney disease (ARPKD) is either detected prenatally or presents with renal masses in the new born period.
- Autosomal dominant polycystic kidney disease (ADPKD) usually presents in late adolescence or adulthood. However, it may be identified in asymptomatic children as an incidental finding or on ultrasound screening of families.
- Multicystic dysplastic kidney (MCDK) is a developmental abnormality of the kidney which is more prevalent in the general population than was previously recognised.

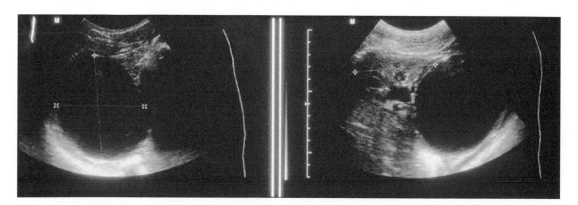

Figure 10.10 Ultrasound appearances of a large simple cyst in the lower pole of the left kidney associated with abdominal pain and a palpable mass. Successfully managed by laparoscopic partial excision/deroofing.

- The practice of "prophylactic" nephrectomy is not supported by the published evidence. Nephrectomy is only indicated for the small minority of MCDKs which give rise to an obvious mass or complications.
- Lifelong monitoring of blood pressure is a prudent precaution (despite removal of a MCDK) in view of the possible risk of hypertension arising in the solitary contralateral kidney.

FURTHER READING

George RP, Greenbaum LA Cystic Renal Disease. In Docimo SG, Canning D, Khoury A, Pippi Salle JL (eds), Textbook of Clinical Pediatric Urology, 6th Edition. Boca Raton: Taylor & Francis 2019: 381–410.

Hollowell JG, Kogan BA. How much imaging is necessary in patients with multicystic dysplastic kidneys? J Urol. 2011;186:785–786.

Thomas DFM, Najmaldin AS. Multicystic Dysplastic Kidney. In: Puri P (ed), Newborn Surgery, 4th Edition. London: CRC Press 2018: 1048–1056.

Wang MK, Gaither T, Phelps A, Cohen R, Baskin L. The incidence and durability of compensatory hypertrophy in pediatric patients with solitary kidneys. Urology. 2019;129:188–193.

Urinary Tract Calculi

ALEXANDER CHO, PATRICK G DUFFY and NAIMA SMEULDERS

Topics covered

Incidence and epidemiology
Pathology/aetiology
Clinical presentation
Diagnostic imaging
Metabolic screening

Minimally invasive surgery: ESWL, PCNL,
  ureteroscopy, PCCL
Open surgery
Follow-up

INTRODUCTION

Urinary stones (calculi) are rare in children but their incidence is increasing in developed countries and they can give rise to significant morbidity.

- **Urolithiasis** is defined as a macroscopic calcification localised anywhere in the urinary tract including the bladder.
- **Nephrocalcinosis** refers to microscopic calcification secondary to calcium salt deposits within the kidney interstitium, the tubules or the tubular epithelium.

A predisposing factor is present in up to 60% of patients – of whom a third have an identifiable metabolic disorder.

A multi-disciplinary team approach including paediatric urologists, interventional radiologists, nephrologists and adult stone urologists, is essential to ensure optimal care for children with stone disease.

INCIDENCE AND EPIDEMIOLOGY

The incidence of stone disease varies widely by geographic region, reflecting differences in the prevalence of environmental, dietary and genetic factors.

A geographical 'stone belt' extending from the North African countries, Turkey, Pakistan, Northern India across to the Philippines is characterised by a higher prevalence of stones especially within the bladder. Chronic malnutrition has been implicated, but relative dehydration associated with the climate and diarrhoeal illness may also be contributory factors. There is also a higher prevalence of endemic metabolic disorders in the same population.

Another stone belt exists in the southern-eastern region of the USA known as the 'North American Stone Belt' with the incidence of urolithiasis being nearly twice that of north-west regions.

The estimated annual incidence of urinary calculi in children in the UK is around 50 per 100,000. The risk of kidney stones appears to be higher amongst boys in the first decade of life, but higher in girls in the second decade. The proportion of stones secondary to infection continues to decline in the UK and is currently around 20%. Infective stones are more common in boys and they present at a younger age.

There has been a recent increase in urolithiasis in the adolescent female population and although a specific cause has not been identified, consumption of animal protein, a high salt intake and obesity have been implicated as possible factors since these are known to be associated with stone formation.

AETIOLOGY

Urinary calculi are composed of crystalline and matrix components in varying proportions. Matrix, a gelatinous glycoprotein, is a particular feature of infective stones which are typically whitish and chalky and crumble easily. The mineral components are mainly calcium, ammonia and magnesium phosphate. Metabolic stones, e.g. cystine and xanthine, are predominantly crystalline and are correspondingly harder.

Factors Involved in Stone Formation

- **Abnormal urinary metabolites or elevated concentration of normal urinary constituents**. When the concentration of stone-forming solutes exceeds the saturation point, crystal deposition occurs which acts as a nidus for stone formation. A low fluid intake and reduced urinary output accelerates this process due to higher urinary concentration of the solute and an unfavourable urinary pH.

- **Reduced urinary inhibitors of crystallisation**. Citrate binds to urinary calcium forming a soluble complex and thereby inhibits formation of calcium stones. Conversely, reduced citrate levels favour stone formation.

- **Urinary infection.** Gram-negative urease-positive organisms such as *Proteus*, *Klebsiella* and *Pseudomonas,* enzymatically split urea to produce ammonia, with consequent alkalisation of the urinary pH and precipitation of ammonium salts – typically combined with magnesium and phosphate. Infection is also a key factor in the production of the proteinaceous matrix component of calculi.

- **Anatomical abnormalities of the urinary tract**. Stasis of urine within a dilated or obstructed urinary tract predisposes to stone formation due to precipitation of stone forming solutes with or without co-existing urine infection. Anatomical or functional abnormalities of the urinary tract can be identified in up to 30% of children presenting with urolithiasis.

- **Foreign materials**. Non-absorbable foreign bodies, usually surgical in origin (stents, fragments of catheters or non-absorbable sutures) act as a nidus of encrustation and stone formation.

- **Prematurity**. Ex-premature children (born <37 weeks' gestation) are at higher risk of nephrocalcinosis and nephrolithiasis This risk is exacerbated by extreme prematurity, co-morbidity and the use of furosemide, thiazides and other drugs. Neonates with intestinal failure due to necrotising enterocolitis (NEC) are at risk of secondary hyperoxaluria. Although up to 40% of neonates <32 weeks gestational age have evidence of nephrocalcinosis this rarely progresses to the formation of discreet stones (nephrolithiasis.

- **Pharmacological agents**. Approximately 1–2% of renal calculi are drug induced as a consequence of increased urinary excretion of solute (e.g. with loop diuretics) or decreased excretion of inhibitory substances (e.g. with topiramate for the management of epilepsy).

- **Genetics**. A positive family history stone disease in a first or second-degree relative represents an important risk factor. However, familial recurrence is not necessarily a consequence of inherited transmission as it may be an effect of shared environmental factors including dietary habits.

Stone Structure

Infective calculi

Infective stones initially comprise a combination of magnesium, ammonium phosphate and glycoprotein matrix in varying proportions. Calcium phosphate and other inorganic constituents then become incorporated into the expanding stone mass. Their consistency is variable, with areas of hard calcified material embedded within softer, less densely calcified matrix. Calcified areas are radio-opaque but the softer matrix component, which may extend throughout much of the collecting system, is radiolucent or only faintly apparent on plain X-ray. The descriptive term 'staghorn' refers to an infective calculus that has adopted the configuration of the renal pelvis and calyces (fancifully likened to the antlers of a stag). Rarely, the infective process progresses to involve the entire renal parenchyma in a chronic inflammatory mass – xanthogranulomatous pyelonephritis.

Metabolic calculi

CALCIUM

Hypercalciuria is the commonest metabolic abnormality and is found in up to 50% of patients with an identifiable metabolic cause. The commonest form is idiopathic hypercalciuria in which the hypercalciuria is not accompanied by hypercalcemia and no other cause is identified. It is thought to represent an autosomal dominant trait with variable penetrance.

Elevated urinary calcium levels are more frequent in premature infants, children on a ketogenic diet and in children being treated with drugs such as furosemide or topiramate. Children with neurological conditions associated with profound physical disability (e.g. severe cerebral palsy) are at greater risk of stones because of skeletal 'demineralisation' induced by their immobility. In newborn infants, the combination of

hypercalciuria and nephrocalcinosis points to an underlying renal tubular defect.

OXALATE

Hyperoxaluria accounts for 10–20% of children with stones, of whom a half have primary hyperoxaluria. This autosomal recessive disorder is characterised by deficiencies of hepatic enzyme resulting in the overproduction of oxalate. Type 1 hyperoxaluria is associated with nephrocalcinosis, recurrent stone formation and 100% progression to end-stage renal failure whereas types 2 & 3 have a less severe clinical course. A combination of renal and liver transplantation has been employed for severe forms and new treatments for the underlying hepatic enzyme deficiency are currently being investigated in clinical trials. Secondary hyperoxaluria occurs in malabsorption states such as Crohn's disease or short gut syndrome. Cystic fibrosis is also associated with higher incidence of renal stones related to hyperoxaluria.

CYSTINE

Cystine is one of four amino acids (the others being lysine, arginine and ornithine), which are excreted in abnormally high concentrations as a result of an autosomal recessive disorder affecting the proximal tubule. The solubility of cystine in urine is low – leading to crystal deposition, recurrent episodes of stone formation and subsequent risk of renal failure.

URIC ACID

Metabolic disorders of uric acid metabolism are rare in children but acute deposition of uric acid crystals within the urinary tract can occur as a result of massive cell breakdown, e.g. following the commencement of cytotoxic treatment for leukaemia or lymphoma. In these conditions, uric acid crystalline debris 'silts up' the collecting systems, leading to anuric renal failure. Uric acid is radiolucent and cannot be directly visualised on plain X-ray.

XANTHINE

Xanthine oxidase deficiency, a rare autosomal recessive disorder, results in the deposition of insoluble, non-opaque xanthine stones within the urinary tract.

Underlying Urological Conditions

Predisposing urological abnormalities can be identified in approximately 20–30% of children with urinary calculi. However, since the majority of children with urinary tract abnormalities do not develop urolithiasis it seems likely that additional factors, notably a concomitant metabolic abnormality are implicated in the small minority of who do develop stones.

Stone formation is a rare complication of pelvic-ureteric junction (PUJ) obstruction and when it does occur the stones are characteristically small and multiple. Although vesicoureteral reflux (VUR) is present in 14% of cases it may be a secondary phenomenon following the passage of uretric calculi rather than being implicated as a primary cause of urinary tract infection (UTI). Neuropathic bladder dysfunction carries an increased risk of stone formation due to incomplete bladder emptying and UTIs.

The use of intestinal segments for bladder reconstruction (enterocystoplasty) is accompanied by a 20–40% risk of bladder stones. This is due to factors which include; urinary stasis, intestinal mucus in the urine acting as a nidus for crystalline deposition and chronic low-grade bacteriuria. The risk can be reduced by the use of regular bladder washouts to promote effective clearance of urinary mucus.

CLINICAL PRESENTATION

Age

Stones may develop from 1 to 2 months of age onwards, with the incidence being higher under 5 years of age – reflecting the relative importance of infective stones (predominantly in boys) in this age group.

Urinary Infection

Although stones typically present in older children with recognisable symptoms the clinical picture in infants may be deceptively non-specific, consisting of vague ill health, low-grade fever and failure to thrive. The isolation of *Proteus* from a child's urine should always prompt investigation for possible stone disease.

Haematuria

Macroscopic or microscopic haematuria is a common feature of calculi, but there is only a poor correlation between its severity and the extent and distribution of stones within the urinary tract. The absence of haematuria on microscopy or reagent strip testing does not exclude the possible presence of stones.

Passage of Stone Material Per Urethra

Occasionally stones come to light when a fragment or some softer matrix material is passed per urethra. Rarely, a urethral stone can cause acute urinary obstruction. In infants the presence of unusual material and streaks of blood in the nappy may be incorrectly ascribed to balanitis.

Pain

Acute renal colic of the pattern and severity encountered in adults is not a prominent feature of the symptomology in children. When pain does occur, it is often a poorly localised symptom in a fractious, unwell child.

Abdominal Mass

Xanthogranulomatous pyelonephritis presents with general ill health, which may be accompanied by a palpable abdominal mass – a clinical picture resembling Wilms' tumour.

Incidental Finding

The presence of stones may occasionally come to light as an entirely incidental finding. Alternatively, they may be identified unexpectedly in a child without urinary symptoms who is being investigated for other symptoms caused by unsuspected stone disease. Stones may also be detected on sibling screening and in our experience a third of cystinuria patients are diagnosed in this way.

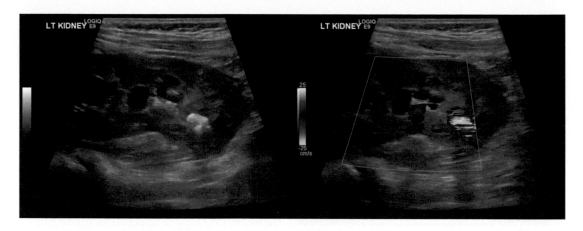

Figure 11.1 Ultrasound appearances of renal calculi with posterior acoustic shadowing (left image) and corresponding 'twinkle artefact' (right image).

DIAGNOSIS

Initial Screening for Calculi

Ultrasound

Ultrasound is the primary diagnostic modality in children because of the quality of the imaging and because it does not entail exposure to radiation. Stones are seen as discrete echogenic foci which cast a posterior acoustic shadow (Figures 11.1 & 11.2). A 'twinkle artefact' is seen with colour Doppler ultrasound due to multi-reflecting rough surface of the stone. Ultrasound has high sensitivity and specificity for the visualisation of renal stones (61–93% and 95–100%, respectively) but these figures are much lower for the detection of ureteral stones.

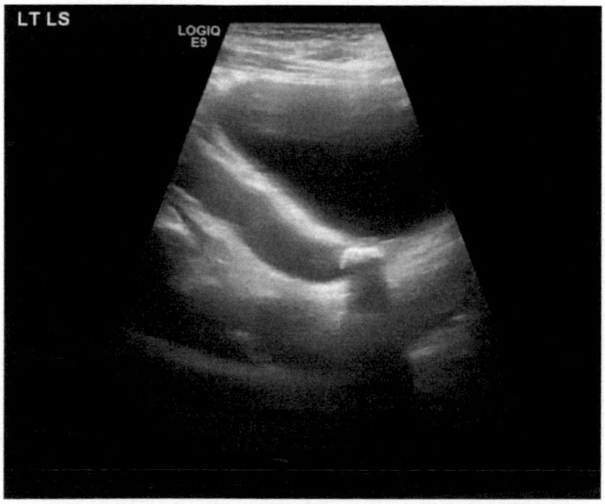

Acute upper tract obstruction caused by the impaction of a stone may only be associated with a misleadingly mild degree of hydronephrosis, with an anterior-posterior diameter of <15mm.

Abdominal X-ray (AXR)

The sensitivity of an abdominal X-ray for detecting radio-opaque urinary stones is only 50% and it is not routinely used for urolithiasis screening.

Unenhanced ultra-low dose spiral computed tomography (CT)

CT is considered the gold standard imaging modality for urolithiasis. In the paediatric age range it is generally reserved for indeterminate cases following ultrasonography or where exact details regarding the stone are necessary for surgical decision-making. With the ultra-low dose Stone Protocol sequences, the radiation exposure has been reduced to <3mSv whilst maintaining sensitivity for urolithiasis at over 96% (Figure 11.3). With dual-energy CT-imaging, the stone density (in Hounsfield units) can be calculated to further aid surgical planning.

Figure 11.2 Ultrasound scan demonstrating a distal ureteric calculus with associated proximal ureteric dilatation and posterior shadowing.

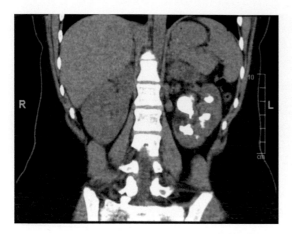

Figure 11.3 Low dose CT image demonstrating complex left staghorn calculus.

Evaluation Prior to Treatment of Proven Stone Disease

DMSA

Differential function in the affected kidney(s) should be documented on a ^{99m}Tc dimercaptosuccinic acid (DMSA) scan before intervention and re-evaluated after treatment. This can be combined with a low-dose unenhanced CT scan of the urinary tract which is co-registered with the DMSA tomographic images (DMSA SPECT-CT) to provide the additional assessment of the renal parenchymal function adjacent to renal stones (Figure 11.4).

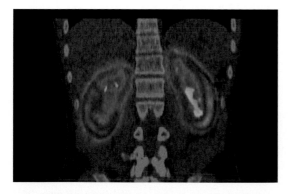

Figure 11.4 DMSA SPECT-CT demonstrating left staghorn calculus and small stones on the right with good functioning surrounding renal parenchyma.

Intravenous urography

Intravenous urography (IVU) can provide additional anatomical information (e.g. on calyceal anatomy) but an ultra low-dose CT scan is usually sufficient to provide the information needed when planning percutaneous nephrolithotomy.

Additional investigations

DYNAMIC RENOGRAPHY

Dynamic renography, e.g. (^{99m}Tc)mercaptoacetyltriglycine (MAG3), is undertaken if obstruction is suspected. However, it is not possible to make a reliable diagnosis of PUJ obstruction when a stone is present in the renal pelvis. The presence of underlying obstruction can only be reliably diagnosed after complete removal of the stone.

MICTURATING CYSTOGRAPHY

Micturating cystography (MCUG) is not performed routinely. Even when VUR is demonstrated it may be a transient phenomenon (secondary to infection and the passage of stone material to the bladder) which resolves once the infection has been treated and stone clearance has been achieved. If indicated (e.g. to exclude posterior urethral valves or other pathology) cystoscopy can be performed at the time of an interventional procedure for the stone(s).

METABOLIC INVESTIGATIONS

If stone fragments are obtained, crystallographic evaluation with infra-red spectroscopy may aid the diagnosis of an underlying metabolic disorder. However, metabolic screening by urinary biochemistry analysis must also be undertaken routinely because underlying metabolic disorders may not always be reflected in the chemical composition of the stones. The presence of urinary infection and/or abnormalities of the urinary tract abnormality does not exclude the possibility of co-existing metabolic disorder and every child with stone disease, regardless of the perceived aetiology, should therefore undergo metabolic screening after the eradication of infection and ideally at least 6 weeks after stone clearance (Table 11.1).

Table 11.1 Metabolic screening protocol

Plasma levels of urea, electrolytes, creatinine, calcium, phosphate, magnesium, uric acid

Early morning urine sample (pH to exclude renal tubular acidosis)

'Spot', i.e. untimed, urine sample 2–5 ml:
- –Ratio of calcium, oxalate, cystine, citrate and urate to creatinine
- –Urine microscopy and culture

24-hour urine collection:
- –Calcium, cystine, creatinine clearance, total urinary volume
- –A separate 24-hour collection is required for oxalate analysis as the sample is acidified during collection

METABOLIC SCREENING

Stone screening can be reliably undertaken on a random 'spot' sample of 2–5 ml of urine, although an early morning specimen may be preferable for some studies. Twenty-four hour urine collections may be indicated depending on the clinical presentation, a positive family history for stones, stone analysis and results from the urinary 'spot' samples. Urine biochemistry analysis is used to monitor the effect of preventative measures where a metabolic cause has been identified.

MANAGEMENT

Children who present acutely with complications should be urgently referred to a paediatric stone unit. Following initial resuscitation, the priority is decompression of the obstructed urinary system. This may be achieved by percutaneous nephrostomy or by retrograde insertion of a JJ stent if this is feasible and the child's condition is stable. Definitive stone surgery should be deferred until the patient has recovered from the acute episode.

The aims of treatment are to achieve complete stone clearance whilst minimising renal tissue damage and complications. Some patients may need a planned, staged approach with a combination of interventions at different intervals to achieve complete stone clearance.

Treatment Modalities

Less invasive techniques have become increasingly applicable for use in children and have consequently reduced the requirement for open surgery in this age group.

Guidelines based on the published literature can be briefly summarised as follows:

- ESWL is the treatment of choice for renal calculi <20 mm in size.
- PCNL is the treatment of choice for renal calculi >20 mm in size.
- Ureteroscopy and lithotripsy with the holmium laser is the treatment of choice for ureteric calculi.

Medical expulsive therapy (MET)

This can be considered for the treatment of an uncomplicated ureteral stone <10 mm if the child's clinical condition is stable. Medical expulsive therapy using alpha-adrenergic antagonists to relax the ureteric smooth muscle has been shown to increase stone expulsion rates in children without causing significant adverse side effects. Tamsulosin and doxazosin are the most commonly used agents. Close follow-up is essential to confirm stone-clearance and assess the possible need to move on to other treatment modalities.

External shockwave lithotripsy (ESWL)

Shockwaves, generated either by piezoelectric energy or by an electromagnetic generator, are transmitted to the patient via a silicon-membrane covered cushion containing a fluid or water film (Figure 11.5). Using in-line ultrasound or X-ray linked to the shockwave generator, this energy is focused on the renal stone(s). Unlike adults, children frequently require general anaesthesia or heavy sedation to ensure they maintain a suitable position throughout the duration of the treatment session.

ESWL is valuable for the treatment of renal stones <2 cm and stones in the upper ureter. The reported success rates range from 49% to 95%. It is less effective for the treatment of very dense stones (>1000 HU) such as those composed of

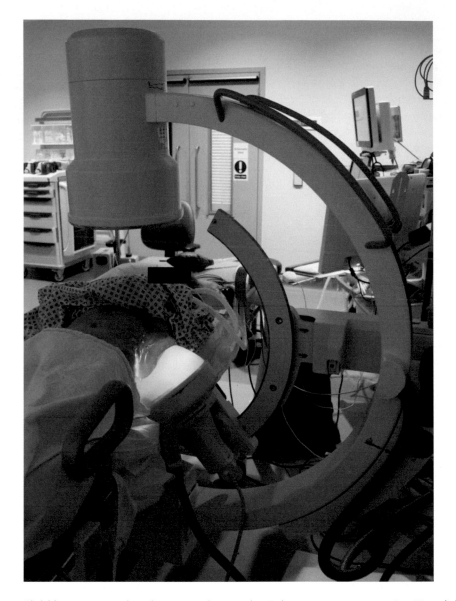

Figure 11.5 Child being treated under general anaesthesia by a current generation Piezolith lithotripter. Stone localisation and imaging during the treatment is achieved by a combination of in-line ultrasound and, if necessary, X-ray C-arm.

cystine or calcium-phosphate, although this is not an absolute contraindication. ESWL also has a role for 'mopping up' residual fragments following PCNL. JJ stents are not routinely placed for ESWL. If the child already has a stent in situ it is removed at the end of the ESWL session under the same general anaesthetic to facilitate the passage of fragments.

Complications

Steinstrasse (the presence of a column of stone fragments in the ureter) occurs in 8% of cases – with the risk being higher in smaller children with large stones. It can be managed by retrograde insertion of a JJ stent, although ureteroscopy may be required for stone clearance.

Children who are thought to be at greater risk of developing steinstrasse are monitored after ESWL with an early ultrasound scan and planned review.

Dermal bruising is common and haematuria occurs in up to 40% of patients. Initial concerns regarding risks of impaired renal growth, renal scarring or hypertension have not materialised and the published data have demonstrated that ESWL is a safe treatment modality in children.

Percutaneous nephrolithotomy (PCNL)

PCNL is typically used for large staghorn calculi, renal stones unsuitable for ESWL or stones persisting following previous intervention. Stone-free rates of up to 98% have been reported and PCNL has largely replaced open surgery for the treatment of large stones in children.

The procedure starts with a cystoscopy and retrograde contrast studies to delineate the ipsilateral renal and ureteric anatomy. Then, with the patient prone, percutaneous needle puncture into the selected calyx is performed under ultrasonographic or fluoroscopic guidance. Serial dilators are passed over a guidewire to widen the tract sufficiently to permit the introduction of an endoscope into the renal collecting system (Figure 11.6). Under direct vision, the stone is

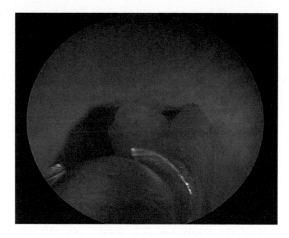

Figure 11.7 Endoscopic view with the nephroscope. Stone fragment removed with a grasper under direct vision after disintegration with a pneumatic probe.

either removed or is disintegrated with an ultrasonic or pneumatic probe (Figure 11.7). The kidney is drained post operatively by a nephrostomy tube or internal JJ-stent.

The "standard" PCNL tract corresponds to 24–30Fr but miniaturised PCNL systems are now available, such as the SuperMini PCNL with tract size of 14F. However, reduced tract size usually comes at the expense of speed of stone clearance. The stone(s) are disintegrated with Holmium YAG laser and removed via active suction along the tract.

Complications

Bleeding requiring transfusion occurs in <10% of cases. Infective/febrile complications occur in up to 15% of cases – highlighting the importance of appropriate peri-operative antibiotic cover. Persistent urinary leakage, hydrothorax, injury to lung/liver/spleen and pelvicalyceal scarring are uncommon but recognised complications.

Ureterorenoscopy (Ureteroscopy) (URS)

Ureteric stones and renal stones in favourable anatomical positions can be treated using semirigid ureteroscopes (4.5/6.5 6.8/8.5 F) or by

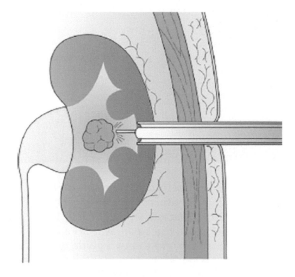

Figure 11.6 PCNL – percutaneous sheath, nephroscope and lithoclast.

flexible ureteroscopy (Figure 11.8a, b). Under direct vision, the stones are fragmented by laser. Small stone fragments can be cleared with an endoscopic basket and sent for stone analysis. The remainder can be further fragmented to dust which passes spontaneously. However, passive dilatation of the VUJ/PUJ by a period of indwelling ureteral stenting may sometimes be necessary to enable the ureteroscope to be negotiated into the ureter and kidney.

A stone-free rate of 90% has been reported in children. Complications occurring in 10% of cases include UTI, haematuria and intra-operative complications such as ureteral perforation or tear. Ureteral strictures are uncommon but it is important that care is taken to minimise trauma to the ureter and VUJ during instrumentation.

Minimally invasive cystolithotomy

Endoscopic treatment is now feasible for the majority of bladder stones. Access can be achieved per urethra, via a Mitrofanoff channel or via a direct percutaneous channel – percutaneous cystolithotomy (PCCL). The stone is fragmented using a lithoclast or laser and fragments can be extracted directly (Figure 11.9a, b). The PCCL route avoids urethral trauma and permits the use of a larger access sheath to deal with larger bladder stones and reduce operative time. Open surgery (cystolithotomy) remains the preferred option for very large stones or if there are a large number of stones of significant size.

Urethra

Urethral calculi are rare in children. They may result from impaction of a calculus (or post-ESWL fragments) during its passage through the urethra, or the formation of a stone within an anatomical abnormality of the urethra such as the remnant of a rectourethral fistula following surgery for an anorectal anomaly.

Urethral calculi can be removed or crushed using rigid endoscopic biopsy forceps. Meatotomy may be required to release a stone impacted within the fossa navicularis.

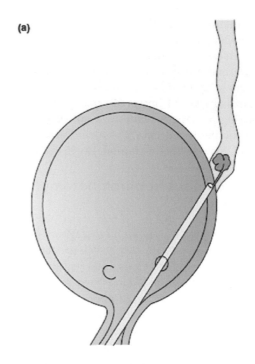

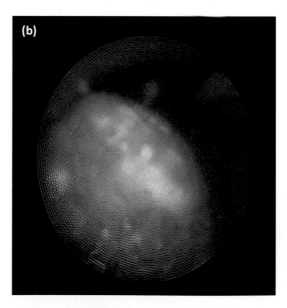

Figure 11.8 (a) Ureteroscopy and laser lithotripsy (left). (b) Ureteroscopic view (right) demonstrating ureteric stone partially laser fragmented. Note the clear laser fibre in the 7 o'clock position and the two guide wires running in 2 o'clock position that aid passage of the ureteroscope. The smaller telescopes limit the optics which reduces the image quality.

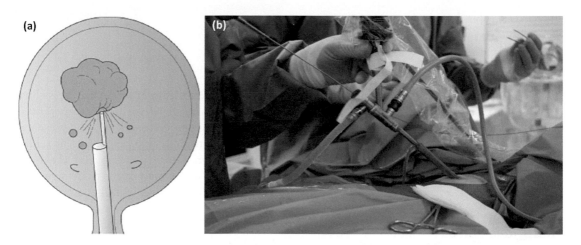

Figure 11.9 **(a)** Endoscopic fragmentation of bladder calculus by lithoclast (left). **(b)** PCCL access into bladder with a nephroscope passed via a clear access sheath.

Laparoscopy

A poorly functioning kidney which has been damaged by stone disease or xanthogranulomatous pyelonephritis can be removed laparoscopically. However, laparoscopic nephrectomy in such cases should only be undertaken by an experienced laparoscopic surgeon because of the extensive perirenal inflammatory adhesions and risk of damage to adjacent organs.

Open pyelolithotomy

Although, largely superseded by ESWL and endoscopic techniques, open surgery still plays a limited role – for example in urolithiasis in congenitally obstructed systems or children with severe skeletal abnormalities which may preclude endoscopic intervention.

Following exposure and mobilisation of the kidney, isolated stones within the collecting system can usually be removed with stone forceps via an incision in the renal pelvis (Figure 11.10). The bulk of a staghorn calculus can also be removed by this approach, but the subsequent removal of fragments impacted in the calyces can be difficult and may require later intervention with ESWL to achieve complete stone clearance.

Complications include haemorrhage, particularly after multiple nephrotomies, retained or displaced stone fragments, prolonged urinary

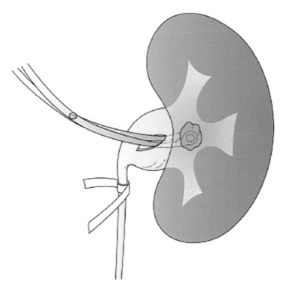

Figure 11.10 Pyelolithotomy. Open removal of a calculus from the renal pelvis.

leakage and parenchymal damage resulting in loss of renal function.

FOLLOW-UP

Recurrence

Stone disease in children is associated with a significant risk of recurrence – with a 20% incidence of further stone formation within 10 years.

This risk can be reduced by appropriate follow up and management – ideally in a joint urology-nephrology clinic.

Infective calculi

The recurrence risk can be minimised by correcting any underlying predisposing anatomical abnormality and by maintaining infection-free urine with antibiotic prophylaxis for 12 months following surgery. A circumcision can be considered in young boys with infective stones.

Metabolic calculi

Following the initial stone episode, the recurrence rate in children with underlying metabolic disorders is around 40% within 5 years.

A high fluid intake is essential for all groups together with dietary modifications dependent on the metabolic abnormality. In addition, a number of specific measures can be utilised as outlined in Table 11.2.

Residual fragments

Even in the absence of infection or urinary stasis, seemingly 'insignificant' residual stone fragments of less than 4mm have a 50% likelihood of increasing in size ('regrowing') in structurally normal kidneys and up to 80% in abnormal kidneys. Achieving complete stone clearance at the time of initial intervention is therefore of the upmost importance.

Table 11.2 Medications commonly used for metabolic stone prevention

Thiazide diuretic	Hypercalcuria – despite diet modification
Potassium citrate	Hypercalcuria, hyperoxaluria, Cystinuria – only with acidic urinary pH
Tiopronin, D-penicillamine	Cystinuria
Pyridoxine	Primary hyperoxaluria

XANTHOGRANULOMATOUS PYELONEPHRITIS (FIGURE 11.11A, B)

This rare manifestation of stone disease is characterised by a destructive inflammatory mass which invades renal parenchyma. The presentation is with chronic sepsis: weight loss, anaemia, elevated inflammatory markers and the presence of a mass which may extend to involve adjacent viscera. Pain is usually dull and persistent. The diagnosis is confirmed by a combination of ultrasound, CT and DMSA, which reveals absent or minimal function in the affected kidney. Open nephrectomy is usually preferred because of the dense perirenal inflammatory adhesions and risk of damage to adjacent organs. Postoperative monitoring of the remaining kidney and aggressive treatment of any further UTIs are essential.

KEY POINTS

- Urinary calculi are becoming more common in children. Urinary infection is still an important aetiological factor but the importance of predisposing metabolic disorders is being increasingly recognised.
- Every child who presents with calculi should be thoroughly evaluated to identify any underlying metabolic disorder or urological malformation – regardless of presumed primary aetiology.
- The initial priorities of management consist of relieving obstruction, treating sepsis and achieving complete stone clearance.
- Urine biochemistry should be combined with stone analysis to diagnose metabolic disorders.
- Minimally invasive modalities such as ESWL, PCNL and endoscopic lithotripsy have now superseded open techniques in the treatment of children's stones.

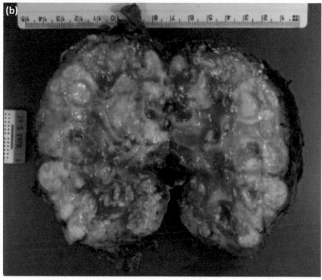
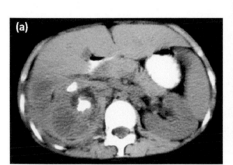

Figure 11.11 (a) CT scan (left): xanthogranulomatous pyelonephritis of the right kidney illustrating calculi embedded within a non-functioning inflammatory renal mass. Normal left kidney. (b) Histopathology specimen of an XPN kidney (right): the kidney has been split open along its long axis.

> - Careful follow-up, with maintenance of sterile urine and appropriate treatment of any metabolic disorder, is essential to minimise the risk of stone recurrence.

FURTHER READING

Bowen DK, Tasian GE. Paediatric stone disease. Urol Clin N Am. 2018;539–550.

Issler N, Dufek S, Kleta R et al. Epidemiology of paediatric renal stone disease: a 22-year single centre experience in the UK. BMC Nephrol. 2017; 18:136

Papageorgiou E, Smeulders N. Renal Calculi. In: Davenport M, Geiger J. (eds), Operative Paediatric Surgery, 8th Edition. Taylor & Francis, [In Press].

Purkait B, Sinha RJ, Bansal A, Sokhal AK, Singh K, Singh V. What is the fate of insignificant residual fragment following percutaneous nephrolithotomy in paediatric patients with anomalous kidney? A comparison with normal kidney. Urolithiasis. 2018;46:285–290.

Rob S, Jones P, Pietropaolo A, Griffin S, Somani BK. Ureteroscopy for stone disease in paediatric population is safe and effective in medium-volume and high-volume centres: evidence for a systematic review. Curr Urol Rep. 2017;18:92.

Velázquez N, Zapata D, Wang HHS et al. Medical expulsive therapy for paediatric urolithiasis: systematic review and meta-analysis. J Ped Urol. 2015;11(6):321–327.

Urinary Incontinence

HENRIK STEINBRECHER

Topics covered

Definitions, epidemiology, classification
Neurology and development of continence
Patient assessment

Structural incontinence
Functional daytime incontinence
Night time incontinence

DEFINITIONS, EPIDEMIOLOGY, CLASSIFICATION

Urinary incontinence can be defined as the "uncontrollable leakage of urine". It is one of the commonest conditions of childhood, with daytime incontinence (diurnal enuresis) affecting around 15% of 4-year-old children and 2% of 9 year olds. Approximately 20% of 4–5-year-old children experience some degree of bedwetting (nocturnal enuresis). Although the incidence declines during the course of childhood, nocturnal enuresis continues to affect 1–2% of adolescents. Urinary incontinence (both diurnal and nocturnal) is classified as "primary" if the child has never been reliably dry and "secondary" when the onset of wetting occurs after a period in which the child had previously been dry.

Urinary incontinence may be classified as either organic or functional in aetiology (Figure 12.1). Organic causes (anatomical or neurological abnormalities) are relatively rare and account for

only 1% of cases. These are described elsewhere in this book. This chapter deals solely with the functional causes of urinary incontinence.

NEUROLOGY AND NORMAL DEVELOPMENT OF CONTINENCE

Normal urinary continence depends on a co-ordinated relationship between bladder filling and detrusor contraction and by coordinated relaxation and contraction of the urethral sphincter. It is also dependent on intact neural pathways and regulation by higher centres in the brain.

During infancy, voiding is a reflex act which occurs in response to involuntary detrusor contractions. Although bladder function is not under voluntary control in infancy, higher centres in the brain have been shown to exhibit arousal activity in response to sensory input prior to voiding. After toilet training, these centres play a far more

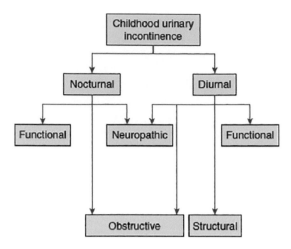

Figure 12.1 Simple classification of childhood urinary incontinence.

significant role in controlling overall bladder function and continence.

The lower urinary tract is supplied by three different nerve groups:

Sacral parasympathetic (pelvic splanchnic) nerves (S2, 3, 4). These comprise both pre and post ganglionic fibres. Acetylcholine is the principal neurotransmitter.

Thoracolumbar sympathetic (hypogastric) nerves (T10–L2). Sympathetic fibres synapse in the paravertebral ganglia of the sympathetic chain before branching out to become the hypogastric plexus, and finally merging with the pelvic plexus supplying the bladder base, bladder neck and proximal urethra. Stimulation of the sympathetic pathways results in relaxation of the bladder detrusor muscle and contraction of the bladder neck and posterior urethral sphincter complex. The main postganglionic neurotransmitter is noradrenaline.

Sacral somatic nerves (S2,3,4). The somatic nerve supply originates within Oluf's nucleus of the anterior horn of S2, 3, 4 spinal segments. These nerves, which are richly supplied with serotonin and noradrenaline receptors, merge to form the pudendal nerves supplying the pelvic floor muscles and external urethral sphincter.

The most important factor in successful toilet training is the development of voluntary inhibition of the voiding reflex. This can be affected by psychological, social and behavioural factors.

During the first year of life, the rate of bladder emptying remains fairly constant at approximately 20 times per day. This decreases to around five times a day by the age of 7 years. This reduction in voiding frequency is due partly to a growth-related increase in bladder capacity (which is disproportionately greater than the volume of urine produced) and partly to the development of sensory C-fibres in the nerves supplying the bladder.

Once a child has been successfully toilet trained, the normal bladder cycle is under voluntary control and consists of the following phases.

1. The bladder fills and the urethra contracts via modulation from T10 to L2 lumbar sympathetic nerves and S2, 3, 4 voluntary somatic innervation.
2. The urethra relaxes under voluntary control mediated by S2, 3, 4 somatic nerves.
3. The pelvic floor relaxes under voluntary control mediated via S2, 3, 4 somatic nerves.
4. The detrusor muscle contracts in response to stimulation via parasympathetic S2, 3, 4 nerves.
5. Voiding occurs to completion.
6. The urethral sphincter contracts under S2, 3, 4 voluntary somatic control.

CLINICAL ASSESSMENT

The initial priority is to exclude an organic (anatomical or neurological) cause of the urinary incontinence. This can usually be achieved with the combination of taking a thorough history, careful physical examination and appropriate investigations (Table 12.1).

History

Three fundamental questions should be asked:

- *Does the wetting occur principally or entirely by night or by day?*
- *Is the incontinence primary i.e. lifelong and predating attempts at toilet training or*

Table 12.1 Organic causes of urinary incontinence

Urinary infection (intermittent leakage)
Neuropathic (continuous/intermittent leakage)
Bladder outflow obstruction (intermittent leakage)
Structural (continuous leakage)
Exstrophy/epispadias
Ureteric ectopia (girls)
Congenital short urethra (girls)
Urovaginal confluence (girls)

secondary ie developing in a child who was previously dry and toilet trained (even if only for a short time)?
- *In the case of daytime wetting, does this occur continuously or intermittently?*

Urinary incontinence which occurs only during the day time is usually functional rather than organic in aetiology. One exception is involuntary leakage from an ectopic ureter which may sometimes only be apparent when the child is upright – and not when they are supine and asleep.

There is virtually never an underlying organic basis to urinary incontinence which occurs solely at night and which is not accompanied by day time daytime symptoms (termed monosymptomatic nocturnal enuresis).

The organic causes of primary daytime urinary incontinence include congenital anatomical abnormalities and certain conditions such as bladder outflow obstruction or neurological impairment. Although the secondary onset of daytime incontinence may also have an organic basis such as late presenting posterior urethral valves or a neurological condition it is almost never due to a congenital anatomical anomaly.

Intermittent daytime wetting (in which the child can remain dry for periods of varying duration) may occasionally have an organic cause (such as bladder outflow obstruction or neurological disease) but it is functional in the overwhelming majority of cases – particularly when the wetting occurs infrequently.

Despite attempts to obtain an accurate history from the child and their parents it may not be possible to form a clear picture of the precise pattern of symptoms and frequency of wetting at the time of the initial consultation.

Typical information to be obtained in a history in a child with wetting is listed in Table 12.2.

A detailed history may sometimes point to a specific form of urinary incontinence. For example, involuntary dribbling of urine in girls which occurs immediately or shortly after voiding is a characteristic feature of vaginal "reflux" – often due to the presence of labial adhesions. This is considered in more detail below.

Giggle incontinence is a distinctive condition in which urinary leakage occurs only when the child (usually a girl) is giggling or laughing but at no other time.

Examination

This should include the abdomen, spine, back, genitalia and lower limbs. It should also include observing the child's gait and performing a limited neurological examination of the lower limbs.

Salient findings include:

Abdomen – Is the bladder palpably enlarged? Are the kidneys palpable? A palpable bladder which can be emptied ("expressed") by applying suprapubic pressure is virtually pathognomonic of neurological disease – particularly in the presence of gross constipation.

Genitalia – Examination of the male genitalia is aimed at identifying conditions such as primary epispadias, Balanitis xerotica and meatal stenosis (including cases of hypospadias). In the female, the examination should look for conditions including primary epispadias (Figure 12.2), common urogenital sinus (Figure 12.3) and labial adhesions (Figure 12.4). The external opening of an ectopic ureter is very occasionally evident on gross inspection, although in some girls urine may be observed leaking from the introital area. It is usual for examination of the genitalia of older girls and adolescents to be performed under sedation or anaesthesia. Examination of genitalia should be performed in the presence of suitable chaperones.

Table 12.2 Information to be obtained when taking the medical history

	Example	Comment
Number of episodes of wetting/day and or night/week	Day = 5/7, 3x/day Night = 7/7, 1x/night (early morning)	An accurate description is essential to permit a reliable assessment. Words such as "Occasional", "often", "sometimes" are insufficient.
Frequency of voiding/day and/night	Day/Night = 7/1	Often children do not visit the toilet during the entire school day (a period of over 6 hours). This should be noted.
Presence of urgency/ Vincent's curtsy sign	Rushes to toilet, drops everything to go, car journeys interrupted,	In Vincent's curtsy, the child crouches down on one heal, pushing upwards on perineum to prevent leakage.
Urge incontinence	Wets on way to toilet	Children may comment they don't know they are wetting until it has happened.
Stress incontinence	Exercise (running, trampolining, jumping), Cough, sneezing	Giggle incontinence is a specific entity.
Stream – onset, presence of hesitancy		Hesitancy may be caused by obstruction. A seemingly normal stream does not exclude obstruction.
Stream characteristic	Stop/start, continuous	This is may represent obstruction or detrusor instability.
Fluid intake, last drink taken, type of drink taken	ml/day, (often a prop such as a cup on the table can be used as a visual aid to estimate intake	Stimulants drinks such as cola or blackcurrent juice can exacerbate detrusor instability.
Bowel habit	Bowels open 1–2x/day, no pain, no blood, normal motions	It is vital to obtain a bowel history in children with urinary incontinence.
Use of shampoos, soaps, etc	Hair wash in bath, child sits in soapy water etc	A recent change in perineal bacterial flora leads to the development of lower tract infection (cystitis) and bladder instability.
Family history of wetting	Parents wet until teens, siblings wet.	
History of urinary tract infection		Recurrent infections can lead to detrusor instability
Drug history, other health history	Asthma, cystic fibrosis, ADHD, autism (altered higher control mechanisms), Trisomy 21 (higher risk of detrusor-sphincter dyssynergia)	Some medical illnesses and their treatment affects bladder function.
Social history	Sleeping arrangements, proximity to toilet	Snoring or inability to wake from sleep may be implicated in nocturnal enuresis.

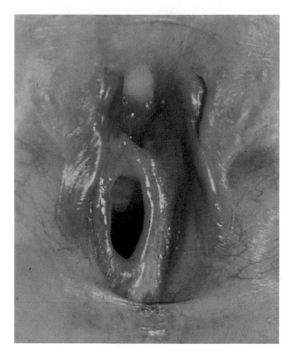

Figure 12.2 Female epispadias. Bifid clitoris with wide urethral meatus. This anomaly in females is invariably associated with sphincter weakness incontinence.

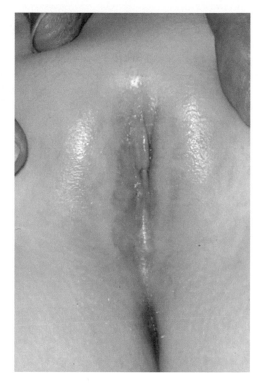

Figure 12.4 Extensive occlusion of the introitus by labial adhesions – resulting in retrograde filling of the vagina during voiding. Symptoms cured by separation of labial adhesions.

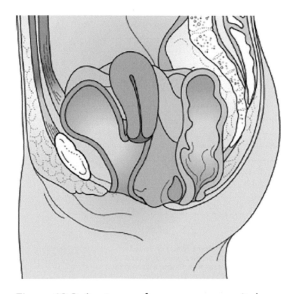

Figure 12.3 Anatomy of common urogenital sinus anomaly.

Neurology – The spine should be carefully examined for cutaneous lesions denoting possible occult spinal dysraphism such as hairy patches, swellings, cutaneous haemangiomata and sinuses. Blind ending pits overlying the tip of the coccyx are not usually of neurological significance but if there is any doubt it is always safer to arrange a neurological referral and/or spinal imaging. Sacral agenesis is not accompanied by cutaneous lesions but there may be a palpable absence of the lowermost sacral segments and flattening of the upper buttocks. Neurological disease is suggested by exaggerated lower limb reflexes (or frank clonus) or by wasting of the calves or deformities of the feet, especially if asymmetrical. The lowermost sacral segments should be examined for motor and sensory integrity. An abnormal gait should always raise the possibility of an underlying neurological condition.

INVESTIGATIONS

Frequency – Volume Chart

There are many types but all charts include a 24-hour time column, a fluid intake column, urine output column and some provision for recording when the incontinence occurs (Figure 12.5). Many charts also record when the child opens their bowels. Continuous charting over as little as 48 hours is often sufficient to provide a reliable assessment of intake and output and the extent of the impact of the incontinence on the life of the child and their family. It will also provide the clinician with some indication of the level of co-operation which might be expected from the child and their parents when planning treatment. However, charts tend to be completed at weekends and may not provide an accurate picture of what happens on school days. A copy of the

Frequency Volume Chart

Name:_____   Hospital Number:_____

Time	Day 1				Day2			
	IN (ml) [Type]	OUT (ml)	WET (tick)	Awoke * To bed †	IN (ml) [Type]	OUT (ml)	WET (tick)	Awoke * To bed †
0000								
0100								
0200								
0300								
0400								
0500								
0600								
0700								
0800								
0900								
1000								
1100								
1200								
1300								
1400								
1500								
1600								
1700								
1800								
1900								
2000								
2100								
2200								
2300								
TOTALS								

Please fill this chart in over 2 consecutive days. Record the nature and volume of fluid drunk in the 'IN' column at the corresponding time and all urine passed in the 'OUT' column at the appropriate time. Any wetting episodes should be marked with a tick at the appropriate time. Please also record waking and sleeping times in the column provided. Bring this sheet with you to your clinic visit as directed by your clinician.

Figure 12.5 Example of frequency/volume chart.

Bristol stool chart may also help the parents to assess constipation.

Urinalysis or Urine Culture

Reagent strip (Dipstick) testing of the urine should include glucose because glycosuria and frequency caused by diabetes can occasionally lead to incontinence. Cultures are usually negative.

Simple non-invasive measurement of flow rate. This should normally demonstrate a flow rate of >15 ml/second with non-staccato voiding pattern. In an older child measurement of flow rate at the bedside or in the out-patient clinic can be combined with a post void ultrasound scan of the bladder to assess bladder emptying.

Urinary tract ultrasound scan. This should be performed in all children with day time wetting. Relevant upper tract findings include:

Duplication anomalies – particularly if there is evidence of dilatation or a congenitally dysplastic upper pole moiety suggesting an ectopic ureter

Dilatation – which may indicate organic outflow obstruction or a neuropathic bladder.

The bladder scan should include measurement of *pre-void bladder volume* and *post-void bladder residual volume* – which should not usually exceed 10% of normal age-adjusted bladder capacity.

Bladder wall thickening is suggestive of either outflow obstruction, neuropathy, idiopathic overactivity or detrusor – sphincter dyssynergia).

Other Investigations

These are only performed for specific indications.

Although **lumbo-sacral spinal X-ray** is still performed in children with possible spinal dysraphism it has been largely superseded by spinal magnetic resonance imaging (**MRI**). This is now regarded as the definitive investigation since it will visualise tethering, syrinxes and intraspinal cord lipomas and epidermoid cysts associated with the spinal cord abnormality.

MR urography is the most sensitive investigation for detecting an occult upper pole duplex system and ectopic ureter as the cause of primary incontinence in girls. Laparoscopy may also be helpful.

Cystourethroscopy is occasionally indicated (mainly in boys) to assess the bladder neck and to look for anatomical causes of outflow obstruction such as late-presenting posterior urethral valves. **Sleep studies** or an **ear, nose and throat (ENT) opinion** may be indicated in some children with nocturnal enuresis.

Invasive Urodynamics/Video Urodynamics

These are only performed on a very selective basis in children with non-neuropathic incontinence because of the need for catheterisation and exposure to radiation (when combined with radiological screening). However, urodynamics can sometimes be helpful in distinguishing between sensory and motor urgency. The video component is valuable in making the diagnosis of genuine stress incontinence by demonstrating leakage induced by increasingly strong valsalva manoeuvres.

ORGANIC CAUSES OF INCONTINENCE

Labial Adhesions/Vaginal Reflux

The term "vaginal reflux" refers to the phenomenon of retrograde filling of the vagina with urine during voiding. Urine then leaks from the vagina after the girl stands up to leave the toilet. It is commonly caused by the presence of labial adhesions but can also occur in girls who sit on the toilet with their legs closed. Treatment consists of conservative or surgical management of any labial adhesions or advising the girl to sit with her legs further apart on the toilet. A gentle cough or valsalva manoeuvre after the completion of voiding may help to expel any urine from the vagina.

Ectopic Ureter

This classically presents with continuous dribbling incontinence. However, there may be a postural element – with the urinary leakage being absent or much less pronounced at night when the child is lying supine.

Genuine Stress Incontinence/Wide Bladder Neck

Strenuous sporting activity in girls (such as gymnastics) is accompanied by a higher incidence of stress leakage than was previously recognised. An empirical trial of an alpha-adrenergic agonist (e.g. ephedrine) may be employed in more severe cases. If genuine stress incontinence (rather than simply a wide bladder neck) is confirmed on video urodynamics it may be necessary to consider a bladder neck sling or similar procedure.

Female Epispadias

Surgical intervention is usually required (see Chapter 15).

Spinal Neurological Disorders

Relevant points in the history include:

> *Urinary incontinence of unusual severity, especially if accompanied by constant dribbling of urine.*
> *Marked disturbance of bowel habit, particularly if associated with fecal soiling.*

Almost 90% of cases of occult spinal dysraphism are accompanied by cutaneous lesions – hence the crucial importance of a careful examination of the spine. It is important to note that some children with neuropathic bladder dysfunction may nevertheless have virtually (or entirely) normal lower limb locomotor function. Urological management is the same as for other forms of neuropathic bladder. (See Chapter 13.)

Bladder Outflow Obstruction

This is far more common in boys – in whom the causes include: posterior urethral valves, urethral stricture (including post hypospadias repair), syringocele, meatal stenosis and exceptionally, pathological phimosis (Balanitis xerotica obliterans). In girls, haematocolpos or hydrocolpos due to imperforate hymen may present with bladder outflow obstruction, generally at or after puberty and with an accompanying history of primary amenorrhoea.

Pelvic tumours and severe constipation can interfere with voiding in both sexes but tend to cause urinary retention rather than incontinence.

Bladder ultrasound typically demonstrates post void residual urine which is often (but not invariably) accompanied by bladder wall thickening. However, the absence of upper tract dilatation does not exclude outflow obstruction. Diagnosis is by cystoscopy and/or micturating cysto urethrography (MCUG). It is not uncommon for the incontinence to persist (sometimes for years) despite successful relief of obstruction and the long-term use of anticholinergic agents may be indicated.

FUNCTIONAL DAY-TIME INCONTINENCE

Around 3% of girls and 2% of boys aged 7 years' experience functional daytime wetting at least once a week. Many also have nocturnal incontinence. A number of different patterns of functional day time incontinence can be identified – with detrusor overactivity being an important feature of most (Table 12.3).

Table 12.3 Functional daytime incontinence

Detrusor instability
Urge syndrome
Uncomplicated
Dysfunctional voiding
Deferred voiding
Lazy bladder
Occult neuropathic bladder
Detrusor instability or central (CNS)
Giggle incontinence
Non-detrusor instability
Diurnal frequency syndrome
Sensory urgency

Simple Treatments

One of the simplest and most rewarding forms of treatment consists of providing the parents and an older child with an explanation of the normal micturition cycle and describing the measures needed to establish a more normal voiding pattern.

These typically comprise a regimen of regular voiding (5–6 times a day at 2–3 hourly intervals) and a regular intake of fluid in volumes which are appropriate for the child's age. As an approximation this corresponds to a minimum intake of 500 ml at age 5 years, 750 ml at age 7 years, 1000 ml at age 10, 1250 ml at age 12 and 1500–2000 ml at age 15+.

Certain drinks should be avoided, especially in children with symptoms of bladder overactivity. These include ; tea, coffee, hot chocolate, cola type drinks and any drink containing blackcurrent. In addition to their diuretic effects they may also provoke detrusor overactivity.

The advice provided to parents and child should be reinforced with regular follow-up, encouragement and support – either by face to face contact or by telephone. Paediatric urology nurse specialists or specialist continence nurses can play a particularly valuable role in providing this service to children and families.

Urinary tract infections (UTIs) are common in children with functional day time incontinence and there is often a causal inter relationship. It is important that UTIs are effectively treated and measures are taken to prevent them from recurring. These may include increasing the child's fluid intake and voiding frequency (to maintain diuresis and bladder emptying) and reducing the use of soap agents such as shampoo and bubble bath which may significantly alter the balance of perineal bacterial flora. Introducing bio-yoghurt into the diet can also be helpful.

It may sometimes be necessary to prescribe a prophylactic antibiotic such as a single daily dose of Trimethoprim at 2 mg/kg/day (or Nitrofurantoin 1 mg/kg/day) until the bladder dysfunction has been adequately treated. Effective treatment of constipation is also essential because of its role in causing both UTI and bladder dysfunction. This typically entails the regular use of laxatives such as Movicol Paediatric (half – 1 sachet/day), lactulose (2.5–5 ml/day) and/or Sennakot (2.5–5 ml/day) to try to ensure the rectum is empty.

OVERACTIVE BLADDER

Medical Treatment

If the symptoms of frequency and urgency do not respond to the simple measures outlined above the next line of treatment consists of anticholinergic agents. **Oxybutynin** is most widely used agent – with a typical starting dose of 2.5 mg twice a day, increasing to 2.5 mg three times a day. The principal alternative is **Tolteridine** (typical dose 1–2 mg twice a day).

If the child is able to take tablets these agents are also available in a slow release form as oxybutynin (5–10 mg, once a day) or slow release Tolteridine (2–4 mg, once a day). Oxybutynin and Tolteridine are both associated with a risk of systemic anti-muscarinic side effects which may include dry eyes, dry mouth, constipation and occasionally, personality/behavioural changes. **Solifenacin**, a newer anticholinergic agent with minimal systemic side effects, is being used increasingly in older children in a typical dose of 5–10 mg once a day. It is not licensed for use in younger children. Likewise **Mirabegron**, a beta3 agonist, is used in older children although it is not yet officially licensed in the UK for use in patients under the age of 18.

These agents should not be used in children with significant post void residual volumes and/or a pattern of infrequent voiding because inhibition of detrusor activity may lead to further impairment of bladder emptying and urinary retention.

Transcutaneous Electrical Nerve Stimulation (TENS)

This technique has been used in some centres with a typical regimen consisting of a 20 minutes session performed three to five times a week over 6 weeks. Transcutaneous electrical nerve stimulation (TENS) is thought to improve bladder control by modifying interneuronal interaction at spinal cord level. Success rates of up to 60% have been reported but the duration of improvement is variable.

Posterior Tibial Nerve Neurostimulation

In this technique a fine needle is inserted into the vicinity of the tibial nerve in the lower leg and an electrode pad is placed over the heel. Electrical impulses are transmitted via the tibial nerve to the spinal cord and sacral plexus. Treatment typically consists of weekly sessions of 30 minutes duration over 12 weeks. Posterior tibial nerve neurostimulation has been approved by the UK National Institute for Clinical Excellence (NICE) for the treatment of refractory detrusor overactivity. Although mainly used in adults it has also been used in children and young people.

Sacral Nerve Stimulation

This is an invasive intervention which entails surgical implantation of a stimulator in the region of the sacral nerves. It has been used more extensively in adults but experience in children is very limited.

Intravesical Botulinum A Toxin Injection

This approach is being increasingly used in children with severe bladder overactivity which has not responded to other forms of treatment. Cystoscopy is performed under general anaesthesia and small doses of Botulinum A toxin are injected into the bladder wall muscle at multiple sites.

Up to 15% of children experience impaired bladder emptying or urinary retention following intravesical Botox injection and for this reason the possible requirement for clean intermittent catheterisation (CIC) must be explained (or even taught) prior to the procedure. The duration of response to intravesical Botox is variable but may be of the order of 6–9 months. One or more further injections may be required.

Nevertheless, intravesical Botox injections may be valuable in conferring a period of symptomatic relief while other measures are being introduced.

OTHER FORMS OF FUNCTIONAL URINARY INCONTINENCE

Urge Syndrome/Motor Urgency

Daytime wetting is accompanied by symptoms of urgency in more than 80% of children. The child only becomes aware of the sensation of needing to void shortly before the act of voiding supervenes. Indeed, many children claim that they do not realise that they are voiding at all.

Urgency tends to occur when the bladder is full rather than during filling. The cause is unknown but it is likely to be a manifestation of delayed maturation of normal bladder control. Children may attempt to prevent impending leakage of urine by contracting their urethral sphincter and pelvic floor muscles. In some children this may be reinforced by additional manoeuvres – notably crouching with the heel pressed into the perineum (Vincent's curtsy sign).

Dysfunctional Voiding

This is characterised by a urinary flow which is of varying intensity or interrupted ("staccato") voiding. Urodynamic studies demonstrate detrusor-sphincter *dyssynergia* with either incomplete relaxation of the sphincter or alternating phases of contraction and relaxation. Voiding is often incomplete. The most likely explanation is that children who have learned to use voluntary contraction of the urethral sphincter to suppress leakage due to detrusor instability then go on to adopt a pattern of behaviour which prevents them from relaxing the sphincter during deliberate voiding. The condition is virtually confined to girls and is accompanied by recurrent urinary infections in more than 90% of cases. Vesicoureteric reflux (with or without renal scarring) is present in around 30% of cases. This is mostly secondary reflux caused by sustained exposure to elevated intravesical pressures generated by a combination of detrusor overactivity and detrusor-sphincter dyssynergia. The treatment of dysfunctional voiding centres on "re-educating the voiding mechanism" – initially with a regular voiding regimen and other simple measures. For those suffering from more severe forms of dysfunctional voiding a range of techniques is now available which can be grouped under the heading "**Urotherapy**" or "**Cognitive Bladder Training**." The key elements involve biofeedback (using uroflowmetry and dedicated computer programmes) to train the child to relax their sphincter mechanism and pelvic floor during voiding in response to visual and sensory signals. High success rates have been reported but these techniques are time consuming, demanding and require the input of a fully trained urotherapist and appropriate equipment.

Non-Neuropathic Neuropathic Bladder/Hinman's Syndrome

This is a rare disorder in which the bladder behaves like a "neuropathic" bladder despite the absence of identifiable neurological cause. The radiological features resemble those of genuine neuropathic bladder – including trabeculation, sacculation and elongation of the bladder ("fir-tree" bladder). Upper tract dilatation and other secondary changes in the upper renal tracts are also present in the majority of cases.

In the classic form (Hinman's syndrome), there is almost invariably a background of domestic turmoil or a history of severe physical or psychological upset occurring at, or shortly after, the time of toilet training. It is thought that some children, who are unusually fearful of wetting themselves, grossly overuse their external urethral sphincter to counteract unstable detrusor contractions in a desperate attempt to stay dry. This leads to elevated intravesical pressure and reduced compliance, with secondary upper tract complications.

The condition typically presents at around 5–8 years of age with unusually severe urinary incontinence which is compounded in most cases by UTIs and marked disturbance of bowel habit. However, this condition may also develop at a later age and, as in younger children, may be accompanied by symptoms of renal insufficiency in severe or longstanding cases. The natural history is variable but, if untreated, the condition carries a very real threat of severe upper tract damage and renal insufficiency. Expectant management is not a safe option. The treatment options are the same as those for the management of true neuropathic bladder (see Chapter 13). Very rarely a child will present with the features of a non-neuropathic neuropathic bladder despite the lack of any history of psychological disturbance. Bowel function is usually normal. The management is the same as for true neuropathic bladder

Sensory Urgency

This poorly understood condition is largely confined to girls. Despite clinical features which are strongly suggestive of detrusor overactivity, urodynamic evaluation reveals a stable bladder. The symptoms of urgency are purely sensory in origin. Sensory urgency in adults is a feature of interstitial cystitis but it is very doubtful whether this condition occurs in children. The use of intravesical oxybutynin has been described.

Diurnal Urinary Frequency

This condition affects mainly boys aged 4–7 years in whom it is characterised by the sudden onset of severe daytime urinary frequency. In some cases this may be as often as every 10–15 minutes. Even when the sensory frequency is severe it is only rarely accompanied by wetting. The symptoms are confined to the day time and there is no corresponding nocturia. Urine culture is negative and ultrasound findings are normal. The aetiology is unknown but is likely to involve a strong behavioural component. The symptoms do not respond to anticholinergics. The condition is always self-limiting – typically over a period of 3–12 weeks. However, a few children experience recurrent episodes over the next 1–2 years.

Deferred Voiding

This is common in both sexes and occurs most often at around 4–6 years of age. The child suddenly becomes aware of an urgent need to void (due to presumed unstable detrusor contraction) and experiences some degree of involuntary wetting if voiding is delayed. This usually occurs because the child is engrossed in other activities, for example playing outdoors, which take precedence over the social demands of continence. No treatment is required in this age group because the condition is self-limiting. Deferred voiding is less common in older children – in whom it may be a manifestation of broader behavioural disturbance. Psychological input may be required in such cases.

Lazy Bladder

Affecting mainly girls in age range 8–10 years, this condition usually presents with daytime incontinence and/or UTI. However, because the bladder remains visibly and palpably distended after voiding the condition may sometimes present with the incidental finding of a lower abdominal swelling.

The upper renal tracts are always non dilated and the urodynamic picture is one of low-pressure retention with detrusor-sphincter dyssynergia and non-sustained detrusor contractions. The condition is almost certainly behavioural in origin. It is usually self-limiting and often resolves quite suddenly during the course of puberty. For children who are troubled by symptoms, cognitive bladder retraining has the best outcome. In severe cases CIC may be indicated – although this may not be tolerated. Anticholinergics should be avoided or used with caution.

Giggle Incontinence

This distinctive form of incontinence occurs mainly in girls – in whom it typically presents at around 9–12 years. Urinary leakage only occurs with giggling or laughing but at no other time. Other aspects of voiding function are entirely normal. Giggle incontinence is a source of considerable embarrassment and distress in older children and teenagers – both at school and during social activities. Urodynamic examination may reveal some mild detrusor instability but the findings are usually normal. Giggle incontinence is generally believed to be a neurological (rather than urological) phenomenon which is analogous to a form of cataplexy disorder mediated via higher neurological centres in which a sudden loss of muscle tone is triggered by emotion. There is often a family history. Whether it is a genuinely self-limiting condition is unclear because apparent improvement in puberty and early adult life may, in reality, represent no more than adaptation to avoid the precipitating circumstances.

Methylphenidate (Ritalin) is the most consistently effective agent. However, it is a regulated drug and should be reserved for severely affected patients. Oxybutynin is helpful in some cases and Imipramine can also be considered.

Night Time Urinary Incontinence (Nocturnal Enuresis)

Nocturnal enuresis (bedwetting) is one of the commonest conditions of childhood. Around 10% of 7-year-old children wet the bed three or more times a week and a small minority experience intractable nocturnal enuresis which persists into late adolescence and adulthood.

Urinary incontinence which only occurs at night is termed "**monosymptomatic**" whereas nocturnal enuresis which is also accompanied daytime wetting is termed "**non-monosymptomatic**" or "**polysymptomatic**".

Nocturnal enuresis is classified as "**primary**" if the child has always wet the bed and "**secondary**" if the child has previously been dry at night.

Butler and Holland postulated a "3 Systems Model" to account for the main causes of nocturnal enuresis (Figure 12.6) i.e.

- *Low release of Arginine Vasopressin (AVP) with overproduction of urine at night*
- *Lack of arousal from sleep*
- *Bladder overactivity and associated daytime symptoms*

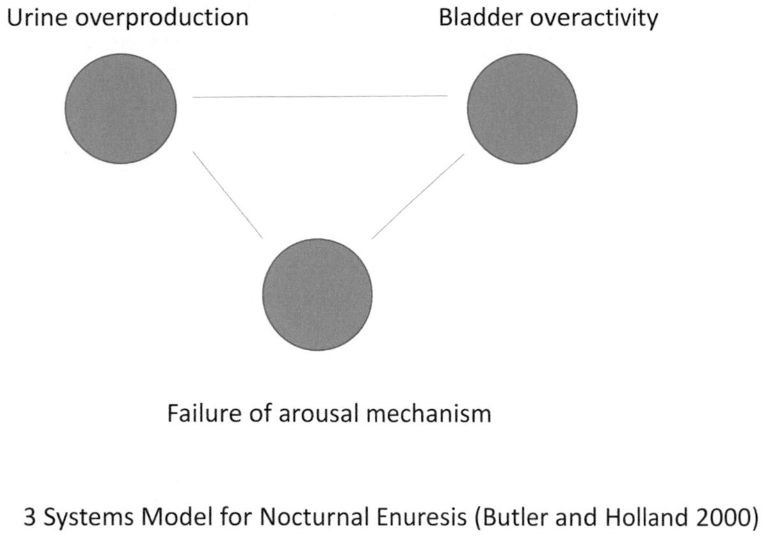

Urine overproduction   Bladder overactivity

Failure of arousal mechanism

3 Systems Model for Nocturnal Enuresis (Butler and Holland 2000)

Figure 12.6 The 3 systems model of nocturnal enuresis.

The aim of management is to identify which of these factors is most likely to be responsible in the affected child and plan their treatment accordingly.

Primary Monosymptomatic Nocturnal Enuresis

This is twice as common in boys as girls. The clinical features are variable and whilst some children wet the bed every night others are less severely affected, with less severe leakage, fewer wet beds or alternating spells of wet and dry nights.

The aetiology is multifactorial and in any individual one or more of the following factors may apply:

A positive family history (in upwards of 75% of cases).

Absence of a circadian rhythm of vasopressin release. Levels of vasopressin normally increase at night. However, vasopressin release is absent or reduced in up to 75% of children who wet the bed (and in an even higher proportion of those with a positive family history). This leads to a nocturnal urinary output which exceeds the functional bladder capacity.

Sleep arousal difficulty. Nocturnal enuresis does not, as is commonly supposed, result from abnormally deep sleep, as bed wetting occurs at all stages of the sleep cycle. However, many affected children lack the arousal from sleep which would normally occur when the bladder fills to the point where it approaches its functional bladder capacity. The child usually sleeps through the episode of incontinence, being unaware that they have wet the bed.

Although nocturnal enuresis is sometimes a manifestation of emotional problems or behavioural disorders, the great majority of children with primary monosymptomatic nocturnal enuresis are normally adjusted. Apart from a urine dipstick test (to exclude glycosuria and diabetes) investigations are rarely indicated. The prognosis is excellent, with spontaneous resolution by the time of physical maturity occurring in 97–99% of affected individuals. The probability of cessation in any 1 year is approximately 1 in 6.

Secondary Monosymptomatic Nocturnal Enuresis

In the majority of cases the onset can usually be linked to some physical or emotional upset.

However, it is important to exclude the possibility of an underlying organic condition – particularly one associated with polyuria such as diabetes mellitus or diabetes insipidus. However, such causes are rare.

Treatment of Monosymptomatic Nocturnal Enuresis

This should not usually be considered until the age of 5 years. The choice of treatment is partly determined by the clinical features. But regardless what treatment is chosen its success will be heavily dependent on the motivation of the child and the family. Although treatment provides a way of managing rather than curing the condition, effective symptomatic relief may help to expedite the resolution of the underlying nocturnal enuresis sooner than might otherwise have been the case.

Parents should be encouraged to adopt a positive attitude to treating the bedwetting. Scolding and punishment are to be avoided at all costs. The management of monosymtomatic nocturnal enuresis is generally undertaken in a community setting by primary care doctors, paediatricians and specialist continence nurses.

Simple Measures to Reduce Overnight Urine Production

The child should not drink after a set time in the evening (e.g. 6 pm) and should try to maintain a steady intake of fluid throughout the day rather than drinking more in the afternoon or early evening. It is also important that the child empties their bladder before going to bed.

The use of star charts, combined with rewards, can be particularly helpful in younger children.

Use of a Vasopressin Analogue Such as Desmopressin

This mimics the circadian rhythm by decreasing the obligatory production of urine by the kidneys overnight. The success rate is up to 70% but the relapse rates after cessation of treatment are relatively high (30–50%). This treatment is more likely to be effective in children with a family history of nocturnal enuresis and those who wet the bed shortly after going to sleep. The

success rate is lower in children who also suffer from day time wetting. Desmopressin nasal spray products are no longer available because of the small risk of serious adverse reactions which included hyponatraemia, seizures and water intoxication.

Oral formulations have a more favourable risk-benefit profile. Currently, these are available as **Desmotabs** (200–400 mg at night) or **Desmomelt** (120–240 mg at night) and are usually taken 1 hour prior to bedtime.

Enuresis Alarm

Children with a deep sleeping pattern are the best candidates for treatment with an enuretic alarm. These alarms are intended to sensitise the child to the feeling of a full bladder and raising their level of awareness whilst asleep. After a while the child acquires the ability to respond appropriately by waking before leakage of urine occurs. The equipment typically consists of an auditory or vibratory alarm connected to a pad placed on the mattress (Figure 12.7). The alarm is activated when the first drop of urine leaks onto the pad. Enuresis alarms are more effective in children aged 7 years and upwards – in whom success rates are typically in the range 60–75%. Subsequent relapse rate are much lower than those after treatment with medication. Alarms are less successful in children who are not motivated to become dry and those who also suffer from daytime wetting.

Nocturnal hypoxia has been identified as a possible cause of nocturnal enuresis in some children with history of snoring and/or poor attention during the day at school. The findings of sleep studies have also been cited by proponents of this possible explanation. Although, tonsillectomy has been reported to cure nocturnal enuresis in selected cases this has not been confirmed by a recent prospective controlled trial.

Non-Monosymptomatic or Polysymptomatic Nocturnal Enuresis

When nocturnal enuresis is accompanied by day symptoms such as urgency, frequency, stress incontinence and constipation, the first priority

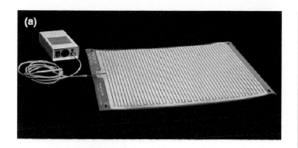

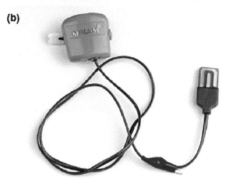

Figure 12.7 (a) Enuresis alarm. The pad is placed under the bed sheet, with bedside battery powered buzzer. (b) Compact enuresis alarm suitable for the treatment of nocturnal enuresis or ambulatory treatment of diurnal enuresis. The buzzer device is pinned to the pyjamas (or clothes when used in the day time) and the sensor worn between two pairs of underclothes.

should be to investigate the possible cause(s) of the daytime symptoms. In practice the nocturnal enuresis is unlikely to respond to measures such as an enuresis alarm until the day time wetting has been effectively treated. When used selectively (principally in children who are also troubled by daytime urgency and frequency) anticholinergic agents such as Oxybutynin are effective in up to two-thirds of cases. A combination of treatments may be required in some children – for example, the use of Desmopressin and an enuresis alarm. Imipramine, a tricyclic antidepressant, is no longer recommended as first-line treatment and should never be prescribed in conjunction with Desmopressin.

KEY POINTS

- The initial priority is to exclude organic causes of urinary incontinence – although these are rare.
- Most organic (anatomical or neurological) causes of daytime wetting can be excluded on the basis of history, examination and ultrasonography.
- Day time wetting in children is most commonly due to detrusor instability. In the majority of children the natural history is one of spontaneous resolution but this can usually be expedited by simple measures.
- Primary monosymptomatic nocturnal enuresis seldom, if ever, has an underlying organic basis.

FURTHER READING

1. Tryggve Nevéus, von Gontard Alexander, Hoebeke Piet, Hjälmås Kelm, Bauer Stuart, Bower Wendy, Jørgensen Troels Munch, Rittig Søren, Walle Johan Vande, Yeung Chung-Kwong, Djurhuus Jens Christian. The standardization of terminology of lower urinary tract function in children and adolescents: report from the Standardisation Committee of the International Children's Continence Society. J Urol. 2006;176:314–324.
2. Butler R, Holland P. The Three Systems: a conceptual way of understanding nocturnal enuresis. Scan J Urol Nephrol. 2000;34:270–277.

NICE Clinical guidelines https://www.nice.org.uk/guidance/cg111 (Bedwetting)

https://www.nice.org.uk/guidance/ipg362/chapter/1-Guidance (PTNS)

Websites:
www.i-c-c-s.org
www.eric.org.uk

Neurogenic Bladder

KYLE O ROVE and CHRISTOPHER S COOPER

Topics covered

Etiology
Pathophysiology
Prenatal intervention
Newborn evaluation and management
Investigations
Treatment and outcomes
Catheterization

Increasing bladder capacity and reducing
  pressure
Bladder outlet procedures
Transition to adulthood
Sexual function
Neurogenic bowel

INTRODUCTION AND DEFINITION

Neurogenic bladder is a non-specific term that implies an abnormality of innervation causing bladder dysfunction. Injury to the nervous system may be congenital or acquired, peripheral or central, isolated or syndromic. As the primary functions of the bladder are to store and empty urine through coordinated activity of the detrusor muscle and urinary sphincter, dysfunction may result in urinary incontinence, elevated storage or voiding pressures, or incomplete emptying. Children and young people with neurogenic bladder are at risk of progressive deterioration in bladder function leading to kidney damage. Appropriate surveillance and management are crucial to maintaining renal function, achieving continence, and improving quality of life for these patients.

ETIOLOGY

Spina bifida is the most common cause of congenital neurogenic bladder. In the United States, approximately 1,500 children with spina bifida are born each year and the worldwide reported incidence is 3.1 per 10,000 births. The incidence has been decreasing over the last two decades but varies considerably by country and ethnicity. Myelomeningocele is the most severe form of spina bifida, accounting for 90% of cases, while the remaining 10% are comprised of lipomyelomeningocele or meningocele. Other congenital causes of neurogenic bladder include closed and occult forms of neural tube defects such as tethered spinal cord, intradural lipoma, and intraspinal cysts. See Table 13.1. The term "spina bifida occulta" may also be applied to an isolated vertebral anomaly consisting of incomplete

Table 13.1 Etiology of childhood neurogenic bladder

Congenital	Acquired
Myelomeningocele	Spina cord injury
Sacral agenesis	Spinal cord infarction
Tethered cord	Spinal cord tumor
Closed and occult forms of neural tube defects	Sacrococcygeal teratoma
Anorectal malformations	Neuroblastoma
	Transverse myelitis
	Cerebral palsy
	Idiopathic causes

formation of the posterior spinous process. This anomaly, which is often an incidental finding, is found in up to 15% of the population. It is confined to the bony elements the vertebrae and is rarely accompanied by any underlying neurological lesion.

The critical period of neurulation (closure of the neural tube from cephalad to caudad) occurs in the first few weeks of pregnancy. Adequate levels of folic acid are important for normal closure of the neural tube and low maternal dietary intake of folate or dysregulated folate metabolic pathways have been implicated as a major risk factor for the development of neural tube defects. In the United States, it is recommended that women should commence folate supplements 2 months prior to conception and women of childbearing age should consume 400 mcg folic acid daily. Other risk factors implicated in the etiology of neural tube defects include maternal obesity, diabetes mellitus, and advanced maternal age.

Survival rates of children born with myelomeningocele have improved dramatically since the 1950s when less than 20% survived beyond 24 months of age. The development of the ventriculoperitoneal (VP) shunt for the control of hydrocephalus led to significantly improved survival and by the mid-1970s the survival rate had increased to over 50%. It is predicted that more than 90% of the infants currently being born with spina bifida will survive, with the majority living into adulthood. The introduction of clean intermittent catheterization (CIC) by Lapides in 1972 was an important advance in the management of neurogenic bladder. Subsequently, the widespread introduction of urodynamic investigations led to recognition of the need for proactive management if the leak point pressure exceeded 40 cm of water or other adverse parameters of neurogenic dysfunction were demonstrated on urodynamics.

Other causes of congenital neurogenic bladder include partial and complete sacral agenesis (caudal regression syndrome) which may occur in isolation or conjunction with anorectal and cloacal malformations. Acquired neurogenic bladder may be due to spinal cord trauma, tumors, extensive pelvic surgery, spinal cord infarction, transverse myelitis, developmental syndromes and cerebral palsy. Finally, certain adverse features of neurogenic bladder may be present in the acquired condition of non-neurogenic neurogenic bladder (or Hinman's syndrome).

PATHOPHYSIOLOGY

Vertebral anomalies in the lumbosacral region account for about 50% of cases with lumbar and thoracic lesions accounting for 28% and 20% of cases respectively. It should be noted, however, that the level of the vertebral abnormality does not correlate closely with the level of the neurological deficit or the outcome for bladder function.

The functions of the normal bladder are to store urine and to empty under voluntary control. These functions are organized at the level of the brainstem and spinal cord. The sympathetic innervation of the detrusor muscle and urethral smooth muscle is mediated through the hypogastric nerve fibers emanating from the lumbar region. The parasympathetic innervation of the detrusor muscle is mediated by pelvic nerve pathways transmitted via the sacral roots S2 - 4 and the striated sphincter is innervated by the pudendal nerves also originating from the sacrum. Upper motor neuron lesions lead to an overactive bladder with no voluntary sphincter control. Contractions of an overactive bladder against the resistance created by a non-relaxing sphincter (termed detrusor/sphincter dyssynergia) typically lead to detrusor hypertrophy and a thick-walled bladder. Lower motor neuron lesions are characterized by an acontractile, flaccid detrusor, small, smooth walled bladder, and denervation of the external sphincter. However, most spina bifida patients have a mixed neurologic picture with features of both upper and lower motor neuron lesions.

PRENATAL INTERVENTION

As a consequence of widespread prenatal detection of myelomeningocele by ultrasonography, fetal surgical intervention for the repair of these lesions has become a clinical reality. One prospective, randomized trial found that fetal intervention reduced the requirement for VP shunts and was associated with improved lower limb function at 12 and 30 months age. However, it did not result in any improvement in urodynamic parameters or any significant reduction in the requirement for CIC. More recent data have suggested, however, that prenatal repair may reduce the need for CIC between 6 and 10 years of age and may perhaps increase the potential for spontaneous voiding. The complications of fetal repair include preterm delivery and uterine dehiscence.

NEWBORN EVALUATION AND MANAGEMENT

Cesarean section is recommended to minimize trauma to the exposed neurologic tissue. At the time of delivery, an open myelomeningocele is immediately apparent as an exposed plaque of neural tissue. Closure of the lesion within the first 24 hours is recommended to minimize the risk of ascending infection (meningitis).

There are currently no standard evidence-based guidelines for urologic management of neurogenic bladder in newborn infants with spina bifida. The timing of commencement of CIC is considered below. A baseline renal and bladder ultrasound scan is performed after 24–48 hours and renal function is assessed with serum creatinine or cystatin c. Following discharge from hospital a voiding cystourethrogram (VCUG) or video urodynamic study is performed after 3 months of age. Baseline urodynamic parameters assessed by this study should include; filling pressures, compliance, presence of detrusor overactivity, sphincteric function, leak point pressures, presence of vesicoureteral reflux (VUR), and configuration of the bladder neck (open or closed). The ultrasound appearances of the kidneys and bladder are abnormal in up to 20% of infants with myelomeningocele.

Spina Bifida Occulta (Occult Spinal Dysraphism)

These abnormalities include lipomeningomyelocele, tethered cord, and sacral agenesis. External signs of the underlying abnormality (prominent sacral dimple, fatty subcutaneous mass, tuft of hair, hemangioma, or skin tag) are present in more than 80% of cases. External evidence of sacral agenesis is less obvious but may be apparent as an asymmetric gluteal cleft. The spine can be evaluated with ultrasound in the first 2 to 3 months of life but thereafter spinal magnetic resonance imaging (MRI) scan is the "gold standard" imaging modality.

Initial Management

CIC is commenced if the bladder is not emptying to completion. However, when adequate bladder emptying is confirmed by clinical observation and ultrasound two options can then be considered;

1. Immediate commencement of clean intermittent catheterization and anticholinergic medication.

   Proponents of the early commencement of CIC argue that this is a logical form of management because at least 80% to 90% of patients with myelomeningocele will have neurogenic bladder dysfunction. In addition, by commencing CIC early it may be possible to prevent or reduce the requirement for bladder augmentation as well as helping to safeguard the kidneys.

2. Monitoring of bladder function with renal and bladder ultrasound scans (and periodic urodynamics) with the onset of clean intermittent catheterization being deferred.

Those who advocate this approach argue that it decreases the burden for the caregivers and carries a lower risk of urinary tract infection (UTI) because bacteria are not being introduced into the urinary tract.

However, monitoring and deferred introduction of CIC are only appropriate for infants who have safe urodynamic parameters of bladder function. CIC should be commenced if the initial urodynamic study demonstrates unfavorable characteristics such as reduced compliance, significant detrusor sphincter dyssynergia, or high-grade VUR. Indications to abandon the observational approach in favor of CIC and anticholinergics include; development of hydronephrosis, worsening parameters of bladder function on urodynamics or recurrent UTIs.

INVESTIGATIONS

Routine follow-up typically comprises ultrasound scans of the kidneys, ureters and bladder every 3 months during the first year of life, then reducing to 6 monthly intervals until 3 years of age, with an annual scan thereafter. A baseline renogram with 99^mTc dimercaptosuccinic acid (DMSA) or 99^mTc dimercaptoacetyltriglycine (MAG3) is performed in the first 6 months of life and repeated according to clinical indications. Renal function is monitored by measurement of serum creatinine (or cystatin c) on an annual basis – or more frequently in children with hostile patterns of bladder function or frequent UTIs. The frequency of video urodynamic studies is determined by such factors as; the results of initial and subsequent studies, the perceived level of risk posed by the neurogenic bladder,

the frequent occurrence of UTIs or the onset of changes in the upper tracts on ultrasound. Urodynamics should be performed prior to possible reconstructive surgery in children expressing the wish to become socially continent.

VIDEO URODYNAMICS

A urodynamic study will provide information on bladder and sphincteric function. The study is performed using a dual lumen catheter inserted into the bladder (for filling and measurement of intravesical pressure) and a balloon catheter placed in the rectum for the measurement of intra abdominal pressure. The bladder is filled at a rate of approximately 10% of the estimated age-adjusted bladder capacity per minute. This is calculated according to the formula (age in years + 2) × 30 mL. For videourodynamics the bladder is filled with a solution of radiographic contrast material. During bladder filling, intravesical pressure (Pves) is recorded. The contribution made by the detrusor muscle (Pdet) to intravesical pressure is calculated by subtracting the intra abdominal pressure (Pabd) from the intravesical pressure ie (Pves – Pabd). Sphincteric function can be assessed by electromyography with patch electrodes placed in the perianal region or by the insertion of needle electrodes (which is believed to be more accurate). However, there are some differences in the use of electromyography. In the UK for example, X-ray screening (videocystography) is used in preference to electromyography for the assessment of sphincter function. At different stages in the study fluoroscopic imaging is performed to visualize the bladder and to demonstrate abnormalities such as trabeculation, diverticula, stones, and/or VUR. Particular attention is paid to the bladder outlet and sphincter, visualizing whether it is open or closed and observing the relationship between sphincter activity and detrusor contractions.

A normal, healthy bladder remains stable during filling with pressures remaining below 15 cm H_2O throughout. At the time of voiding, the detrusor muscle contracts after relaxation of the external sphincter allowing the bladder to empty to completion. Points of interest during the filling phase include the maximum intravesical pressure, the involuntary leakage of urine (incontinence), and the pressure at which the leakage occurs. A high detrusor leak point pressure (DLPP) of >40 cm H_2O is regarded as unsafe. Bladder compliance is calculated as volume over pressure and a figure of <20 mL/cm H_2O denotes reduced compliance (inability of the bladder to accommodate physiological volumes of urine at safe pressures). If the patient is capable of voiding, attention is paid to possible detrusor-sphincter dyssynergia (contraction of the detrusor muscle against sphinteric resistance), voided volume, post-void residual, flow rate, and characteristics of the flow curve (bell-shaped, staccato, intermittent, flat). It is important to note, however, that interpretation of urodynamic findings is relatively subjective and is influenced by a number of factors including inter observer variations, limited reproducibility, technical artifacts and patient anxiety.

A "safe" neurogenic bladder is one which does not pose a threat to the upper tracts and renal function. However, maintaining a safe pattern of bladder function is often dependent on the use of regular CIC. The type of bladder in which CIC is most likely to protect the upper tracts and help the child to achieve continence is one which is capable of storing physiological volumes of urine at safe pressure and in which sphincter resistance is sufficient to prevent urinary leakage for periods of 3–4 hours between catheterization (Figure 13.1).

Urodynamic studies often demonstrate abnormalities of detrusor function, notably detrusor overactivity. Detrusor overactivity combined with a sphincter which fails to relax in response to detrusor contraction (detrusor sphincter dyssynergia) is regarded as an "unsafe" or "hostile" pattern of neurogenic bladder dysfunction. Without appropriate intervention, over 70% of patients with detrusor sphincter dyssynergia will experience urinary tract deterioration, including the development of hydronephrosis, within 3 years. In such cases, the functional bladder capacity is reduced and the bladder is typically thick walled and trabeculated (Figure 13.2). The finding of detrusor sphincter dyssynergia demands prompt intervention – initially by the introduction of CIC. However, this is often insufficient and further measures (notably bladder augmentation) may be required to safeguard the upper tracts and enable the child to achieve continence.

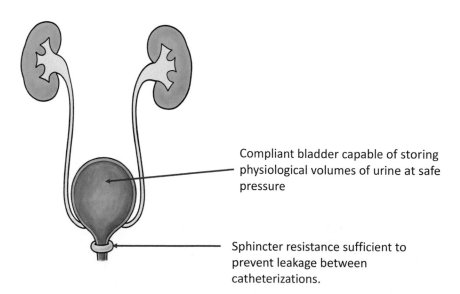

Compliant bladder capable of storing physiological volumes of urine at safe pressure

Sphincter resistance sufficient to prevent leakage between catheterizations.

Figure 13.1 This is the type of neurogenic bladder which is most amenable to CIC. The bladder is capable of storing urine at "safe" pressures and sphincter resistance is adequate to retain physiological volumes of urine in the bladder for periods of 3–4 hours between catheterizations.

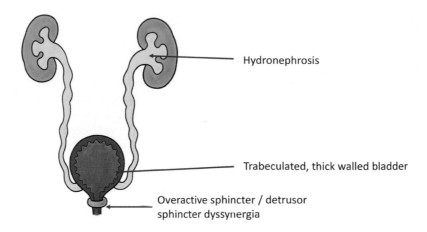

Figure 13.2 Hostile characteristics. Overactive sphincter and/or detrusor sphincter dyssynergia causing functional outflow obstruction. Detrusor overactivity. Unfavorable urodynamic parameters, thick walled bladder and upper tract dilatation.

A different abnormality of sphincter function is sphincter weakness due to denervation (typically associated with lower motor neuron lesions). This is a safe pattern of neurogenic bladder dysfunction because the impaired sphincter resistance effectively acts as a "safety valve" preventing the bladder from generating sustained elevated pressures. Functional capacity is reduced due to low pressure urinary leakage. Intermittent catheterization is not an effective means of achieving continence because the bladder is incapable of storing urine without leakage for a sufficiently long period between catheterizations (Figure 13.3).

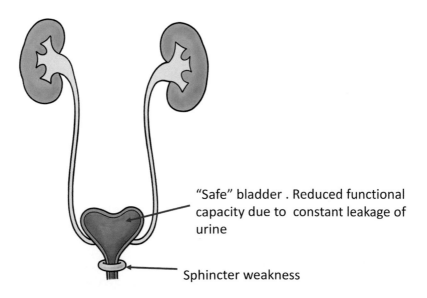

Figure 13.3 Sphincter weakness (typically associated with lower motor neuron lesions). This is a safe bladder but functional capacity is reduced because of low pressure leakage of urine. CIC does not achieve continence because the bladder is incapable of storing adequate volumes of urine between catheterizations.

Opinion differs on whether children with neurogenic bladder should routinely undergo annual urodynamic evaluation or whether it should be performed on a more selective basis in response to changes in clinical status (e.g. recent onset of UTIs, new or worsening urinary leakage, new or worsening upper tract dilation). Proponents of regular annual urodynamics argue that it is not sufficient to rely on monitoring the upper tracts because hydronephrosis is not a sensitive indicator of deteriorating lower tract function. Those who favor a selective approach cite the greater financial cost of annual studies and the larger number of studies which have to be performed in order to detect those cases of deteriorating bladder function for which intervention might be required. Regardless of differing policies regarding the frequency of urodynamic studies there is a strong consensus that all patients with neurogenic bladder should remain under urologic surveillance to safeguard the upper tracts, ensure adequate emptying of the bladder, and minimize the risk of UTI.

TETHERED SPINAL CORD

This is common feature of closed variants of spina bifida (occult spinal dysraphism). Up to 60% of children have normal urodynamic findings during early infancy but this figure has fallen to 20% by 3 years of age. These findings have been cited as evidence that this is a progressive neurologic lesion for which early surgical intervention to untether the spinal cord is indicated in order to improve urodynamic outcomes. However, this does not obviate the requirement for continuous monitoring and follow-up because there is a 25% incidence of retethering after surgery. Some care is required when interpreting and the published data on pre and postoperative urodynamic studies in children undergoing surgery for tethered cord. Whereas neurosurgical intervention for tethered cord in infants is widely performed by pediatric neurosurgeons in the United States a more conservative, selective policy is generally favored by British Pediatric Neurosurgeons.

Children with a tethered spinal cord mostly have a much better prognosis than those with meningomyelocele.

TREATMENT AND OUTCOMES

The primary aim is to safeguard renal function and minimize the risk of UTIs by ensuring that urine is stored at low pressures and the bladder empties completely every 3–4 hours. Once this has been achieved the secondary aim is to try and provide a socially acceptable degree of urinary continence if this is a priority for the child and their family.

Bladder emptying can be achieved by spontaneous voiding in some cases, or more often by intermittent catheterization (via the urethra or a catheterizable channel) or by a cutaneous vesicostomy or urinary diversion. Reduced functional capacity of the bladder and/or unsafe intravesical pressure can be managed by intravesical injections of Botox or by bladder augmentation. Finally, bladder neck procedures to increase bladder outlet resistance children can be performed to treat incontinence caused by sphincter weakness.

CATHETERIZATION

Clean intermittent catheterization (CIC) is usually initially performed via the urethra but for some young patients this may not be feasible or acceptable in the longer term. This may be because of body habitus, inability to catheterize the urethra or the preference of the child and/or family. In these circumstances it becomes necessary to create an alternative route for catheterization, namely a continent catheterizable channel.

The introduction of the Mitrofanoff appendicovesicostomy was a significant advance in the management of neurogenic bladder dysfunction (Figure 13.4). It usually provides patients with a much greater degree of personal independence and has been shown to be durable with a high long-term success rate. The

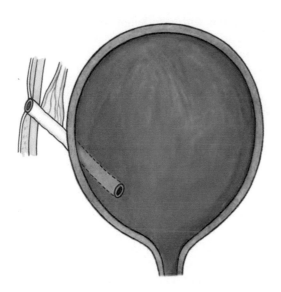

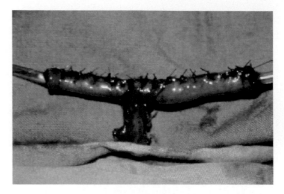

Figure 13.5 Monti tube fashioned from ileum. This is the most satisfactory alternative to the appendix for creating a continent catheterizable channel.

Figure 13.4 Appendicovesicostomy (Mitrofanoff procedure). The appendix is disconnected from the caecum and mobilized on its blood supply. The tip is excised to create a tube which is implanted into the bladder using a submucosal (anti reflux) tunnel. The other end of the appendix is brought out as a discreet stoma on the skin of the abdominal wall (or umbilicus).

commonest complication is stenosis of the cutaneous stoma – with a reported incidence varying between 15% and 40% over a 5-year period. This is usually amenable to simple revision, although more than one revision may be required. The Mitrofanoff procedure is particularly beneficial for young females – especially those confined to a wheelchair.

If the appendix is not available because it has been removed, is unusable, or reserved for another channel (such as appendicocecostomy) the main alternative is a channel created from the wall of the ileum or colon – eponymously named as Monti or Yang-Monti channel (Figure 13.5). However the appendix is the preferred source of a continent catheterizable channel because it provides the most reliable access for the passage of catheters and has a lower complication rate compared with the alternatives.

Intermittent catheterization is a clean rather than sterile procedure and some bacteria are inevitably introduced into the bladder with the passage of the catheter. Approximately 70% of patients on CIC have asymptomatic bacteriuria but fewer than a third of these experience symptomatic UTIs. The risk of UTIs can be lowered by increasing the frequency of CIC to minimize the opportunity for bacteria to multiply within static bladder urine. Where possible, the use of antibiotics should be kept to a minimum to reduce the risk of bacterial resistance.

CIC is typically performed at 3–4 hourly intervals throughout the day. Night time management is often more problematic because children and parents may (understandably) be reluctant to have perform CIC late at night or the early hours of the morning. This is of particular relevance in those neurogenic bladders which exhibit "hostile" characteristics since this may lead to sustained high-pressure storage of urine and consequent deleterious effects on both the kidneys and bladder. As in children with posterior urethral valves, overnight drainage with an indwelling catheter has been shown to be beneficial in protecting bladder and renal function and reducing the frequency of UTIs.

INCREASING BLADDER CAPACITY AND REDUCING INTRAVESICAL PRESSURE

The options for achieving this include: pharmacological agents, intravesical injections, and surgical reconstruction.

Pharmacological Agents

Oxybutynin is currently the only anticholinergic drug approved by the American Food and Drug Administration (FDA) for the treatment of neurogenic bladder in children. Anticholinergics act by suppressing overactivity of the detrusor muscle but have the disadvantage of causing anticholinergic side effects such as dry mouth, constipation, flushing, and impaired concentration. Alternative agents for the treatment of detrusor overactivity include other anticholinergics and **Mirabegron** – a beta-3 adrenergic agonist. Although none of the currently available alternatives to oxybutynin are approved for use in children by the FDA, clinicians may decide to prescribe them on an "off-label" basis for young patients those who are unable to tolerate first-line agents such as oxybutynin. Alpha-adrenergic blockers (such as **doxazosin** and **tamsulosin**) which act on receptors at the bladder neck smooth muscle can be used for the management of functional outflow obstruction in children with both non-neurogenic and neurogenic voiding dysfunction. Studies in small series of patients have been reported to demonstrate improved flow rates and reduced post void residual volumes in those capable of voiding spontaneously. However, there are conflicting data and the published studies are of varying quality. The side effects of alpha-adrenergic blockers include orthostatic hypotension, reflex tachycardia, syncope, dizziness, and palpitations.

INTRAVESICAL BOTOX INJECTIONS

Botulinum A toxin is a neurotoxin produced by *Clostridium botulinum*. When injected into the detrusor muscle, it inhibits the release of acetylcholine from the presynaptic neuron at the neuromuscular junction. Intravesical Botox is used for the treatment of detrusor overactivity to improve bladder compliance and increase functional capacity. Injections into the bladder wall muscle are performed at multiple sites via a cystoscope. The standard dosage is 10 international units (IU) per kg up to 300 IU in adults. Although it is not approved by the FDA, numerous studies have shown intravesical Botox injection to be a safe and effective treatment of neurogenic bladder in both children and adults. The duration of effect is approximately 6–12 months. In one study in children with spina bifida 73% of patients were enabled to become dry between intermittent catheterizations for 4 months after intravesical Botox injection and 88% experienced symptomatic improvement. Intravesical Botox injections can administered repeatedly without giving rise to tolerance (loss of effectiveness) or causing fibrosis in the bladder wall. The principal side effect is impaired bladder emptying and patients should therefore be prepared for the possibility that they may need to perform CIC – if they are not already doing so. UTI is another potential complication but systemic side effects are rare.

BLADDER AUGMENTATION (ENTEROCYSTOPLASTY)

This is a reliable means of increasing bladder capacity, improving bladder compliance, and reducing intravesical pressure. The urodynamic profile of children being considered for augmentation is characterized by reduced functional bladder capacity, elevated absolute detrusor filling pressures (P_{det} >40 cm H_2O), elevated detrusor leak point pressures (>35 cm H_2O), and poor compliance (<10 mL/cm H_2O). In addition, there are often upper tract changes such as hydronephrosis, hydroureteronephrosis, or secondary VUR. Bladder augmentation is most frequently indicated in children with thoracic and lumbar meningomyelocele and less commonly in those sacral spina bifida and lipomeningocele. It is rarely required in cases of tethered spinal cord.

The technique consists of opening the bladder and incorporating a vascularized segment of intestine (ileum or sigmoid colon) into the bladder wall. It is usually performed as an open surgical procedure but a minimally invasive approach has also been reported. The simplest (and probably most widely performed) technique is the "Clam" ileocystoplasty (Figure 13.6).

a)   b)   c)

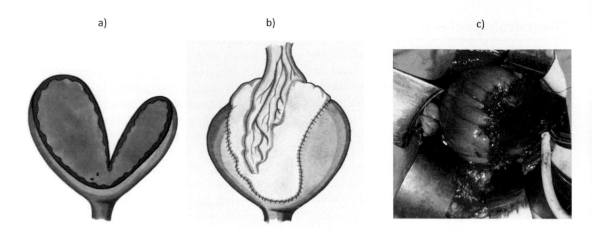

Figure 13.6 Clam ileocystoplasty. (a) Bladder opened and incised down to the trigone creating a "clam" configuration. (b) Segment of ileum isolated on its mesentery, opened (detubularized) and sutured to the bladder. (c) Intraoperative photograph.

By adopting Enhanced Recovery after Surgery protocols developed in adult patients undergoing radical cystectomy it has been possible to reduce the duration of hospital stay for children undergoing bladder augmentation in the authors' institution from 8 to 5.4 days. In addition the average number of complications per patient has been reduced from 2.1 to 1.3 ($p = 0.035$).

Augmentation cystoplasty is associated with a significant incidence of long-term complications, with approximately one-third of patients requiring some further surgery within 13 years of the original operation (Table 13.2). Introducing intestine into the urinary tract carries a risk of hyperchloremic hypokalemic metabolic acidosis and possible implications for growth. Vitamin B_{12} deficiency is an additional risk following augmentation with distal ileum. Asymptomatic bacteriuria is almost universal as a result of bacterial colonization of the reconstructed bladder and the presence of mucus in the urine. Symptomatic infections also occur in up to a third of patients. Other complications may include bladder stone formation (10–20%) (Figure 13.7) and spontaneous bladder perforation (5%). This is serious and potentially lethal complication if it is not diagnosed promptly. A high index of suspicion is required because the initial presentation of bladder perforation may consist of no more than

Table 13.2 Complications of bladder augmentation

Mucus production
Catheter blockage
Urinary tract infection
Bladder stones
Metabolic changes
Hyperchloremic metabolic acidosis
Electrolyte disturbances
Spontaneous perforation
Metaplasia, malignancy
Bowel problems
Diarrhea
Vitamin B_{12} deficiency
Hematuria-dysuria syndrome (gastrocystoplasty)

vague abdominal pain. A computed tomography (CT) cystogram is the most accurate diagnostic investigation. Adhesive intestinal obstruction occurs in approximately 5% of patients within 15 years of bladder augmentation.

The high rates of late malignancy in patients following ureterosigmoidostomy and the findings of studies demonstrating bacterial-derived carcinogens in the urine following enterocystoplasty raised initial concerns that the use of bowel for bladder reconstruction would carry a significant long-term

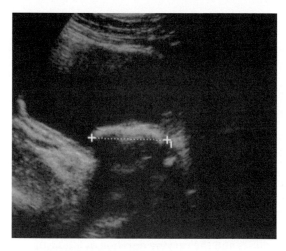

Figure 13.7 Ultrasound scan demonstrating 3.5 cm bladder stone in an augmented bladder.

cancer risk. However, it has now become clear that these concerns were largely unfounded. Long-term studies have found that the risk of bladder cancer in patients with spina bifida who had undergone bladder augmentation is not significantly higher than in age matched spina bifida patients whose bladders had not been augmented. The overall long-term incidence of bladder cancer has been reported to lie between 1% and 4%, with no significant differences between augmented and non-augmented patients in terms of age at diagnosis or survival rates.

Although cystoscopic surveillance and biopsy commencing 10 years after augmentation was previously advocated this has been discontinued in most centers because it not been shown to be helpful or cost effective.

Experimental Research

Because the complications of augmentation are largely attributable to the use of intestine, a number of research programs have tried to address this problem by devising experimental techniques to augment the bladder with materials derived from tissue engineered autologous urothelium or acellular matrices (serving as scaffolds for regenerative cellular infiltration). Clinical experience of this approach is very limited. Following an initial report in a small series of meningomyelocele patients, a subsequent Phase II study of the use of autologous seeded biodegradable scaffolds for bladder augmentation in spina bifida patients found that it did not result in any improvement in bladder compliance or capacity. In addition there was a relatively high rate of serious adverse events – including bladder rupture. On the basis of this study, the authors concluded that the technique could not be recommended for clinical use.

VESICOURETERAL REFLUX

Up to 20% of infants with neurogenic bladder have VUR. Because this VUR is often secondary to the unfavorable urodynamic features of the neuropathic bladder it will resolve in approximately 50% of cases once bladder dynamics have been improved by CIC and anticholinergic medication. If the VUR persists despite these measures and the child is suffering recurrent UTIs it is reasonable to consider correcting the reflux by ureteral reimplantation. However, this is most unlikely to succeed unless it is also accompanied by other measures to address the underlying bladder dysfunction. Endoscopic correction by sub-ureteric injection of bulking agents has a lower success rate in neuropathic bladders – although success rates of 60% to 70% have been claimed by some authors. Ureteral reimplantation can combined with bladder augmentation but is technically more difficult than in a normal bladder. However, ureteral reimplantation is often unnecessary because secondary VUR has a high tendency to resolve once the unfavorable characteristics of the neurogenic bladder have been corrected by bladder augmentation.

BLADDER OUTLET PROCEDURES

Although a number of different surgical procedures are available for increasing bladder outlet and sphincteric resistance, no single technique has proved sufficiently reliable to have gained widescale acceptance. When considering any of these procedures it is essential to ensure that the patient has the physical ability and motivation to perform intermittent catheterization. Preoperative evaluation includes imaging of the upper tracts and video urodynamics. If possible, bladder compliance and detrusor activity should be assessed with the bladder outlet occluded to try and predict how the bladder will behave following surgery. Unless there is good evidence that the bladder will function as a safe low pressure reservoir, strong consideration should be given to performing bladder augmentation at the same time as the surgery to increase outlet resistance.

The surgical procedures can considered in three broad categories (Figure 13.8):

- Operations designed to increase fixed outflow resistance by narrowing the bladder outlet and/or increasing the length of the urethra e.g. Kropp, Pippi Salle procedures.
- Operations designed to enhance outflow resistance by compressing or angulating the bladder neck and/or urethra, e.g. artificial urinary sphincter, colposuspension, or sling.
- Closure of the bladder neck.

Closure of the bladder neck is the most effective means of achieving continence but is usually kept in reserve as a second line approach.

There is considerable variation between different published studies in the reported continence rates following the different procedures. Published continence rates typically average around 60% to 70% but the published results are difficult to compare because of differences in the definition of what constitutes "continence" adopted in different studies and the varying duration of follow-up.

Injection of bulking agents into the bladder neck and sphincter region has also been reported as a method of increasing fixed outflow resistance.

a

Detrusor Tube

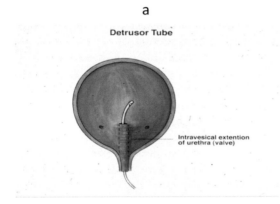

Intravesical extention of urethra (valve)

b

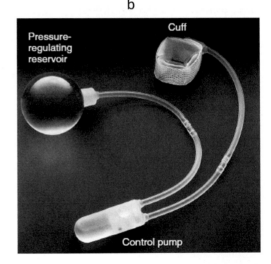

Pressure-regulating reservoir

Cuff

Control pump

c

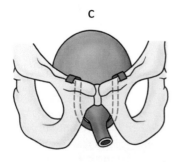

Figure 13.8 Some of the procedures available for increasing sphincter/outflow resistance. (a) Urethral lengthening (e.g. detrusor tube) to increase static outflow resistance. (b) External compression by an artificial urinary sphincter cuff implanted around the urethra. The pump is implanted in the scrotum and the pressure regulating balloon is implanted in a plane between the peritoneum and abdominal wall musculature. (Reproduced by permission from American Medical Systems). (c) Sling procedure. Slings created from autologous or allograft tissue are preferable to synthetic materials.

The continence rates are generally inferior to those achieved by open surgical techniques but a success rate of 25% with one or two injections has been reported.

Complications of the various different procedures include outflow obstruction ("hypercontinence"), tissue erosion, infection, and malfunction of artificial sphincter devices. A further complication is the relatively high incidence of bladder stones – particularly in patients who have also undergone enterocystoplasty.

Closure of the bladder neck is generally seen as a reliable last resort when other techniques have failed. Nevertheless, some pediatric urologists favor bladder neck closure sooner rather than later. The principal drawback of bladder neck closure is that the bladder becomes an enclosed system, with emptying being entirely dependent on a catheterizable channel or indwelling suprapubic catheter or drainage device.

Cutaneous urinary diversion (ileal conduit) was once the mainstay of management of neurogenic bladder but is now rarely used because of the availability of better alternatives. Specific complications include stomal stenosis, long-term upper tract changes and the adverse impact on body image and quality of life imposed by the stoma and urine collection bag.

TRANSITION TO PUBERTY IN ADULTHOOD

Unfortunately, there is a tendency for myelomeningocele patients to become less compliant with regular CIC and other aspects of their care when they progress into adolescence and adulthood. In the United States over 50% of adult spina bifida patients whose neurogenic bladders were previously managed by intermittent catheterization will cease to perform CIC, contrary to medical advice. Factors implicated in poor compliance with treatment and follow-up include obesity, immobility, developmental delay and alcohol and drug dependence.

Those patients who comply with measures to manage their neuropathic bladder appropriately and who remain under urologic surveillance have a very low long-term risk of severe renal impairment

(2%). Indeed, they more likely to die from infection, shunt complications, and pulmonary embolism than renal failure. However, the risks of renal impairment and urological complications are significantly higher in adult spina bifida patients who do not comply with recommended treatment or are lost to urologic surveillance.

Spina bifida patients require multispecialty healthcare throughout their lives and it is important that they receive the help they need to make a successful transition from the care of pediatric specialists to the care of adult specialists in the relevant disciplines.

SEXUALITY AND REPRODUCTIVE HEALTH

The early onset of menarche is more common in female myelomeningocele patients than the general population (12% and 0.6% respectively) and they are less likely to use contraception when they become sexually active.

Pregnancy creates specific problems – particularly in women who have previously undergone reconstructive procedures such as bladder augmentation or the creation of catheterizable channels. Obstetric care should be provided by multidisciplinary team including obstetrician-gynecologist, urologist and other clinicians. Elective caesarian section is often more appropriate than vaginal delivery.

Males may experience erectile dysfunction (ED) of varying severity and 80% of men with spina bifida have been demonstrated to have improved erectile function with the use of sildenafil.

One-quarter to one-third of adolescents and young adults with meningomyelocele between 14 and 23 years of age report having had sexual encounters but only half of meningomyelocele patients state that they are satisfied with their sexual lives.

NEUROGENIC BOWEL

The majority of children with neurogenic bladder also suffer from neurogenic bowel dysfunction. This is unsurprising since the lower urinary tract and rectum share similar innervation pathways via the sacral nerve roots (S2–S4).

For children experiencing difficulty with evacuation the initial treatment options include increasing dietary fiber, fecal softeners, bulking agents such as polyethylene glycol (MiraLAX), oral laxatives (bisacodyl), and suppositories. More active measures include conventional enemas, with water or saline- with or without irritant additives to stimulate defecation. Commercially available rectal washout systems (e.g. Peristeen) are also available. Alternatively, enemas can be administered into the proximal colon via a catheterizable channel (appendicocecostomy) or indwelling caecostomy tube. First described by Malone, this technique (commonly known as the **ACE procedure – antegrade continence enema**) has made an important contribution to the management of neuropathic bowel dysfunction. Complications of the ACE procedure include stomal stenosis and false passage. For many spina bifida patients (particularly those with physical disabilities, the practical difficulties surrounding the independent management of the neuropathic bowel are often more challenging than their neuropathic bladder.

KEY POINTS

- Children with neurogenic bladder require life-long urologic monitoring because urinary tract function can change with time, with adverse consequences for the upper urinary tract and quality of life.
- Eighty percent of patients with a neurogenic bladder will require some form of catheterization (usually clean intermittent catheterization) to ensure effective bladder emptying. Depending on their type of neurogenic bladder, CIC may also enable them to achieve a socially acceptable degree of urinary continence.
- The urinary tract should be regularly monitored with regular renal and bladder ultrasound scans and a baseline urodynamic study should be performed in infancy. Thereafter, urodynamic studies can either be performed on a regular

(e.g. annual) basis or more selectively according to clinical indications.
- Surgical intervention is often necessary to safeguard renal function, achieve a socially acceptable degree of urinary continence and provide an improved quality of life. When considering whether to recommend surgery and when selecting the most appropriate procedure(s), clinicians should take account of any co morbidities and the potential long-term consequences of surgery.

SUGGESTED READING

Austin PF, Bauer SB, Bower W, et al: The standardization of terminology of lower urinary tract function in children and adolescents: update report from the Standardization Committee of the International Children's Continence Society. J Urol 2014; **191**: 1863–1865.e13.

Higuchi TT, Granberg CF, Fox JA, et al: Augmentation cystoplasty and risk of neoplasia: fact, fiction and controversy. J Urol 2010; **184**: 2492–2496.

Husmann DA: Long-term complications following bladder augmentations in patients with spina bifida: bladder calculi, perforation of the augmented bladder and upper tract deterioration. Transl Androl Urol 2016; **5**: 3–11.

McGuire EJ, Woodside JR, Borden TA, et al: Prognostic value of urodynamic testing in myelodysplastic patients. J Urol 1981; **126**: 205–209.

Routh JC, Cheng EY, Austin JC, et al: Design and Methodological Considerations of the Centers for Disease Control and Prevention Urologic and Renal Protocol for the Newborn and Young Child with Spina Bifida. J Urol 2016; **196**: 1728–1734.

Rove KO, Brockel MA, Saltzman AF, et al: Prospective study of enhanced recovery after surgery protocol in children undergoing reconstructive operations. J Pediatr Urol 2018; **14**: 252.e1–252.e9.

Urologic Anomalies in Anorectal Malformations and Renal Ectopia

SARAH L HECHT and DUNCAN T WILCOX

Topics covered

Classification and workup of anorectal
    anomalies
Associated anomalies – urogenital, spinal,
    syndromes
Lower urinary tract dysfunction

Outcomes
    Renal function
    Continence
    Psychosexual
Renal ectopia

ANORECTAL ANOMALIES

Anorectal anomalies comprise a spectrum of congenital malformations in which the anus fails to open normally on to the perineum. At one end of this spectrum are minor anomalies in which the anal canal is present but the anus is anteriorly displaced or covered by perineal skin. With severe malformations, the rectum fails to reach the perineum and instead connects to the genitourinary tract.

Incidence and Etiology

Anorectal malformations occur in approximately 1 in 5000 live births, with a slight male to female preponderance of 3 to 2. The embryological cause is incompletely understood but involves failed division of the primitive cloaca. More recent studies indicate that subdivision of the cloaca is a largely passive process related to the "unfolding" of the caudal body axis.

Genetic determinants of anorectal anomalies are similarly complex and poorly understood. It is unlikely that the varied spectrum of anorectal malformations will prove to be the outcome of a simple gene mutation, although knockouts of certain genes including *ephrin B* and *Sonic Hedgehog* do lead to anorectal anomalies in mice. A high incidence of anorectal malformations has been described in patients with chromosomal abnormalities, such as Down syndrome, trisomy 18, and cat eye syndrome. Various teratogens have also been associated with anorectal malformations.

Classification

The earliest classification divided anorectal malformations into "high" and "low" types based on

183

Table 14.1 Peña classification of anorectal malformation

Male	Female
Rectovesical fistula	Cloaca
Rectourethral fistula	>3 cm common channel
Prostatic	<3 cm common channel
Bulbar	Rectovestibular fistula
Imperforate anus (no fistula)	
Perineal fistula	

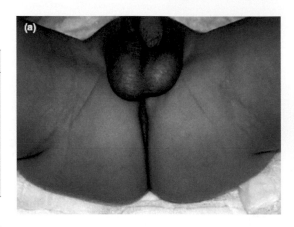

Figure 14.2 Perineum of male infant with a high anorectal malformation with absent anus. Note area of decreased pigmentation at the site where the anus should be.

whether the rectum terminated above or below the levator musculature. A more detailed classification system is based on the location of the rectal fistula. (Table 14.1)

Perineal fistulae represent minor defects in which the rectum opens anteriorly to the center of the anal sphincter. The orifice is usually stenotic, and the sphincter complex is intact.

Imperforate anus without fistula is rare – except in infants with Down syndrome, in whom most anorectal malformations are of the imperforate anus type. In such cases there is no fistula, just a blind-ending rectum that is usually located within 2 cm of the perineal skin. The sacrum is usually well formed and there is a functional anal sphincter complex (Figure 14.1).

A recto-vestibular fistula is the most common defect in girls. The rectum opens by a narrowed connection with the vestibule of the vagina, usually at the posterior fourchette.

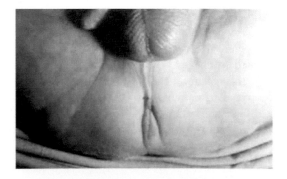

Figure 14.1 Characteristic appearance of a perineum in an infant with a low anorectal anomaly. Note the distinct dimple at the site where the anus should be.

Rectourethral fistulae are the most common defects in males. There are two types. In the bulbar type the rectum opens into the anterior (bulbar) urethra whereas in the prostatic type the rectum opens into the posterior (prostatic) urethra. Prostatic recto urethral fistulae are more severe malformations and are accompanied by a higher incidence of sacral dysplasia and poor anal sphincter musculature.

Rectovesical or recto-bladder neck fistulae represent the most severe form of high anorectal malformations in boys and are typically associated with sacral dysplasia, abnormal pelvic floor musculature, and a poor anal sphincter complex. This type of malformation is also accompanied by a higher incidence of other coexisting congenital anomalies (Figure 14.2).

In a persistent cloacal malformation the vagina, rectum, and urethra are combined into a single common channel. In the case of vaginal or uterine duplication, the rectum opens in the midline at the confluence of the Müllerian structures. Patients with a long common channel (>3 cm) are more likely to have sacral dysplasia and additional congenital anomalies, poor rectal and urinary sphincter musculature. These patients may require more complex surgical reconstruction including vaginal reconstruction (Figure 14.3).

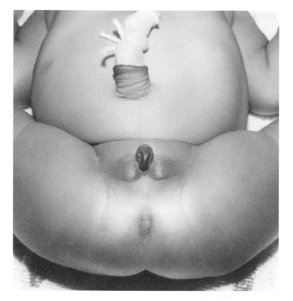

Figure 14.3 Cloacal anomaly with single perineal orifice draining the urinary, genital, and lower gastrointestinal tracts in a female infant.

ASSOCIATED CONGENITAL ANOMALIES

The close embryologic association of the developing anorectal, genital, and urinary systems explains the high incidence of genitourinary anomalies seen in patients with anorectal malformations (Table 14.2).

Table 14.2 Other anomalies associated with anorectal malformations

Anomaly	Incidence (%)
Vertebral	25–40
Cardiac	20
Tetralogy of fallot	
ASD/VSD	
Gastrointestinal	15
Tracheo-esophageal fistula	
Duodenal atresia	
Hirschsprung's disease	
Genitourinary	60

Associated Syndromes

VACTERL

VACTERL is an acronym for **v**ertebral anomalies, **a**norectal anomalies, **c**ardiac anomalies, **t**racheo-**e**sophageal fistula, **r**enal anomalies, and **l**imb anomalies. Most cases are sporadic rather than hereditary. Not all components of the VACTERL association are expressed in every patient. The most common are vertebral, anorectal, and renal abnormalities.

Caudal regression syndrome

Caudal regression syndrome, also termed sacral agenesis, results from failure of formation of part or all of the coccyx, sacrum, and occasionally the lumbar spine and their corresponding spinal cord segments. It is commonly associated with anorectal malformations (27–48%) and genito-urinary anomalies. Caudal regression syndrome is strongly associated with maternal diabetes; mothers with insulin dependent diabetes are 200–400 times more likely to have a child with caudal regression syndrome than nondiabetic mothers (Figure 14.4).

CHARGE

CHARGE is an acronym for **c**oloboma of the eye, **h**eart anomalies, choanal **a**tresia, growth **r**etardation, **g**enital, and **e**ar anomalies. In one series of 32 children with CHARGE, the overall incidence of genitourinary tract abnormalities was 69% (Table 14.3).

Upper Urinary Tract Anomalies

Coexisting anatomical anomalies of the upper and lower urinary tract occur in 50–60% of patients with anorectal malformations, the commonest being vesicoureteral reflux (Figure 14.5). The spectrum of abnormalities encountered in one series of patients is illustrated in Table 14.4.

In addition to structural anomalies, up to 6% of children develop renal impairment, an incidence which increases to nearly 50% of girls with cloacal anomalies. Consequently, early detection of renal impairment is an important aspect of management.

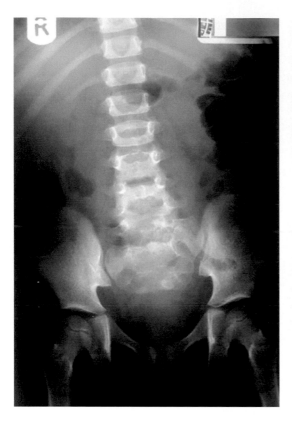

Figure 14.4 Plain radiograph demonstrating sacral agenesis.

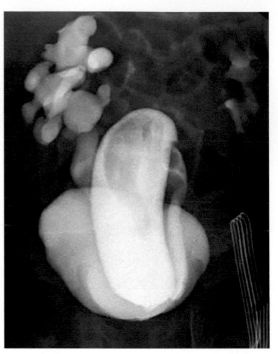

Figure 14.5 Coronal view of a distal loopagram. Contrast passes into the bladder and shows bilateral vesicoureteral reflux (grade IV on the right).

Lower Urinary Tract Dysfunction

In one series, 25% of children with anorectal malformations were found to have severe lower urinary tract dysfunction which was primarily related to a sacral abnormality. The children with severe bladder dysfunction were mostly incontinent, and one-third had reflux nephropathy. In addition, 20% of children in this series experienced deterioration of bladder function following surgical repair of the anorectal malformation. These findings highlight the importance

Table 14.3 Genitourinary malformations in the CHARGE association

	Incidence (%)
Genital anomalies	56
Hypospadias/micropenis	
Undescended testis	
Vaginal and uterine atresia	
Urinary tract anomalies	42
Duplex kidney	
Vesicoureteral reflux	
Renal agenesis	
Hydronephrosis	

Table 14.4 Pattern of structural anomalies of the urinary tract in 45 children with anorectal malformations

Urinary anomaly	Patients (n = 45)
Vesicoureteral reflux	16
Hydronephrosis	6
Crossed fused ectopia	3
Dysplastic kidney	3
Bladder diverticulum	2
Renal agenesis	1
Horseshoe kidney	1
Megaureter	1
Prune-belly syndrome	1

of investigating the lower urinary tract in children whose anorectal anomaly is accompanied by a sacral abnormality.

Genital Anomalies

Abnormalities of the male external genitalia are commonly present, including undescended testes (20%), bifid scrotum (15%), and penile anomalies (25%) – including hypospadias and (less commonly) chordee, epispadias, penile duplication, and (rarely) absence of the vas deferens. Anomalies of the female genital tract are less readily apparent, but Müllerian abnormalities, such as vaginal septa or bicornuate uterus occur in 30–45% of girls with anorectal malformations.

Spinal Anomalies

The incidence of vertebral anomalies in children with anorectal malformations has been reported to be as high as 40%. Many children have associated intraspinal pathology (e.g. tethered cord), which can lead to urological, neurological, and orthopedic complications. It is important to identify cord tethering at an early stage because of the possibility that early neurosurgical intervention may have the potential to avert progressive neurological deterioration. Routine investigation of the spine is required in all patients with anorectal anomalies, with more detailed investigation of the spinal cord being performed where indicated (Figure 14.6). Initial imaging should include both anteroposterior and lateral radiological views of the sacrum. The most commonly identified lesions are partial and complete sacral agenesis (Figure 14.4).

If the sacrum is radiographically normal, significant intraspinal pathology is unlikely. In infants under 4 months of age, spinal ultrasound has proved very sensitive in identifying intraspinal anomalies, although it is less accurate than magnetic resonance imaging (MRI).

Prenatal diagnosis is largely limited to the more serious anorectal anomalies and usually results

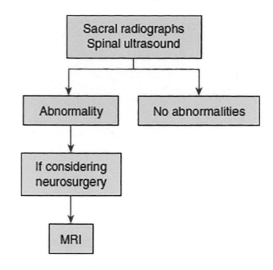

Figure 14.6 Diagnostic algorithm for the investigation of the spine in an infant with an anorectal anomaly.

from the detection of concurrent anomalies – which are more common in severe anorectal malformations. Clues on prenatal ultrasound include dilated bowel, calcified meconium, lack of meconium in the rectum, hydrocolpos (usually identified as a pelvic cystic structure and a poorly visualized bladder), renal anomalies, neural tube defects, and absent radius, among others. Abnormalities of multiple systems may strengthen suspicion for VACTERL or another syndrome with anorectal anomalies. The vast majority of anorectal malformations are still diagnosed postnatally on physical examination. Initial examination of the perineum will reveal an absent anus but a more detailed evaluation should be undertaken to look for features such as the presence and position of an anal dimple, anal skin tag or membrane, flattened buttocks, and gluteal cleft. In girls, it is also important to determine whether there are separate urethral and vaginal openings.

INITIAL MANAGEMENT AND WORKUP

Initial management of the newborn focuses on the gastrointestinal tract. Primary surgical repair can be considered for those infants who pass

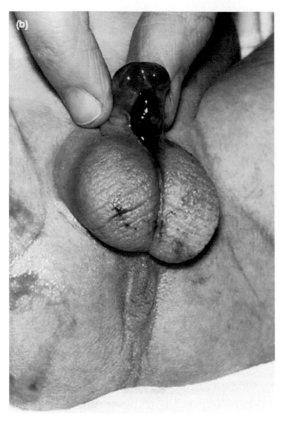

Figure 14.7 Meconium discharging from the urethral meatus of a male infant with a rectourethral fistula. A tract of meconium extending to the perineum would suggest a perineal fistula covered with skin. Note also the presence of hypospadias.

retrograde filling with urine in the obstructed vagina. Historically, hydrocolpos was managed by vaginostomy drainage and/or vesicostomy performed at the time of the diverting colostomy but more recently it has been shown that it hydrocolpos can usually be managed safely by intermittent catheterization of the common channel.

Associated Anomalies

In addition to spinal imaging (ultrasound and MRI when indicated) a urinary tract ultrasound scan should be undertaken to evaluate any structural renal anomalies. Renal scintigraphy with 99^{m}Tc dimercaptoacetyltriglycine (MAG3) to assess drainage and relative renal function can usually be deferred until >3 months of age to allow time for maturation of renal function. The role of routine preoperative voiding cystourethrography (VCUG) is debatable, and, in practice, it may be difficult to identify a suitable anatomical route to catheterize the bladder.

meconium via a perineal or rectovestibular fistula but a diverting colostomy is required in more severe cases where there is no external fistula or internal fistula to the urinary tract (Figure 14.7). Visualizing the passage of meconium can help to identify the location of a fistula which is present. But because it can take up to 24 hours for a newborn infant to pass meconium this period should be allowed to elapse before any surgical intervention is undertaken. An end colostomy is preferable to a loop colostomy and is typically performed at the level of the descending colon to preserve an adequate length of distal colon for surgical reconstruction.

Hydrocolpos is present in 30% of cases of persistent cloaca and is caused by accumulation of secretions, which may be combined with

SURGICAL MANAGEMENT

In general, children undergo definitive repair of their anorectal anomalies at around 3 months of age.

Pre-operative planning includes contrast studies (distal colostogram) to evaluate the length of distal colon available for a pull-through procedure and define the relationship of the rectum to the sacrum and coccyx. Cystovaginoscopy is an essential part of the preoperative evaluation of cloacal malformations and is ideally undertaken when the diverting colostomy is performed. At the time of endoscopy information should be sought on the length of the common channel, the bladder neck, bladder, and ureteral orifices.

A detailed account of the reconstruction of anorectal anomalies is beyond the scope of this chapter. The technique most widely employed is the posterior sagittal anorectoplasty originally described and popularized by Peña (Figure 14.8). Colostomy closure is usually performed several months following anorectoplasty.

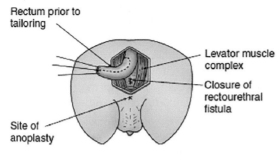

Figure 14.8 Posterior sagittal anorectoplasty. With the patient prone, the rectum is approached via a sagittal incision. The rectourethral fistula is divided and the rectum tailored before being positioned through the levator complex and external sphincter and brought down onto the perineum.

UROLOGIC FOLLOW-UP

Routine clinical follow-up (including renal and bladder ultrasound) should be continued until urinary continence has been established. Urodynamic studies should be performed post-operatively in all patients to establish baseline bladder function. Urodynamics should be repeated if there are new or worsening urinary symptoms (e.g. leakage, frequency, urgency). Further urodynamic evaluation is also required if there are changes in the upper urinary tract (worsening hydronephrosis or deteriorating renal function) or other signs of neurologic deterioration.

Hydronephrosis and vesicoureteral reflux should be managed in the same way as for patients without anorectal anomalies. In boys, urinary reflux into the vas deferens may also be identified. Unfortunately, this is a risk factor for recurrent epididymo-orchitis, which is common in males with anorectal anomalies and may require occlusion of the vas deferens to prevent recurrent episodes of epididymo orchitis.

OUTCOMES

RENAL

Severe and minor anorectal malformations both carry a risk of renal failure, although the incidence is higher with more severe malformations. In one series, 80% of patients with cloacal anomalies developed long-term renal impairment. Another large review of patients with cloacal anomalies found that half of the patients developed chronic renal failure by 5.7 years of age, and 17% went on to develop end-stage renal failure. Between 2% and 6% of patients with high anorectal malformations die from renal insufficiency compared with 1.1% of patients with low lesions. This reflects the higher incidence of associated renal anomalies including renal dysplasia, reflux nephropathy, and bladder dysfunction in those with high anorectal malformations. The management of chronic renal failure and end-stage disease in children with anorectal malformations can be challenging and peritoneal dialysis and subsequent renal transplantation can be difficult because of the previous abdominal operations.

Fecal Continence

Fecal continence after anorectoplasty depends on the functional integrity of the anal sphincter complex, anorectal sensation, and bowel motility. Patients with severe malformations and associated sacral anomalies have a poorer long-term prognosis. Fecal continence rates after reconstructive surgery are closely correlated with the location of the rectourinary fistula. Whereas the continence rate in patients with a perineal fistula is around 90%, the corresponding rates vestibular, bulbar, prostatic and bladder neck fistulas are 70%, 50%, 30% and 12% respectively. Persisting fecal incontinence is managed by a combination of enemas and motility agents. Urologists managing these patients should take into account their fecal continence status, as many patients with fecal incontinence are less motivated to become continent of urine and may therefore forgo interventions such as bladder neck reconstruction or closure, which would provide them with a greater degree of urinary continence. Moreover, bowel dysfunction may predispose these patients to recurrent urinary tract infection.

Urinary Continence

While fecal incontinence is primarily a quality of life issue, urinary incontinence may represent underlying bladder dysfunction which can lead to renal deterioration and morbidity from urinary tract infections. Recurrent urinary tract infection may be overlooked or attributed to coexisting vesicoureteral reflux or renal anomalies, which are prevalent in a high proportion of these children. The importance of lower urinary tract evaluation in these patients cannot be overstated. Urinary continence is dependent on the function of both the bladder and the urethral sphincter complex. Bladder management focuses on bladder emptying and maintaining low pressures. This may require catheterization, treatment with anticholinergic agents, intravesical injections of botulinum toxin and/or bladder augmentation. In these respects the management of bladder dysfunction is essentially the same as for neurogenic bladder (see Chapter 13).

Many patients with a cloacal anomaly have a competent bladder neck – which will enable them to remain dry between intermittent catheterization. By contrast, patients with spinal anomalies more often have an incompetent bladder neck and sphincter complex with resultant urinary leakage despite optimal bladder management. In these cases, various procedures are available to increase outflow resistance including injection of bulking agents and formal bladder neck reconstruction. Bladder neck closure is a further option but this must be accompanied by Mitrofanoff procedure to create a catheterizable channel for bladder emptying.

There is relatively limited published information on urinary continence rates in the anorectal population. A retrospective study of 90 patients in the Netherlands found that nearly all (91%) of anorectal malformation patients with evidence of bladder-sphincter dysfunction on urodynamics had associated urinary incontinence. With only one exception, all these patients had an underlying spinal anomaly. A subsequent study of over 300 patients found a correlation between incontinence rates and the type of malformation, i.e. cloacal anomalies 46% incontinence rate, bladder neck fistula 25%, urethral fistula 25%, vaginal fistula 20%. In those patients who did not have a fistula the urinary incontinence rate was much lower – only 4%.

ADULT OUTCOMES

Very little research has so far been undertaken on sexual function in adults with anorectal malformations. However, they do express an interest in sexuality and sexual function and it is important that these patients receive advice and support from appropriate specialists.

Sex and Fertility

Males

Impaired erectile, ejaculatory, and sensory function have been reported in adult male patients who underwent surgical procedures in the prostatic area at the time of anoplasty. The posterior sagittal approach is thought to be associated with better sexual functional outcomes by reducing the risk of iatrogenic damage to the relevant pelvic innervation. Indeed, one study examining sexual function in 41 males with rectourethral fistulae who had been treated by the PSARP procedure found that 90% of these patients had normal erections and ejaculation and 80% experienced normal orgasms. Outcomes for sexual function are much less satisfactory in men who underwent abdominoperineal procedures for the correction of their anorectal anomaly – particularly in those men with associated spinal anomalies. Psychological factors may also contribute to sexual dysfunction even in patients with normally preserved neurologic and anatomical function.

Fertility in these patients has invariably been assessed in relation to paternity but the published literature is very sparse. Infertility or subfertility may be due to cryptorchidism, genital anomalies, sacral anomalies, recurrent epididymo-orchitis, or iatrogenic injuries.

Females

Adolescent females with anorectal malformations who previously underwent surgery which included vaginal reconstruction will require evaluation as they near puberty. It has been reported that only one-third of these patients menstruate normally and it is important to ensure that the vagina is not obstructed. There are reports in the literature of normal pregnancy in patients with anorectal malformations. However, women with uterine anomalies, such as didelphys are at higher risk for preterm labor and miscarriage. Although some women may be capable of normal vaginal delivery, Caesarian section delivery is necessary in those who have undergone complex vaginal reconstruction or replacement.

Sexual dysfunction appears to be more common in females than in males. One recent study found 50% of women with an anorectal malformation reported sexual dysfunction or distress independent of continence and quality of life. Moreover, 35–45% of female patients surveyed had not been sexually active. Potential problems include inadequate vaginal length or caliber, dyspareunia, poor sensation, and psychosocial distress.

Psychology

Anorectal malformations carry significant psychological morbidity which is reflected in impaired self-esteem, decreased quality of life, and psychosexual dysfunction. Urinary and fecal incontinence are associated with poorer sexual wellbeing and quality of life. Ongoing multidisciplinary care is important for these patients, and ideally this should include the input of a psychologist with knowledge of issues facing patients with anorectal anomalies.

ABNORMAL MIGRATION AND FUSION OF THE KIDNEY

Renal Ectopia

Renal ectopia results from abnormal renal migration and/or fusion during embryologic development. Ectopic kidneys can be classified as simple, horseshoe, or crossed.

Simple ectopic kidney

An ectopic kidney may be located anywhere along the embryological path of ascent from the pelvis to the renal fossa (or rarely, within the thorax). Pelvic kidneys are the most common form of renal ectopia, accounting for 60% of all cases. The majority (90%) are unilateral and they occur more commonly on the left. A pelvic kidney is frequently hypoplastic and irregular in shape (Figure 14.9).

Genital and contralateral urinary abnormalities are often associated with ectopic kidneys and include; absence of the vagina, retrocaval ureter, bicornuate uterus, supernumerary kidney, and

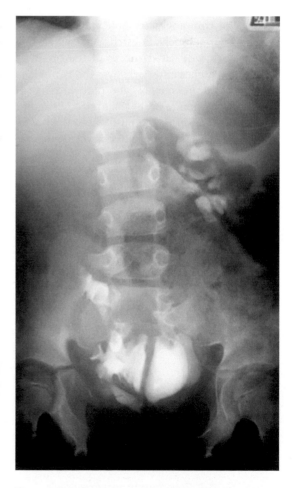

Figure 14.9 Intravenous urogram demonstrating a right pelvic simple ectopic kidney.

ipsilateral ectopic ureter. The ectopic kidney can be a component of more complex syndromes, such as the Mayer–Rokitansky–Küster–Hauser syndrome, Fanconi's anemia or conjoined twins.

Horseshoe kidney

Horseshoe kidneys are encountered in 1:400 and 1:1800 autopsies with male predominance. In 95% of cases, the lower poles of the two kidneys are joined by an isthmus of renal tissue, which may consist of normal parenchyma or dysplastic or fibrous tissue. In about 40% of cases, the isthmus lies at the level of L4 where it is trapped beneath the origin of the inferior mesenteric artery during renal ascent. (Figure 14.10). A small proportion of horseshoe kidneys are fused at their upper poles. The commonest complication horseshoe kidney is ureteropelvic obstruction, which may be due to the deviated course of the proximal ureter as it arches anteriorly over the isthmus or extrinsic compression by aberrant vasculature (or a combination of both) (Figure 14.11a and b). Horseshoe kidney is commonly found in association with other abnormalities or syndromes

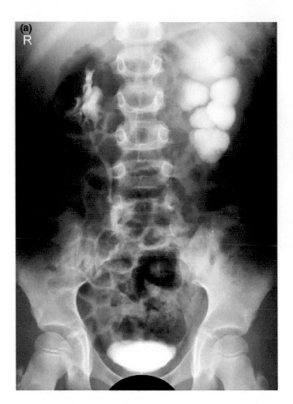

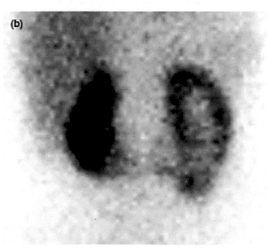

Figure 14.11 (a) Intravenous urogram demonstrating dilatation due to obstruction in the left side of a horseshoe kidney. (b) DMSA scan in the same patient demonstrating reduced isotope uptake in the central part of the left kidney (dilated collecting system) and functioning tissue outlining the isthmus connecting the right and left kidneys.

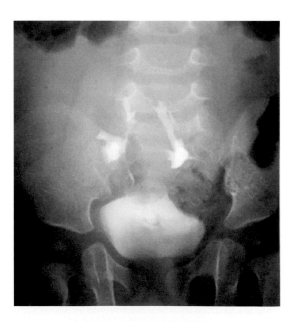

Figure 14.10 Intravenous urogram – pelvic horseshoe kidney.

(notably Turner's syndrome) and abnormalities of the central nervous system, the gastrointestinal tract and the skeletal and cardiovascular systems.

Crossed renal ectopia

A crossed renal ectopic kidney crossed the midline during migration. There are four varieties of crossed renal ectopia:

- With fusion to the contralateral kidney (85% of cases)
- Without fusion (<10%)
- Solitary
- Bilateral

There is a slight male predominance, and crossing from left to right occurs more frequently than from right to left. The point of fusion is usually between the upper pole of the crossed kidney and the lower pole of the normally positioned kidney (unilateral fused type) (Figure 14.12). Associated anomalies are commonly found with renal ectopia. In addition, renal ectopia may also be a component of more complex syndromes.

Presentation and investigation of abnormalities of ascent and fusion

Abnormalities of ascent and fusion are most commonly incidental findings, typically on prenatal or postnatal ultrasound examinations. Conversely, non-dilated pelvic ectopic kidneys may be difficult to visualize on ultrasound, and absence of the kidney in the renal fossa may be misinterpreted as renal agenesis. In such cases, the presence of ectopic functioning renal tissue is best demonstrated by renography with 99^m Tc dimercaptosuccinic acid (DMSA). Crossed fused renal ectopia may sometimes present clinically as an incidentally discovered mass during the course of abdominal examination. The occurrence of pain or symptoms associated with urinary infection generally denotes additional pathology, such

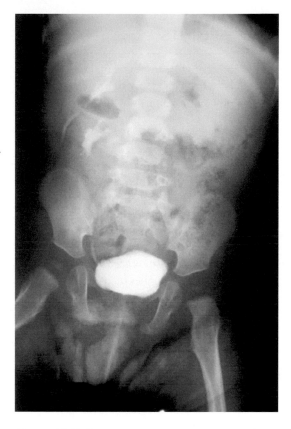

Figure 14.12 Intravenous urogram – crossed fused renal ectopia. Two collecting systems are visualized on the right. No kidney is present on the left side.

as vesicoureteral reflux or ureteropelvic junction obstruction. Investigation of an uncomplicated ectopic or horseshoe kidney can reasonably be limited to ultrasound and a renogram. Additional investigations are indicated if there is hydronephrosis or a history of documented infection raising concerns about possible vesicoureteral reflux. It is important to stress that the majority of patients are untroubled by their abnormally placed kidney, and surgical intervention should be confined to correcting coexisting pathology, obstruction or reflux. When surgery is warranted it should be borne in mind that the anatomy may be abnormal and that the blood supply can have an aberrant course.

KEY POINTS

- Children with anorectal malformations have a high incidence of urinary tract abnormalities and functional urinary problems.
- Early recognition and effective management of urological problems is essential to minimize the risks of renal failure and urinary tract infection.
- Higher rectourinary fistula in males and longer common channels in females represent more severe anorectal malformations. More severe defects are more likely to be accompanied by associated anomalies including spinal defects and renal anomalies.
- Psychosocial and sexual concerns are common as these patients reach adulthood.
- Anomalies of ascent and fusion, including pelvic kidney, horseshoe kidney, and crossed ectopia, are mainly asymptomatic incidental findings. Surgical intervention is only required when there is complicating pathology, such as obstruction or reflux.

FURTHER READING

Bischoff A, Bealer J, Wilcox DT, Peña A. Error traps and culture of safety in anorectal malformations. Semin Pediatr Surg. 2019;28(3):131–134.

Boemers TM, Beek FJ, Bax NM. Guidelines for the urological screening and initial management of lower urinary tract dysfunction in children with anorectal malformations – the ARGUS protocol. BJU Int. 1999;83:662–671.

Caldwell BT, Wilcox DT. Long-term urological outcomes in cloacal anomalies. Semin Pediatr Surg. 2016;25(2):108–111.

Kyrklund K, Taskinen S, Rintala RJ, Pakarinen MP. Sexual function, fertility, and quality of life after modern treatment of anorectal malformations. J Urol. 2016;196(6):1741–1746.

Peña A. Anorectal malformations. Semin Pediatr Surg. 1995;4:35–47.

Thomas DFM. The embryology of persistent cloaca and urogenital sinus malformations. Asian J Androl. 2020;22(2):124–128.

Bladder Exstrophy and Epispadias

PETER CUCKOW and KEVIN CAO

Topics covered

Embryology and anatomy
Bladder exstrophy: Management and outcomes
Cloacal exstrophy: Management and outcomes

Primary epispadias: Management and outcomes
Other bladder conditions; diverticula and
    urachal remnants

INTRODUCTION

This chapter covers one of the most challenging conditions in paediatric urology. As well as requiring complex reconstructive surgery to correct their severe bladder and genital abnormalities, children born with bladder exstrophy encounter continuing problems throughout childhood and adolescence and face possible long-term risks of renal failure and infertility. The relative rarity of bladder exstrophy and related conditions previously made it difficult for paediatric urologists to acquire adequate experience in treating them because even major regional centres received only one or two new referrals a year. To overcome this problem, the United Kingdom adopted a policy whereby the management of bladder exstrophy is confined to two supraregional centres. This has enabled paediatric urologists in these two centres to acquire and maintain a high level of experience and specialist expertise. It has also helped to facilitate the development and assessment of innovative approaches to the management of exstrophy aimed at improving the outcome for

children born with this condition. Although the treatment of bladder exstrophy is provided in a greater number of centres in the Unites States there is nevertheless a considerable degree of collaboration and sharing of expertise between some of the major children's hospitals. In addition to bladder exstrophy, this chapter also considers some of the other congenital disorders of the bladder.

EMBRYOLOGY AND ANATOMY

Three distinct anomalies constitute the exstrophy–epispadias complex (EEC): classic bladder exstrophy, epispadias and cloacal exstrophy. They are thought to constitute a spectrum of abnormalities arising from failure of development of the lower abdominal wall during early gestation.

Bladder Exstrophy

Similarities between the three anomalies comprising the exstrophy–epispadias complex point to a similar embryological origin in the early stages of gestation. However, the precise mechanism remains unclear. The cloacal 'rupture' hypothesis proposes that a failure of integration of the mesodermal, endodermal and ectodermal components of the cloacal plate causes it to rupture – leading to exposure of the bladder plate and urethra. This is supported by animal models in which surgical disruption of the membrane replicates the exstrophy morphology. The alternative 'wedge-effect' hypothesis postulates that overgrowth of the cloacal membrane acts as a mechanical wedge, which has the effect of separating the mesodermal components of the umbilical body wall. This explanation also has some empirical support. Neither of these hypothetical models adequately explains the existence of 'late rupture' and 'covered' variants of EEC anomalies.

Bladder exstrophy is characterised by an open bladder plate and urethra occupying a triangular infra-umbilical space above an open pelvic ring with the rectus abdominis muscles lying on either side. In the male, the penile roots are attached to the lower border of the inferior pubic rami and the two corpora traverse the intervening gap in the bony pelvis (the pubic diastasis) to join each other to form a foreshortened penile shaft. The exposed bladder mucosa lies in continuity with the exposed urethral plate with the openings of the ejaculatory ducts being located at a level equivalent to the verumontanum. The exposed urethral plate extends over the dorsal surface of the corpora and glans (Figure 15.1). The testes are usually descended. Failure of

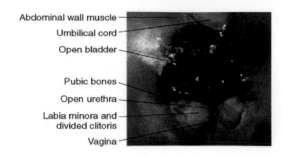

Figure 15.2 Newborn female infant with bladder exstrophy.

development of the lower anterior abdominal wall and pelvic ring results in the anus being located in a relatively anterior position. In females, the bladder component is identical to males and the clitoral corpora are separated with a short urethral plate between the open bladder and vagina (Figure 15.2).

Cloacal Exstrophy

Cloacal exstrophy is a more severe embryological variant, which is accompanied by defective subdivision of the cloaca. Both the bladder and bowel components of the anomaly are exteriorised, with a central area of bowel lying in the midline between two separated halves of the bladder. There is extensive prolapse of the proximal colon and ileum and one or two appendices. A second inferior opening corresponds to a rudimentary loop of distal hindgut. The anus is imperforate.

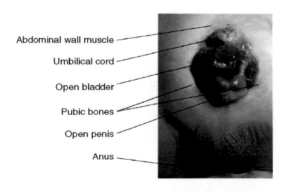

Figure 15.1 Newborn male infant with bladder exstrophy.

Table 15.1 Worldwide incidence and sex distribution of the exstrophy–epispadias complex

	Incidence per live births	Male to female ratio
Bladder exstrophy	1:50 000	2:1
Primary epispadias	1:120 000	5:1
Cloacal exstrophy	1:300 000	0.6:1[a]

[a] Because of the rarity of cloacal exstrophy and limitations in methodology there is considerable variation in the published figures for incidence and sex ratio.

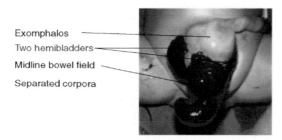

Exomphalos
Two hemibladders
Midline bowel field
Separated corpora

Figure 15.3 Newborn male infant with cloacal exstrophy.

The sacrum is foreshortened and there is a high incidence of spinal dysraphism. The pubic diastasis (gap between the anterior pubic rami) may be so wide that the penile corpora are completely separated. In addition, the testes are often undescended and absent from the scrotum or hemiscrotum. Cloacal exstrophy is often accompanied by an exomphalos located above it (Figure 15.3).

Primary Epispadias

The embryological origins are poorly understood. Primary penile epispadias is accompanied by a variable degree of bony pelvic diastasis – although this is usually less severe than in bladder exstrophy. In less severe forms of the anomaly the pelvic ring may be complete, with an apparently normal abdominal wall. The anus is sited normally and the scrotum also appears normal. A variable length of the urethra lies exposed on the dorsal aspect of the penis. According to the degree of severity of the epispadias, the urethra may open distally on the glans (glanular epispadias), on the shaft (penile epispadias) or proximally at the junction with the anterior abdominal wall (pubic or penopubic epispadias) (Figure 15.4). Underlying deficiencies of the bladder neck, proximal urethra and striated sphincter complex give rise to varying degrees of urinary incontinence – which is more severe in proximal and penopubic cases. In severe forms of epispadias, the posterior urethra merges with the bladder neck, and the verumontanum is either located at this level or within the bladder itself. The ureteric orifices often lie close together and can be normal or narrow in calibre, contrasting with the wide refluxing orifices seen in exstrophy.

In female primary epispadias, an abnormally wide section of urethra lies open and exposed on its dorsal surface and the clitoris is divided (bifid). The urethra is short and wide, with a deficient bladder neck, leading to severe stress-type incontinence in all patients (Figure 15.5).

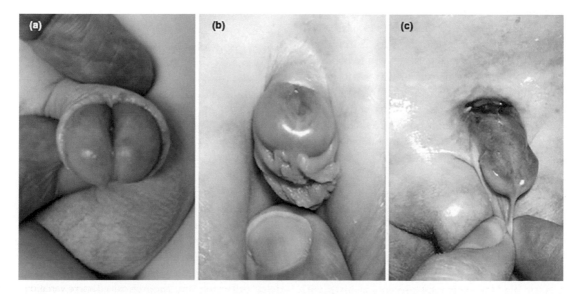

Figure 15.4 Male primary epispadias: (a) glanular; (b) penile; and (c) penopubic.

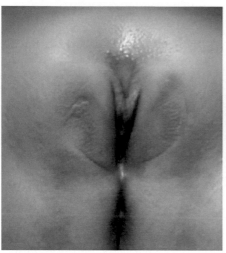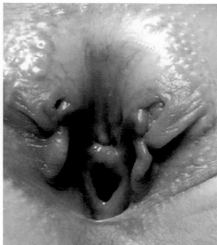

Figure 15.5 Female primary epispadias.

Approximately, 50% of cases of bladder exstrophy are now detected antenatally and in a further 20% of cases the diagnosis can be made retrospectively upon further review of the antenatal scans. Diagnostic features include; lack of urine in the fetal bladder, low-set umbilical cord, short, wide penis and bulging bladder plate. Maternal levels of serum alpha feto protein (AFP) are elevated as a result of exposure of bladder mucosa to amniotic fluid. The antenatal detection rate of cloacal exstrophy is even higher because of the coexisting anomalies. However, these sometimes lead to confusion with abdominal wall defects such as gastroschisis.

Antenatal diagnosis provides an opportunity for parents to consider termination of pregnancy, but counselling should take into account the improving outcomes of intervention, particularly in classic bladder exstrophy.

CLASSIC BLADDER EXSTROPHY

Presentation and Clinical Features

Classic bladder exstrophy presents at birth with a visible bladder plate below a low-set umbilical cord. The mucosa may be inflamed and polypoid, due to exposure in-utero or following delivery. The penile shaft is usually short and thick, with a good sized glans. The scrotum is present in boys with the distinctive upwards direction of the rugae and the testes are normally palpable.

Most affected infants are born at term and are usually otherwise well at birth. The incidence of other congenital anomalies is low, with the exception of inguinal herniae which are present in 80% of males and 15% of females.

Neonatal Management and Primary Closure

Following delivery most newborns can be put to the breast normally. Vitamin K should be given (particularly if surgery is planned within the first few days) and the exposed bladder plate protected with plastic film inside the nappy. Antibiotics or intravenous access are not routinely required at this stage.

Urgent transfer to the specialist centre is rarely indicated and it is preferable for the baby to remain with the mother in the first few days to establish breastfeeding and promote bonding. This enables feeding to be established to help ensure better post-operative nutrition. The benefits of a slight delay outweigh any theoretical concerns regarding decreasing flexibility of the pelvis because, in practice, the abdomen and bladder can usually be closed effectively without the need for osteotomies in the first two to three weeks of life. A baseline renal ultrasound scan is performed to evaluate the upper urinary tract prior to surgery. In premature infants, a longer period of stabilisation is preferable and it is not unreasonable to delay closure for several weeks if medically indicated.

Surgical technique (Figure 15.6)

The surgery is performed under intravenous antibiotic cover and whenever possible an epidural catheter is inserted at the outset to ensure optimal postoperative analgesia. Following catheterisation of the ureters the bladder plate is mobilised and dissected free of the skin and rectus muscles. Any large mucosal polyps are excised and the resulting mucosal defects repaired. At this stage any hernial sacs which are present can be identified and ligated. Mobilisation of the bladder plate is performed by extraperitoneal dissection, which is then continued inferiorly on both sides of the proximal urethral plate down to the level of the verumontanum. In girls, this dissection is continued to just above the vaginal opening. Following deeper dissection around the bladder neck, the bladder and proximal urethra can be mobilised sufficiently to permit midline closure with interrupted 4/0 absorbable sutures. The pelvic floor muscles are divided anterolaterally to enable the urethral/bladder neck complex to be repositioned to lie behind the closed abdominal wall. The ureteric catheters are brought out through the bladder to emerge lateral to the midline muscle and skin closure. The bladder is drained via a silicone stent emerging from the urethral opening. Unless the diastasis is wide,

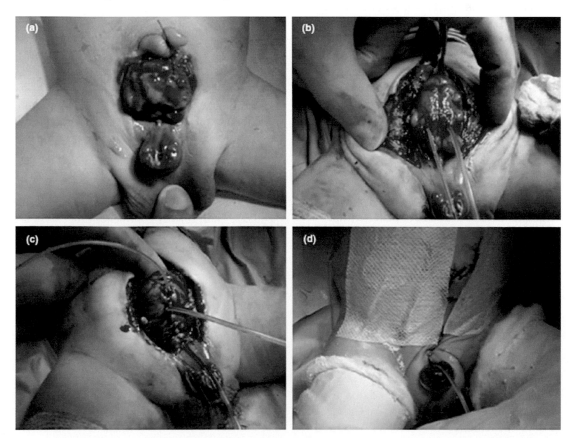

Figure 15.6 (a) Primary closure of a newborn male exstrophy. (b) Separation of the bladder plate. (c) Closure of bladder with ureteric catheters. (d) Appearance after abdominal wall closure with plaster cast (no longer used routinely).

pressure applied to the iliac crests will bring the soft tissues of the abdominal wall together in front of the bladder neck. However, this may not be sufficient to bring the pubic rami completely together in the midline. The pubic rami are approximated as far as possible by use of interrupted horizontal mattress sutures of heavy-gauge polydioxanone (PDS) and the rectus muscles are approximated with interrupted absorbable sutures. During the first few weeks of life it is nearly always possible to achieve successful primary closure without any requirement for pelvic fixation.

Feeding is recommenced postoperatively and oral prophylactic antifungal and antibiotic agents are continued. When all the catheters have been removed an ultrasound scan is performed prior to discharge from hospital to assess bladder emptying and the appearances of the upper tracts.

Complications (including wound breakdown and partial or complete bladder dehiscence) occur in around 10% of cases. Factors predisposing to wound infection and dehiscence include pooling of urine at the new urinary meatus, the use of stents emerging through the midline closure, and retention of the umbilical stump (a focus of potential infection). The risk of dehiscence is also increased by tissue ischaemia if the closure has been performed under tension. Partial dehiscence which does not involve exposure of the bladder can be allowed to heal by secondary intention. However, a more extensive dehiscence with exposure of the bladder plate or prolapse of the bladder will require re-closure, for which pelvic osteotomies are usually indicated.

In classic bladder exstrophy the ureters usually enter the bladder without the oblique transmural tunnel that would normally confer an anti reflux mechanism. For this reason, some degree of vesicoureteric reflux is almost invariably present following primary bladder closure. Any degree of outflow obstruction consequent upon tight urethral closure can pose a risk of upper tract dilatation and renal damage – particularly if infection supervenes. Close ultrasound surveillance is therefore essential to detect possible upper tract dilatation and if this does develop a period of intermittent catheterisation may be required.

Role of pelvic osteotomy

The pelvis in newborn exstrophy patients is sufficiently flexible to allow closure of the bladder without osteotomy in 95% of cases. But where the pubic diastasis is wide or when closure is delayed, pelvic osteotomy is usually required to increase pelvic mobility and facilitate a tension-free closure of the midline. The standard technique consists of division of the bony pelvis between the anterior superior iliac spine and the greater sciatic notch on both sides. The drawbacks include, prolonged operating time, increased blood loss and longer postoperative immobility. Osteotomy is best reserved for revision cases and the correction of cloacal exstrophy. Postoperative fixation of the bony pelvis in small infants can be effectively achieved by the use of frog-leg plasters and mermaid dressings but a period of external fixation is mandatory in older children because of the greater density of their pelvic bones.

Secondary Procedures for Continence and Genital Reconstruction

In girls, primary closure can occasionally be sufficient to impart continence and create a satisfactory cosmetic appearance without the need for further surgery. In the overwhelming majority of exstrophy patients, however, additional procedures will be required to achieve continence and to reconstruct functionally and cosmetically acceptable genitalia. Until further continence procedures are performed, the low bladder outlet resistance leads to dribbling incontinence. Although urinary tract infections are uncommon, some paediatric urologists prescribe prophylactic antibiotics.

Continence Surgery

There are three accepted surgical strategies for the management of bladder exstrophy.

Staged reconstruction

Popularised by Jeffs and Gearhart, this is a well-established standard approach (now termed the 'modern staged repair of bladder exstrophy') in which conventional bladder closure is performed in the neonatal period followed by correction of the epispadiac component at around 2 years of age and bladder neck reconstruction around the age of five. If continence is not achieved because of inadequate bladder capacity, further bladder neck reconstructions may be undertaken – possibly in conjunction with augmentation enterocystoplasty and a Mitrofanoff procedure.

Complete primary repair

This strategy was devised by Mitchell with the aim of creating continence by combining full anatomical reconstruction with the initial bladder closure. In addition to mobilisation of the exposed bladder and urethral plate the penile corpora are also extensively mobilised to facilitate complete penile reconstruction during the same operation. This approach has been reported to give good results whilst requiring fewer surgical procedures. However, the complete primary repair is a technically challenging operation in a newborn infant and it is of particular importance to safeguard the blood supply to the penis.

Kelly operation

This is the procedure of choice at Great Ormond Street Hospital for Children. After successful neonatal bladder closure, examination under anaesthetic to assess the bladder and bladder outlet is undertaken around 3 months later.

The Kelly operation is then performed from around the age of 6 months onwards. The bladder is reopened in the midline and both ureters are reimplanted using the Cohen technique. The soft tissues, including the urethra, penile corpora and pelvic floor, are then fully mobilised before reconstructing the bladder outlet, urethra, sphincter and penis. Detachment of the penile corpora from the lower border of the inferior pubic rami is combined with release of the pudendal pedicles, which lie beneath the pelvic floor muscles and run from the greater sciatic notch to the base of the penis in Alcock's canal. Once the base of the penis is freely mobile the two corporeal bodies can be brought together in the midline, thus eliminating the effect of the pubic diastasis and greatly increasing penile protrusion and apparent length

(Figure 15.7a). The urethral plate is dissected off the corpora and the glans and tubularised over an 8 Fr stent. The bladder neck is delineated at a level between the verumontanum and the ureteric orifices and mucosal triangles are then removed on either side. The bladder neck and bladder are then closed in sequence. The tubularised urethral plate is relocated between the penile corpora, to come to lie in hypospadiac position where the muscles at the base of the corpora are then wrapped around it with loose sutures in a position corresponding to the site of the physiological sphincter in normal males just below the veromontanum. The corporeal bodies are joined in the midline with external rotation to eliminate the dorsal chordee and to secure the position of the urethra below them with the new urinary meatus being sited on the ventral surface of the reconstructed penis. Abdominal wall closure can be combined with an umbilicoplasty if required. The Kelly procedure can be completed with either a glans plasty procedure to advance the urinary meatus on to the glans or, alternatively by two-stage distal urethral reconstruction (analogous to hypospadias repair), using posterior auricular skin grafts at some stage in the following 12 months.

In the senior author's experience, the Kelly operation provides a superior penile cosmetic outcome to the conventional staged repair (Figure 15.7b).

The Kelly procedure can also be performed in girls in whom the two components of the bifid clitoris are mobilised, with their pudendal pedicles being preserved and the labia minora remaining attached. Reconstruction of the bladder neck and urethra is undertaken in a similar fashion to males. The mobilised clitoral corpora are brought together in the midline to reconstruct the clitoris. Genital reconstruction can be successfully completed in a single stage in girls.

Continence Outcomes

Considerable controversy has surrounded the published continence rates following surgical reconstruction of bladder exstrophy. Published results vary considerably and continence rates as high as 70% have been claimed by some groups. Although the differences in reported continence rates can be partly explained by differing selection

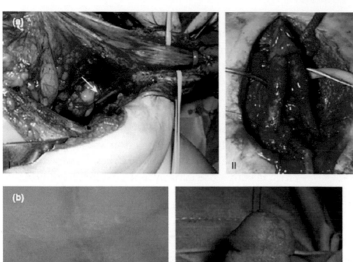

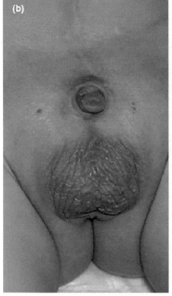
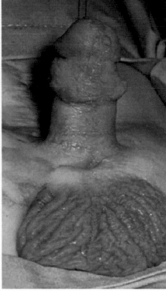

Figure 15.7 (a) The Kelly operation. (I) From the right of the patient, the penile corpora and urethral plate are dissected and the bladder is held to the left, the base of the corpus is separated from the pubis and moved medially, the pelvic floor has been released and the pudendal pedicle is seen (arrowed). (II) From below the penis, the urethra has now been detached, tubularised and brought between the mobile corpora; muscle is being wrapped around it. (b) Kelly operation: postoperative appearances.

criteria for surgery they also reflect the tendency for authors to assess their results according to their own definitions of what constitutes urinary continence. Moreover, authors do not always differentiate between continence with spontaneous voiding and continence (or dry intervals) in children being managed by clean intermittent catheterisation (CIC) following bladder augmentation.

Meaningful comparisons between surgical results and functional outcomes can only be obtained if a standardised definition of what constitutes 'continence' can be agreed and applied equally to all patients and treatment modalities. This does not exist at present. The senior author has proposed the simple grading system for continence which is illustrated in Table 15.2. Using this schema, the senior author has assessed the outcome of 101 patients (70 male and 31 female) operated between 1999 and 2014. Of these, 56 children were followed-up for at least 5 years

Table 15.2 Grading system for continence

Grade	Description
0	Dribbles urine all the time with no control
I	Able to retain urine with a 'dry interval'; some control but still wearing protection
II	Sufficient dry intervals by day; in underwear and not needing protection; wet at night
III	Dry by day and night; no protection or accidents; 'normal child'

and an additional 23 were followed-up over 10 years. In the cohort who had been followed-up for 10 years 81% of males achieved dryness by day (grade II) and 44% were dry at night (grade III). Overall, 13% of males required bladder augmentation surgery. Sixty-seven percent of females were dry by day (grade II) and 33% were dry by day and night (grade III). Bladder augmentation was required in 33% of females. Our experience indicates that the Kelly procedure provides a relatively predictable degree of outflow resistance and that continence is then dependent on the bladder's ability to increase its capacity in response to this enhanced outflow resistance. Persisting incontinence may be due either to inadequate outflow resistance and/or inadequate bladder capacity. Some degree of spontaneous improvement can usually be expected with further growth – particularly around puberty. In children with severe incontinence, however, it is usually necessary to perform a repeat bladder neck reconstruction in combination with ileocystoplasty and the formation of a Mitrofanoff catheterisable channel. Ideally this should be timed to enable the child to become continent by around the age of 6 years. Incontinence which is due to poor outlet resistance can sometimes be reduced by cystoscopic injection of a bulking agent such as Deflux (dextranomer/hyaluronic acid copolymer) into the region of the bladder outlet. If the incontinence persists despite this and similar measures the only remaining option may be surgical closure of the bladder neck.

Late Outcomes

Woodhouse has documented the late outcomes of reconstructive surgery in exstrophy patients and although some of the findings relate to outdated forms of surgical management, such as ureterosigmoidostomy, they nevertheless highlight the importance of long-term follow-up. Renal damage (due to a combination of lower tract obstruction, vesicoureteric reflux and urinary infection) was identified in 25% of patients. Follow-up data indicate that patients who achieve continence following a tight bladder neck procedure in childhood may be at increased risk of decompensation and detrusor failure in later adolescence. Intermittent catheterisation is indicated in such cases – either via the urethra or via a Mitrofanoff catheterisable conduit (which is usually accompanied by augmentation cystoplasty). Stone formation has been reported to occur in up to 25% of patients. The risk of malignancy in the reconstructed exstrophy bladder has been estimated to be in the region of 4% after 30 years of follow-up.

Males have normal sexual libido and 90% can achieve erections, although some require corrective surgery for severe persistent dorsal chordee. The majority can experience orgasm but may have slow or retrograde ejaculation due to abnormalities of the proximal urethra. Fertility is reduced, probably as a result of disruption of the ejaculatory ducts during bladder neck surgery or the consequences of episodes of epididymo-orchitis, which occur in up to one-third of men. The fertility rate in men with exstrophy is around 20%. However, recent studies of quality of life scores in relation to sexual function are comparable to the normal population.

For females, surgery to the introitus may be required to facilitate intercourse but the prospects for fertility are normal. Pregnancy is often complicated by vaginal prolapse although this may prove to be less problematic following contemporary surgical procedures. Delivery by caesarean section is recommended and it is prudent to have a urologist in attendance for patients who have previously undergone bladder augmentation.

Unfortunately, there are some exstrophy patients who have a history of multiple failed operations which is sometimes accompanied by loss of penile corpora and compromised renal function. For these patients, major and complex revisional surgery is required. (See also Chapter 24.)

CLOACAL EXSTROPHY

Initial Presentation and Management

Cloacal exstrophy is more likely to be diagnosed prenatally than bladder exstrophy because of the associated anomalies, which are listed in Table 15.3. Affected infants are frequently born

Table 15.3 Associated anomalies in cloacal exstrophy

Anomaly	Cases affected (%)
Renal anomalies	7
Ectopic kidney, agenesis, hydronephrosis	
Sacral agenesis	60
Spinal dysraphism	50
Myelomeningocoele, lipoma, tethered cord	
Orthopaedic deformity	40
Club foot, hip and pelvic deformity	
Small bowel defects	65
Malrotation, duodenal atresia, short gut	
Cyanotic heart disease	<10

prematurely and cloacal exstrophy may be only one of many problems. Primary closure is usually delayed, often for several months, while other medical conditions affecting the gastrointestinal tract and cardiorespiratory systems are evaluated and managed. Pending surgery, the exposed bladder/bowel plate is protected with plastic film and barrier creams are applied to the surrounding skin. In very low birth weight babies, enteral feeding is established with a target weight of 2.5–3 kg being set before closure is undertaken. If an exomphalos is present, this can usually be managed expectantly since it tends to contract spontaneously without the need for surgical intervention.

Preoperative evaluation includes ultrasound scans of the urinary tract and spinal cord. Iliac pelvic osteotomies are invariably required because of the delay in closure and the wider pelvic diastasis in these patients. Although osteotomies help to facilitate tension-free closure of the abdominal wall this may not be achievable if the abdominal contents cannot be accommodated within the abdominal cavity. In this situation, a plastic silo or mesh is attached over the upper abdomen to reduce tension and is then gradually reduced and removed over the following days. At operation, the bladder/bowel plate is dissected free from the skin and rectus muscles superolaterally and the abdominal cavity is entered. The proximal and distal loops joining the midline bowel plate are identified and separated from the two hemibladders. A tubularised distal hindgut tube is created, which is usually brought out in the left iliac fossa as an end colostomy (in preference to an incontinent anal canal). The hemibladders are joined and closed prior to reconstruction of the bladder outlet and proximal urethra (Figure 15.8).

Gender of Rearing

Historically, males with cloacal exstrophy were often assigned to female gender because of the severity of their genital anomaly and difficulty in reconstructing a functioning penis. This approach is no longer generally practised in the UK because of greater understanding of the role of hormonal

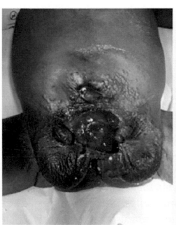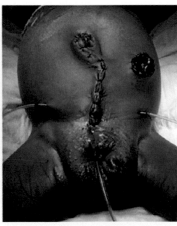

Figure 15.8 Male cloacal exstrophy, closed at three months. Osteotomies enable the bladder plates and hemiphalli to be brought together in the midline. In addition, there has been an end colostomy and umbilicoplasty.

factors responsible for male gender imprinting in intrauterine life.

Initial Outcomes

Although prematurity, severe cardiac anomalies and complications relating to short bowel and parenteral nutrition pose an increased risk of early mortality, the majority of affected newborns now survive into childhood. Careful surveillance of the upper urinary tracts is important in safeguarding long-term renal function. Magnetic resonance imaging (MRI) is used to assess the need for neurosurgical intervention for spinal dysraphism and orthopaedic input may also be required for the correction of any limb abnormalities. Colostomy complications occur in around 50% of patients and it is occasionally necessary to remove the reconstructed hindgut and replace it with an ileostomy.

Continence and Long-Term Outcomes

The combination of exstrophy and neuropathic dysfunction inevitably means that all patients will require enterocystoplasty if they are to achieve continence and storage of urine at safe pressures. Augmentation of the bladder may be difficult if only a short length of small bowel is available and there is no usable appendix. Nevertheless, most children can be successfully managed with ileocystoplasty and Mitrofanoff or Monti procedure. If there is insufficient small intestine, the alternatives for augmentation include a patch of stomach or a hindgut segment. The more complex forms of reconstruction carry the highest risk of failure and any coexisting renal insufficiency will also contribute to greater overall morbidity.

Some individuals with severe forms of cloacal exstrophy will suffer lifelong urinary incontinence regardless of advances in reconstructive surgery. Although male infants are now almost invariably assigned male gender at birth they may be destined to encounter serious difficulties relating to sexual function in adulthood. Moreover, the combination of reduced penile size and surgical damage to vasa deferentia and ejaculatory mechanisms result in high rates of infertility.

Presentation

Primary epispadias is rarely identified prenatally but is usually detected at birth. In milder (glanular) forms of the anomaly, however, the prepuce is intact and the condition may not become apparent until the prepuce becomes retractile.

In girls, the diagnosis of primary epispadias is often considerably delayed because most junior paediatricians are unaware of this rare anomaly and fail to identify it on routine neonatal examination. The classic presentation is with a history of dribbling or stress incontinence and failed toilet training. The diagnosis is readily apparent when examination is undertaken by someone with knowledge of the appearances of the genitalia in this condition (Figure 15.5).

Management

Males

The widely used Cantwell–Ransley epispadias repair can be performed in the first year of life. In this operation the exposed urethral plate is left attached distally to the glans but the entire length of the exposed urethral plate is otherwise mobilised from the penile corporeal bodies before being tubularised and relocated to lie in a ventral position inferior to the corpora. Approximation of the two corpora in the midline then has the effect of eliminating the dorsal curvature (chordee) of the penis. A Heineke–Mikulicz type glans plasty procedure is performed at the distal end of the tubularised urethral plate to create a more ventrally located meatus.

For patients with good penile length this operation is usually successful in creating a terminal urethral orifice and achieving a satisfactory cosmetic outcome. Where the penis is smaller, the phallus may appear shorter with a rather buried appearance. In these patients, penile mobilisation provided by the Kelly operation enables its length to be enhanced, particularly if there is a pubic diastasis.

Epispadias is commonly associated with incontinence due to sphincter weakness and deficiency of the bladder neck. Although it is not possible to reliably assess continence in infants who are still in nappies, some indication can be provided by the penile anatomy (severity of epispadias) and the cystoscopic findings. The Cantwell–Ransley repair is indicated in boys with more distal epispadias if the penis is of good size, the verumontanum is distal to the bladder neck and they appear to void without dribbling. For those with more severe primary epispadias the Kelly procedure is more appropriate. The technical aspects are the same as those employed in bladder exstrophy.

Outcome

The long-term outcome for sexual function is usually good with normal fertility unless there have been urethral complications or epididymo-orchitis. However, ejaculation may be slow or even retrograde. Patients who have only undergone penile reconstruction (the majority) will require additional bladder neck/sphincter surgery if their continence is impaired. Injection of a bulking agent into the bladder neck may improve continence in the short term but the benefit is not sustained. The surgical options then comprise a bladder neck repair or implantation of an artificial urinary sphincter. In some patients it may be necessary to progress to bladder augmentation and a Mitrofanoff conduit. Although the Kelly operation offers enhanced penile length, it remains unclear whether the sphincteric reconstruction included in the procedure will lead to improved continence in due course.

Girls

Since the majority of girls with epispadias are incontinent, reconstructive surgery must be directed at treating the incontinence as well as correcting the genital abnormality. Good results have been reported following distal urethral reconstruction, but more proximal bladder neck surgery may also be required. The Kelly procedure offers the prospect of a favourable prognosis for continence combined with a satisfactory external cosmetic outcome. There should be a few implications for sexual function or fertility.

Other Bladder Disorders

Bladder diverticulum

A diverticulum is an outpouching or 'herniation' of the bladder lining, which protrudes through the bladder wall into the peri vesical space. Diverticula can be classified as primary or secondary. **Primary bladder diverticula** are congenital abnormalities of the bladder, which occur mainly in boys. Connective tissue disorders such as Ehlers Danlos syndrome and Menke's syndrome are also associated with bladder diverticula – as is Williams syndrome. Primary paraureteric diverticula are located adjacent to a ureteric orifice and may be accompanied by VUR. **Secondary bladder diverticula** of varying size develop as a consequence of exposure of the bladder wall to grossly elevated intravesical pressure. Small diverticula are termed 'saccules'. Conditions giving rise to severe outflow obstruction, such as posterior urethral valves, syringocele and urethral strictures are often accompanied by secondary diverticula – as are functional bladder disorders causing grossly elevated intravesical pressure, such as neuropathic bladder and severe dysfunctional voiding with detrusor-sphincter dyssynergia (Hinman syndrome).

Diagnosis

Small, secondary diverticula are generally identified as asymptomatic findings on bladder ultrasound or MCUG during routine evaluation of urological conditions, such as posterior urethral valves. Primary diverticula are usually diagnosed when they are identified on an ultrasound scan performed during initial investigation of children (mainly boys) presenting with voiding symptoms or urinary tract infection.

Management

Secondary diverticula rarely require treatment and tend to resolve or reduce in size after appropriate treatment of outflow obstruction or bladder dysfunction. By contrast, surgical intervention is often indicated for large congenital primary diverticula, particularly when they are located in the region of the bladder neck and give rise to obstructed voiding. Diverticulectomy is also indicated for a large diverticulum with a narrow communication to the bladder lumen in which stasis of urine poses a risk of infection, stone formation and possible late malignancy. Surgery (which can be performed by either an open or laparoscopic approach) consists of removing the diverticulum and repairing the defect in the bladder wall.

Urachal Anomalies

The urachus (communication between the bladder and amniotic cavity) normally closes around the 12th week of gestation to leave a fibrous cord (median umbilical ligament).

A number of abnormalities can result from incomplete or aberrant closure.

In around 10% of cases, the urachus remains open along its entire length to constitute a **patent urachus**. This may occur in conjunction with congenital abnormalities of the bladder, such as prune-belly syndrome or as an isolated anomaly. Typically, a patent urachus presents in the neonatal period with oozing of clear fluid from the umbilicus or periumbilical infection and/or granulation tissue.

Urachal sinus accounts for approximately 50% of cases. In this variant, the portion of urachus that was connected to the bladder closes normally but the rest of the urachus remains patent and in communication with the umbilicus. Presenting features may include; purulent umbilical discharge, fever, lower abdominal pain and tenderness.

Urachal cysts account for approximately 30% of cases. Both ends of the urachus close normally but a central section remains patent to leave an isolated, non-communicating cystic cavity. Urachal cysts present at a later stage in childhood than other urachal abnormalities – typically as a lower abdominal mass, which may be complicated by infection. Very rarely a blind-ending length of patent urachus remains in communication with the bladder to create a non-obstructive diverticulum, which is discovered as an incidental finding on an ultrasound scan or micturating cystourethrogram (MCUG).

Investigation and management

Depending on the presentation, this may involve ultrasound, MCUG and magnetic resonance imaging (MRI). Additional contrast studies (sinography) may also be required to delineate the anatomy. Management is aimed initially at treating any infection with antibiotics and surgical drainage if necessary. Once infection has been eradicated and the anatomy has been established, treatment usually consists of surgical excision. Asymptomatic cysts should also be excised because of the documented long-term risk of adenocarcinoma.

KEY POINTS

- The exstrophy–epispadias complex encompasses a group of rare anomalies, which occur more commonly in males.
- Cloacal exstrophy is usually detected antenatally, as are more than half of all cases of bladder exstrophy. Epispadias, however, is almost invariably diagnosed at birth.
- Most infants with uncomplicated or classic bladder exstrophy are otherwise healthy, and surgical correction can be undertaken safely within the first few days or weeks of life. The cosmetic and functional results obtained with the one-stage Kelly operation may prove to be superior to those achieved with conventional staged repair.
- Late morbidity is common in exstrophy patients and may include incontinence, sexual dysfunction and renal impairment. It is hoped that newer techniques will offer better long-term results.
- Cloacal exstrophy is often associated with prematurity or other medical problems, which take priority over early surgical correction. Reconstruction presents a formidable challenge. Although it is usually possible to create a urinary reservoir, most patients are left with a permanent

colostomy. It may be necessary to consider gender reassignment in severely affected males.

- Primary epispadias is commonly associated with incontinence due to deficiency of the bladder neck and sphincter complex.

FURTHER READING

Gearhart J P, Jeffs RD. Exstrophy–epispadias complex and bladder anomalies. In: Walsh PC, Retik AB, Vaughan ED, Wein AJ (eds), Campbell's Textbook of Urology, 7th Edition. Philadelphia: WB Saunders, 1998: 1939–1990.

Kelly JH, Eraklis AJ. A procedure for lengthening the phallus in boys with exstrophy of the bladder. J Pediatr Surg. 1971;6:645–649.

Siffel C, Correa A, Amar E, et al. Bladder exstrophy: an epidemiologic study from the international clearinghouse for birth defects surveillance and research and an overview of the literature. Am J Med Genet C Semin Med Genet. 2011;0(4):321–332.

Woodhouse CRJ. Exstrophy and epispadias. In: Long-Term Paediatric Urology. London: Blackwell, 1991:127–150.

Woodhouse CRJ. Genitoplasty in exstrophy and epispadias. In: Stringer MD, Oldham KT, Mouriquand PDE (eds), Paediatric Surgery and Urology: Long-Term Outcomes. Cambridge: Cambridge University Press, 2006:583–594.

Hypospadias

NADIA V HALSTEAD, PIERRE D E MOURIQUAND and DUNCAN T WILCOX

Topics covered

INTRODUCTION

Hypospadias is an association of three anatomical anomalies:

- an abnormal ventral opening of the urethral meatus;
- ventral curvature (chordee) of the penis;
- a dorsal hooded foreskin with ventral deficiency.

However, not all three of these features are present in every case.

Hypospadias is better defined as a hypoplasia of the tissues forming the ventral aspect of the penis beyond the division of the corpus spongiosum. It is characterized by a ventral triangular defect whose apex is the division of the corpus spongiosum; the sides are represented by the two pillars of atretic spongiosum and the base is the glans.

ETIOLOGY AND INCIDENCE

The incidence of hypospadias is generally quoted at 1 in 300 live male births (0.33%). However, data from different countries show considerable variation, with reported incidences ranging from 0.006–0.7% in Asia to 0.2% in Europe to 0.34% in North America. Hypospadias appears to be increasing in frequency. The apparent increase in the incidence of hypospadias, coupled with the increasing incidence of testicular cancer and declining semen quality, have been cited as examples of the possible impact of estrogenic environmental pollutants ("endocrine disruptors") on normal virilization of the male fetus. Phthalates, phytoestrogens (found in soy), and mycoestrogens have been identified as some of the environmental pollutants associated with hypospadias. In addition, endocrinopathy, low birth weight, maternal hypertension, maternal vegetarianism, conception via intracervical semination and in vitro fertilization, and advanced maternal age (possibly mediated by placental insufficiency) have been identified by some studies as possible etiological factors.

GENETICS

By contrast to the uncertainty surrounding the extent of the role played by environmental factors, the importance of genetic factors has been reliably documented in numerous studies. The incidence of hypospadias in first degree relatives is of the order of 7–10%, rising to 20% in the siblings of boys with severe hypospadias. There is also an association with certain genetic syndromes including WAGR, Denys-Drash, and Opitz. However, genetic factors apply mainly to the more severe forms of proximal hypospadias whereas distal forms are more likely to occur as sporadic (non-inherited) anomalies. Defects in genes expressed during development of the genital tubercle and urethral plate have been implicated in the etiology of hypospadias. These include SHH, GL1, GL2, GL3, FGF8, FGFR2, WT1, BMP 7, WNT5A, and DGKK. Mutations in homeobox genes (HOXA13, HOXA4, IRX5, IRX6), genes involved in androgen production and signaling (HSD3B1, HSD17B3, SRD5A2, AR), and estrogen production and signaling (ESR1, ESR2, ATF3, VAMP7) have also been identified in some patients and have also been studied experimentally in "knock out" mouse models.

DISORDERS OF SEX DEVELOPMENT (DSD) AND ASSOCIATED ANOMALIES

Severe forms of hypospadias can present with similar appearances to disorders of sex development (DSDs), especially when severe hypospadias is associated with undescended testes and a prostatic utricle. In some series, up to 50% of patients with both hypospadias and cryptorchidism have been found to have an underlying genetic, gonadal, or phenotypic sexual abnormality. It is essential that all patients with hypospadias who have undescended testes are fully investigated so that DSD can be excluded. Apart from an increased overall incidence of undescended testis, other anomalies in patients with isolated hypospadias are rare. Abnormalities of the urinary tract are uncommon, occurring in approximately 2% of patients. For this reason, routine ultrasound screening is unnecessary. The overall incidence of undescended testis is in the range 5–10%, rising to 50% in those with severe perineal or penoscrotal forms of hypospadias. These severe forms are also associated with a persistent prostatic utricle in 20% of cases. When this is present it can create difficulties with urethral catheterization of the bladder. But since it is rarely necessary to remove a prostatic utricle, cystography, or cystoscopy to look for a possible utricle are not routinely required and need only be performed if the child is symptomatic.

CLASSIFICATION

Although many classifications have been described based on the position of the ectopic urethral meatus (Figure 16.1), the level of division of the corpus spongiosum may provide a more accurate means of distinguishing anterior hypospadias with little or no chordee from posterior hypospadias with chordee and hypoplasia of the tissues forming the ventral aspect of the penis (Figure 16.2). In approximately 70% of cases, the urethral meatus is located on, or adjacent to, the glans or on the distal penile shaft. In the remaining 30% of cases, the meatus is more proximal (midshaft to perineal) and the anatomy is more complex.

The authors' classification, therefore, recognizes three main types of hypospadias.

1. Hypospadias with a distal division of the corpus spongiosum with little or no chordee.
2. Hypospadias with a proximal division of the corpus spongiosum with a marked degree of hypoplasia of the ventral tissue and a significant degree of chordee.

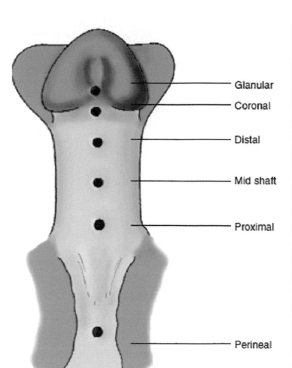

Figure 16.1 Standard classification of hypospadias.

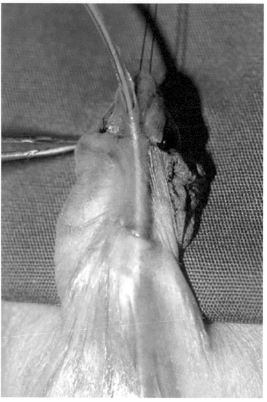

Figure 16.2 Deceptively severe case illustrating the potential pitfalls of classification based on the position of the urethral meatus. The urethra terminates with an opening on the glans but the entire urethra is "paper thin" and this case is, in effect, a proximal form of hypospadias with chordee.

3. Hypospadias which persists despite multiple previous operations. (Patients with this condition were previously termed "hypospadias cripples").

SPECIFIC SURGICAL PRINCIPLES

Although more than 300 different techniques have been described for the repair of hypospadias, the last decade has seen the emergence of a growing consensus amongst specialist hypospadias surgeons. For most patients this comprises either tubularization of the urethral plate or a two-stage repair – usually involving a free flap. This chapter will concentrate on these two techniques, but other methods that are still in current use will also be described.

Regardless of the repair, there are three specific components to the surgical correction of hypospadias:

- Correction of the penile chordee
- Reconstruction of the urethra (urethroplasty)

- Skin coverage of the penis aimed at achieving a normal cosmetic appearance

In general, surgical correction is recommended between 6 months and 18 months of age with the aim of achieving an optimal cosmetic and functional outcome.

Correction of Penile Chordee

Penile chordee can result from several factors including ; abnormal tethering of the penile shaft skin on to the underlying structures, tethering of the urethral plate to the corpora cavernosa or atretic corpora spongiosum tissue extending

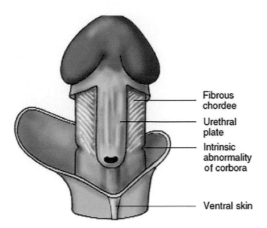

Figure 16.3 Causes of penile curvature associated with hypospadias.

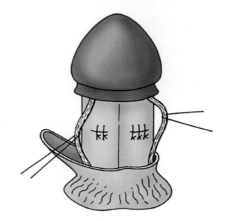

Figure 16.4 Correction of intrinsic chordee by plication on the dorsal aspect of the corpora, following mobilization of the overlying neurovascular bundles.

from the abnormal meatus to the glans. Finally, chordee may be due to an intrinsic flexion deformity of the corpora cavernosa (Figure 16.3). Correction of penile chordee should be addressed in the following order:

1. Degloving the penis by fully mobilizing the overlying skin. In most patients (80%), this will correct the chordee.
2. Excision of the atretic and fibrous corpora spongiosum proximally and distally to the abnormal meatus.
3. Dissection of the urethral plate, which is carefully elevated off the corpora cavernosa. (Not all surgeons perform this step, opting instead to go straight to a dorsal plication.)

In some patients ventral curvature of the penis persists despite these steps, in which case it is necessary to plicate the dorsal aspect of the tunica albuginea (Figure 16.4). Unfortunately, despite dorsal plication there is a tendency for ventral curvature to recur at puberty. If dorsal plication is insufficient to correct the degree of ventral curvature or where the surgeon's preference dictates, a more extensive corporal procedure (corporoplasty) may be indicated.

Urethroplasty

Reconstruction of the urethra can be performed in a single stage or in a two-stage procedure.

Generally, a single-stage repair is appropriate for distal, mid shaft, and proximal hypospadias without significant chordee. A two-stage repair is generally reserved for severe proximal or perineal hypospadias with chordee and for "hypospadias cripples." Most surgeons now perform tubularization of the urethral plate as their preferred one-stage method.

Tubularizing the urethral plate (Figure 16.5)

The most widely used single-stage repair is a Duplay-type tubularization incorporating a vertical incision in the urethral plate, as described by Snodgrass. This allows the urethral plate to be tubularized without tension. In addition, it has been asserted that epithelialization of the urethral plate incision may contribute to the circumference of the neourethra.

In this procedure, the urethral plate is marked and then deeply incised (Figure 16.5a, b); its width is then assessed. The urethral plate is incised and then rolled into a tube (Figure 16.5d). Some surgeons favor a modification in which a free graft of preputial skin is inlaid into the incision in the urethral plate in the hope of reducing the risk of contraction and stenosis of the neourethra (Figure 16.5b, c). If the urethral plate is wide and sufficiently supple to be tubularized

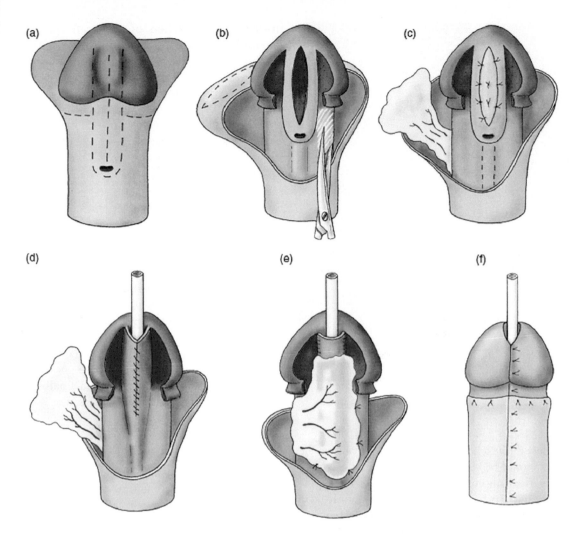

Figure 16.5 **(a)–(f)** Key steps in tubularized incised plate (Snodgrass) repair (see text for explanation).

over an 8 Fr catheter, it can be rolled into a tube without the need for a urethral plate incision (Duplay procedure) (Once the neourethra is formed, a vascularized de-epithelialized pedicle of tissue is placed over the anastomosis to reduce fistula formation (Figure 16.5d, e). The glanuloplasty is performed by reapproximating the glans wings in two layers. The skin is then reconfigured, ensuring that there is adequate coverage on the ventral surface so that penile chordee does not recur (Figure 16.5f). A dripping stent can be left draining for 7 days. The authors have found that a stent is rarely needed in children under 12 months of age.

Two-stage repair (Figures 16.6 and 16.7)

The type of severe hypospadias for which a two stage repair is most appropriate is illustrated in Figure 16.6.

The first stage of the operation involves correcting the chordee as described above (Figure 16.7a, b) followed by preparing the glans and harvesting the free flap (Figure 16.7c). Once the chordee has been corrected, a midline ventral incision is made from the most dorsal part of the new meatus on the glans to the current meatus. Glans wings are created so that the glans opens

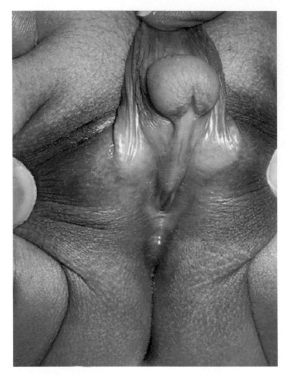

Figure 16.6 Severe proximal hypospadias – unsuited to single-stage repair.

widely ("like a book"). The ideal material for the flap should be easy to harvest, without leaving a long-standing cosmetic defect. It should be supple and non-hair bearing. The most commonly used graft material is inner preputial skin. However, postauricular Wolfe skin grafts can also be used for primary repair. Buccal mucosa and bladder mucosa are less frequently used for standard two-stage repairs but do have a role in "salvage" hypospadias repairs.

When the donor graft has been taken, the fat and subepithelial tissue are removed to enhance graft revascularization (Figure 16.7c). The graft is then placed into the glans and tacked with absorbable sutures; "windows" are made in the graft to allow hematomas to escape and a few midline quilting sutures are placed to anchor the graft to on its base (Figure 16.7d, e). A firm dressing is applied, with a catheter, which holds the graft in place and minimizes hematoma formation. After 1 week the dressing and catheter are removed. The second stage of the repair is usually performed after 6 months. This step

involves tubularization of the graft into the neourethra (Figure 16.7f, g) and then placing a second vascularized layer over the anastomosis (Figure 16.7h). Once this is completed the glans is reconstructed and the penile skin closed (Figure 16.7i).

Other techniques which are still in current usage are described below.

Urethral repositioning

The MAGPI procedure (Figure 16.8) is an acronym of "meatal advancement and glanuloplasty incorporated". It is only suitable for cases in which the urethra is mobile – which can be confirmed if simple traction can move the meatus to the tip of the glans. A vertical incision between the tip of the glans and the meatus is created (Figure 16.8a, b) and then closed transversely, thereby advancing the meatus. A circumferential incision is made in the skin below the corona and the meatus. The glanuloplasty is then performed in two layers (Figure 16.8c, d), and finally the penis is circumcised and the skin closed.

Pedicle flaps

Two types of pedicle flap are commonly used, the meatal-based flap and the preputial flap. Both procedures utilize skin flaps which remain attached at some point to the urethral plate.

Meatal-based flap (Mathieu procedure) (Figure 16.9)

The urethral plate is incised (Figure 16.9a) and the glans flaps developed. A vascularized flap of proximal penile skin is created using the meatus as the base (Figure 16.9b). The flap is then placed on to the urethral plate and both lateral edges are sutured to it. Adjacent subcutaneous tissue is used to cover ("waterproof") the suture line (Figure 16.9c). Once the neourethra is created, the glanuloplasty is performed (Figure 16.9d). As a rule, the maximum length of this flap should be no more than three times the width of the base and in practice, this technique is unsuited for a urethroplasty exceeding 1.5 cm.

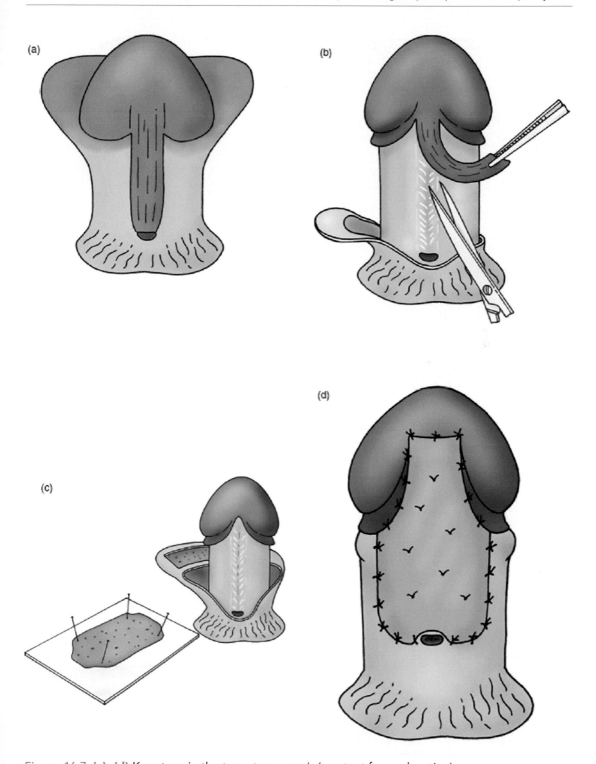

Figure 16.7 (a)–(d) Key steps in the two-stage repair (see text for explanation).

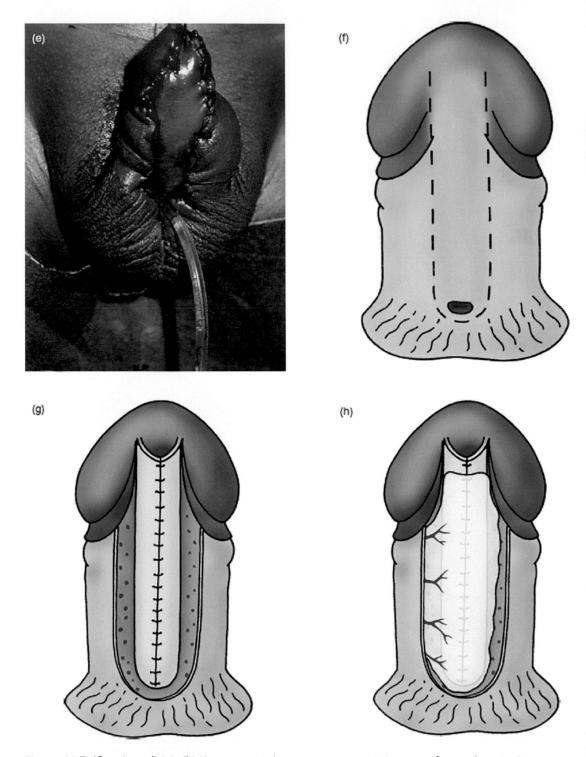

Figure 16.7 (Continued) (e)–(h) Key steps in the two-stage repair (see text for explanation).

(i)

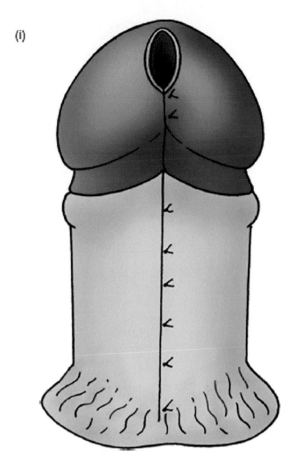

Figure 16.7 (Continued) **(i)** Key steps in the two-stage repair (see text for explanation).

Preputial flap (onlay island flap procedure) (Figure 16.10)

The urethral plate is incised vertically using two parallel incisions. The penis is then degloved back to its base using a circumferential subcoronal incision. The glans flaps are then created and the proximal thin urethra is cut back until normal urethral tissue is found. A pedicle flap is then created out of the inner prepuce, as shown in Figure 16.10a. The preputial flap is brought around the side of the penis to its ventral surface and sutured to the urethral plate (Figure 16.10b, c). Once the neourethra has been created, the subcutaneous pedicle is anchored to the tunica albuginea lateral to the urethral anastomosis (Figure 16.10d). Occasionally, it is necessary to divide the urethral plate in order to correct the chordee. In these rare cases, the preputial flap can be tubularized, thereby creating the neourethra alone. The lateral glans wings are then approximated in two layers to recreate the glans, and the skin is closed (Figure 16.10e).

The Koyanagi procedure and its variants are alternative procedures for severe proximal hypospadias. It aims at using the urethral plate and the neighboring strip of ventral tissues along with the inner aspect of the preputial hood, which is transferred ventrally with its pedicle. This large and well-vascularized material is freed from the ventral aspect of the corpus spongiosum down to the base of the penis. This allows the penis to straighten and to build an extended plate, which is subsequently tubularized.

Covering the Penis

When the urethra has been reconstructed, it is necessary to recreate the meatus, glans, and occasionally the foreskin. Glanuloplasty is performed by bringing the two wings of the glans around to cover the urethra; the glans is then closed in two layers. The distal end of the neourethra is sutured to the new meatus, thereby creating a slit-like opening. The residual inner preputial skin adjacent to the coronal sulcus is brought around the ventral side of the penis to create a circumferential mucosal "cuff" or "collar" surrounding the glans. If parental preference is for preservation of the foreskin, a prepucioplasty may also be performed to construct a foreskin. Skin coverage is provided by moving the excess skin from the dorsal side to the ventral side. There are no significant differences in complication or revision rates when comparing hypospadias repair with circumcision or prepucioplasty.

Common Variants of Hypospadias

Chordee without hypospadias (Figure 16.11)

In most cases this is a misnomer since they do in fact represent a form of hypospadias in which the distal penile urethra is flimsy, despite the presence

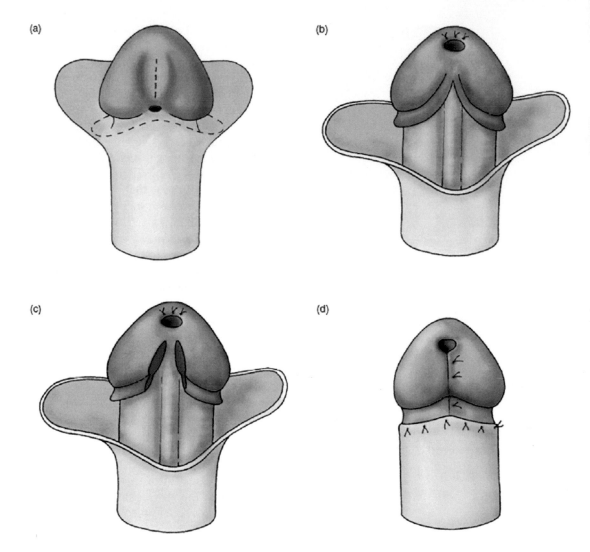

Figure 16.8 Urethral repositioning, key steps in the MAGPI repair (see text for explanation).

of a glanular meatus and circumferential prepuce. It may be possible to achieve good correction by degloving the shaft and excising chordee tissue while preserving an intact urethra. However, this may not be possible if the urethra is flimsy and cannot be preserved intact. In such cases it is necessary to excise the abnormal urethral tissue back to healthy spongiosum-supported urethra and proceed to perform a urethroplasty as if it were the corresponding degree of true hypospadias.

Megameatus intact prepuce (Figure 16.12)

Because there is no external clue to the presence of this variant it sometimes comes to light for the first time in a boy who is about to undergo circumcision for cultural or medical reasons. In this situation a planned cultural circumcision should be completed. If the circumcision is being performed for medical reasons the

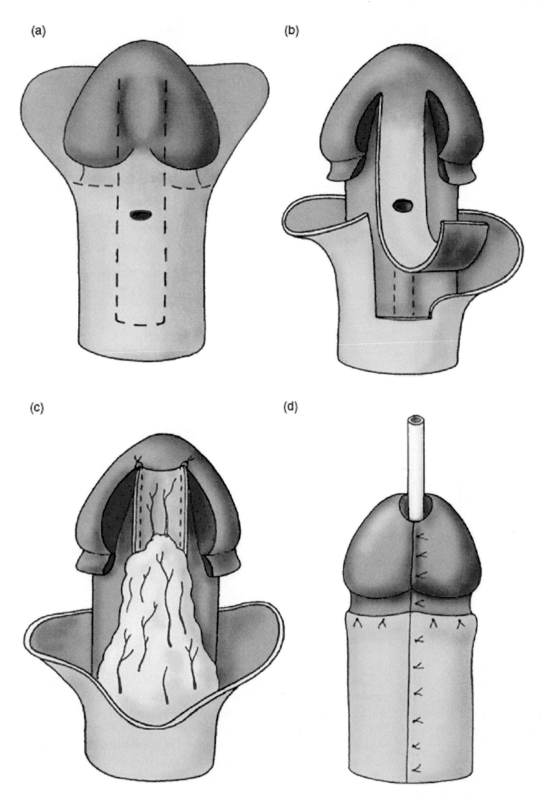

Figure 16.9 Key steps in the perimeatal-based flap (Mathieu) repair (see text for explanation).

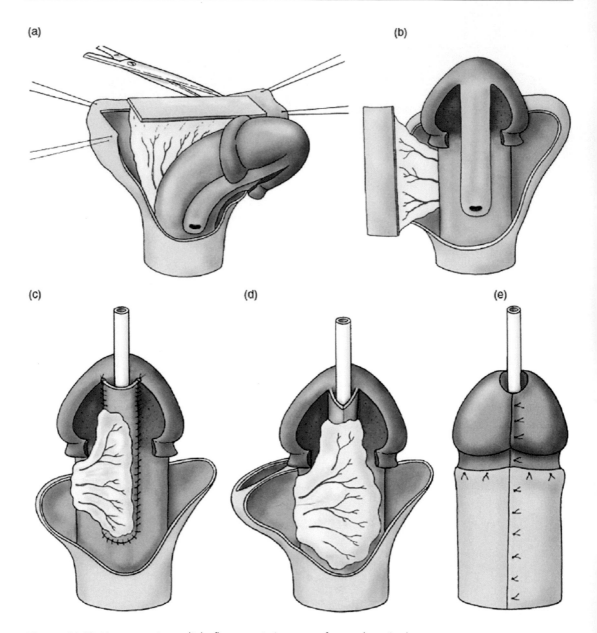

(a)

(b)

(c)

(d)

(e)

Figure 16.10 **Key steps in pedicle flap repair (see text for explanation).**

surgeon should ideally explain the findings to the parents and seek their guidance before proceeding. If the parents opt for surgical correction of the glanular defect, referral to a specialist is advisable.

"Salvage" or "redo" surgery often calls for ingenuity and familiarity with a number of different techniques. Where the neourethra is largely intact and the surrounding skin is healthy, a procedure using locally available skin may suffice, but where there is extensive scarring and, particularly in the presence of residual chordee, it is usually preferable to abandon the unhealthy existing neourethra and perform a substitution procedure with an onlay or tubularized free graft. Postauricular skin is suitable, but buccal mucosa, harvested from the lower lip (Figure 16.13) or cheek, is more widely used for this purpose.

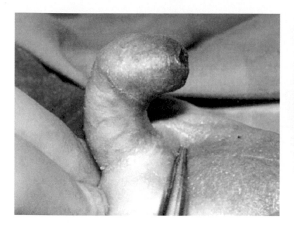

Figure 16.11 Chordee without hypospadias.

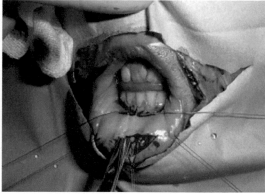

Figure 16.13 Buccal mucosa graft – site on buccal aspect of the lower lip marked out prior to harvesting of the buccal skin graft for salvage repair.

GENERAL SURGICAL PRINCIPLES

Magnification

Most surgeons now use standard operating loupes, which are easy to use and provide magnification in the range 2.5–4.5×.

Hormone Administration

Anatomic factors such as glans width and development of the urethral plate have been shown to correlate with surgical outcomes with a glans width ≤14 mm being associated with an increased risk of complications. Some surgeons administer

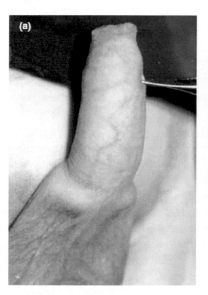

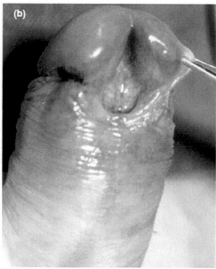

Figure 16.12 Megameatus intact prepuce variant (a) normal external appearances before the prepuce is retracted, (b) glanular anomaly revealed by retraction of the prepuce, deep glans groove with "fish mouth" megameatus.

preoperative testosterone to increase penile length, glans circumference, and tissue vascularity. However, due to paucity of literature and insufficient evidence, we do not advocate its use.

Sutures

The suture material should be fine gauge, absorbable, and easy to use. We currently prefer 7-0 or 6-0 polydioxanone (PDS): these fine absorbable monofilament sutures provide excellent strength and are absorbed before suture tracts are formed.

Hemostasis

A bloodless operating field is essential for hypospadias surgery. It can be achieved by using one of the three following techniques:

- A tourniquet at the base of the penis. Care must be taken not to leave the tourniquet for too long because of the theoretical risk of reperfusion injury.
- Adrenaline 1:100 000 can be used, up to a maximum dose of 10 mg/kg. Although there is a theoretical risk that excessive vasoconstriction might compromise the vascularity of skin flaps, there is no evidence that this occurs in practice.
- Bipolar diathermy is generally preferred, but the safe use of modern monopolar diathermy has been described. Diathermy may be inadequate to control bleeding from the glans. It is currently our policy to use a tourniquet followed by a compressive dressing at the end of the operation.

Antibiotics

Practice varies with respect to the use of prophylactic antibiotics. Whilst some surgeons do not routinely use any covering antibiotic, others favor a course of prophylactic antibiotic for the period while the catheter or stent is in situ. Recent published evidence suggests that prophylactic antibiotic coverage may be unnecessary.

Urinary Drainage

The indications for postoperative urinary diversion depend upon the type of reconstruction and patient's age. No stent is necessary in many infants under 12 months of age undergoing surgery for distal hypospadias. Stenting can also be avoided after the most minor type of repair.

In general, however, postoperative drainage takes the form of a 6–8 Fr dripping stent. Use of a standard Foley indwelling urinary catheter carries the concern that the deflated balloon might distend or disrupt the delicate suture lines of the anastomosis when the catheter is being withdrawn.

Dressing

The dressing serves many purposes, which ideally include gentle compression of the penis to reduce hemorrhage and edema, immobilization, protecting the penis from contact and reducing postoperative pain. Many dressings are available and are subject to preference of the surgeon. The dressings stay in place for between 2 and 7 days, depending on the complexity of the repair.

OUTCOME

The results of hypospadias repair reflect the severity of the original defect and the type of operation performed.

Tubularization of the Urethral Plate

The technique of tubularization, as originally described by Duplay, has an overall secondary operation rate of around 10%, principally for urethral fistula. It has the advantage of creating a slit-like meatus, with a more normal and acceptable cosmetic appearance. The functional and cosmetic outcomes following the Snodgrass repair (tubularized incised plate, TIP) appear to be at least as good. Re-operation rates following correction of distal hypospadias are approximately 5%

but rise to 50% for proximal hypospadias and 23% following secondary repairs. Urethrocutaneous fistula is the commonest complication but the incidence can be significantly reduced with technical modifications such as the use of "waterproofing" flaps and two layer closure. Concerns have been expressed about the potential long-term risk of stenosis as a consequence of scarring and contraction in the incised portion of the urethral plate. However, emerging long-term data indicate that although urinary flow rates may be somewhat reduced, clinically significant stenosis is relatively rare and only a small percentage of patients will require dilatation.

Two-Stage Repair

Bracka has reviewed his personal series of 600 patients managed by two-stage repair. In the majority of cases the neourethra had been fashioned from a free graft derived from inner preputial skin. The first-stage operation required revision in 4% of patients for persistent chordee or to increase the area of meatal skin. The overall fistula rate following the second procedure was 6%, with "redo" or "salvage" repairs having a higher fistula rate of 10% (compared with 3% for primary procedures). A higher fistula rate was encountered in patients operated on in the earlier part of the series before the use of a vascularized dartos flap between neourethra and the skin to "waterproof" the suture line. Urethral stenosis occurred in 7% of patients. This figure was attributable, in part, to balanitis xerotica obliterans. Long-term functional outcomes in patients following a two-stage repair have recently been reported by a number of centers. Up to 40% of patients report spraying of the urinary stream and some described having to "milk" the penis following voiding to empty the neourethra to avoid postvoid dribbling. In one study of the functional outcome in 43 adults following reconstruction with buccal mucosal grafts, seven (16%) had urinary symptoms, of whom two had experienced severe urinary symptoms. In all, 26% of patients described problems with urinary spraying. This technique does, however, give an excellent cosmetic result.

Urethral Advancement

Duckett reported his experience with the MAGPI procedure for the correction of glanular hypospadias in his series of over 1000 patients. Of these, only 1.2% required a secondary procedure. Partial meatal regression is, however, a relatively common problem with this procedure and leads to an inferior cosmetic result.

Pedicle Flaps

In the Mathieu repair distal strictures are rare (1%) and fistulae occur in approximately 4% of cases. However, the meatus is often crescentic in appearance, giving a poor cosmetic result. Wide glans mobilization and a midline dorsal incision of the urethral plate may reduce this problem.

Preputial Flaps

This method of repair is often reserved for the more complex cases of hypospadias: consequently, the rate of complications is higher. There is wide variability in the published fistula rate, from 4% to 69%.

Psychosexual Outcome

Sexual function following successful hypospadias correction should be unaffected, with normal erectile function and normal prospects of fertility, providing the patient does not have coexisting undescended testes. Studies have found that the majority of men (80%) report satisfactory sexual function, but they may be more apprehensive to seek out sexual contact. The literature on long-term psychosocial and psychosexual outcome of men who have undergone hypospadias surgery is generally reassuring, with >70% satisfied with the cosmetic appearance. However, this figure is reduced by comparison with normal controls. There are only very limited data comparing psychosexual outcomes of men who had undergone correction of their hypospadias in childhood with men whose hypospadias remained uncorrected.

Men who had no recollection of their surgery had an improved body image and greater satisfaction with their overall appearance when compared with men who could remember having undergone hypospadias surgery. Awareness of the genitals may begin at 18 months, which is why surgical correction is generally recommended before this age.

COMPLICATIONS

Distal hypospadias repair has a quoted complication rate ranging from 5–10%. By contrast, complication rates following surgery for proximal hypospadias can range from 15% to as high as 90%. Even in high volume centers treating large numbers of hypospadias patients this statistic holds true. For example, a recent study published from the Children's Hospital of Philadelphia reported a 45% complication rate following correction proximal hypospadias. Every subsequent redo urethroplasty is associated with a higher risk of complications.

Early

Because of the vascularity of the penis, postoperative hemorrhage can often be a concern. For this reason, most surgeons favor the use of some form of compressive dressing or bandage to reduce the risk of bleeding and hematoma formation and to alleviate postoperative edema. It is particularly important to minimize hematoma formation, as this can act as a focus for infection and subsequent fistula formation. Most complications following hypospadias surgery arise within the first year, with a reported 64% of complications being already present at the first postoperative visit. Complete dehiscence of the repair is fortunately rare, but when it does occur the subsequent secondary or "salvage" repair is a daunting task.

Late

The long-term complications of hypospadias surgery are well known and, sadly, all too common. Their incidence is determined by the initial severity of the hypospadias, the choice of procedure and the skill and experience of the surgeon.

Fistula

Fistulae are the most common complications following hypospadias surgery and can occur in up to 4–50% of patients. Some fistulae are immediately apparent following removal of the catheter but others may not develop until many years after the repair. The location of a hypospadias fistula varies, but it is often just proximal to the junction of the glans and penile shaft. The occasional occurrence of large or multiple fistulae usually indicates that the original urethroplasty was unsatisfactory and will need to be repeated.

Before attempting to repair a fistula, it is imperative to exclude meatal and/or distal urethral strictures since the presence of distal obstruction will predispose to recurrence of the fistula. Fistulae are sometimes associated with urethral diverticula, which should be excised at the time of the fistula repair.

Repair of hypospadias fistulae should not be dismissed lightly and some published series have reported a 50% recurrence rate after fistula closure. The timing of surgery is important and although early closure was favored in the past it is now recommended that an interval of at least 6 months should be allowed to elapse between the original repair and fistula closure. Many techniques have been described. Simple closure, consisting of freshening and then closing the fistula edges and the overlying skin, is associated with a high recurrence rate and is not recommended by the authors. A flap-based repair has also been described, in which the fistula is dissected down to the urethra and the urethral defect closed by inserting absorbable sutures. A flap of skin is then formed – from which a vascularized subcutaneous layer is created and placed over the urethral repair. Once the urethra is covered, the skin flap is advanced to close the skin defect. Although more complex, this technique is more effective, with a 90% success rate.

In some cases, the fistula is very large and represents a failure of the original urethroplasty. Surgery which is limited to fistula closure in these cases is generally doomed to failure, and a formal repeat urethroplasty is required to achieve a satisfactory result. Whether is necessary to use a urinary catheter following fistula repair is much debated and the reported success rates seem similar regardless of whether or not a catheter was used to divert the urine postoperatively. Therefore, unless there is some doubt about postoperative voiding it is usually possible to perform a fistula repair without leaving a urethral catheter for postoperative drainage of the bladder.

Meatal Stenosis

Meatal stenosis (<8 Fr caliber) can result from; ischemia of glans flaps, an inadequately mobilized glans wrap or extending the tubularization of the neo urethra too far distally on the glans. It typically presents with difficulty voiding, a narrowed urinary stream or spraying. In some patients, however, it may present with urinary tract infections secondary to incomplete bladder emptying due to obstructed voiding. Meatal stenosis can be treated initially with gentle dilatation of the meatus. Although this can be accomplished as an outpatient procedure using a fine-tipped catheter in minor degrees of stenosis, dilatation under general anesthesia is required for moderate or severe degrees of stenosis. When dilatation alone will not suffice, formal meatotomy is generally successful – although published outcome data following this procedure are limited.

Urethral Stenosis

Urethral stenosis has become a rare complication because modern procedures avoid a circular (circumferential) anastomosis. Although strictures can occur at any point along the length of the urethroplasty they most commonly occur at the distal and proximal ends of the neourethra. Distal stenosis is often associated with a fistula and can usually be treated with regular dilatation but in severe cases a formal surgical repair is necessary.

Proximal stenosis is a serious complication which, if severe, often requires complete reconstruction of the urethra. An obstructive pattern can frequently be seen on urinary flowmetry after tubularized incised plate (TIP) urethroplasty but this does not necessarily denote clinically significant obstruction.

Persistent Chordee

The persistence of penile chordee after hypospadias repair may be due to inadequate correction at the time of the original repair. In rare cases, however, it may be the consequence of postoperative fibrosis. In the correction of persistent chordee the first step is to deglove the penis completely to exclude skin tethering as the cause. If true chordee is found to be present after this maneuver, dorsal plication of the tunica albuginea is usually sufficient to correct it.

Balanitis Xerotica Obliterans

This rare complication caused by chronic inflammation and fibrosis of the glans and meatus results in scarring and meatal stenosis. Topical steroids help in some patients, but the majority requires a formal meatoplasty to correct the stenosis.

Urethrocele

This term refers to a dilated, "baggy" section of neourethra, often resulting from distal obstruction that gives rise to "back pressure" distension of the proximal neourethra. It may also be secondary to an absence or deficiency of supportive corpus spongiosum tissue. The various presentations of a urethrocele include; poor urinary stream, postvoid dribbling, urinary tract infections, swelling of the ventral aspect of the penis at the time of voiding and urethral calculi secondary to stasis. Surgical treatment requires excision of the redundant urethral tissue and treatment of any distal stenosis as necessary.

KEY POINTS

- Despite advances in technique, instrumentation and aftercare, the correction of hypospadias remains one of the most technically challenging aspects of pediatric urology.
- There is no place for the "occasional" hypospadias surgeon, even in the correction of so-called "minor" hypospadias. Surgeons should have a detailed understanding of the various concepts and surgical techniques and maintain a clinical workload that is sufficient to obtain consistently good results.
- Preservation of the urethral plate is the keystone of modern single-stage procedures. However, there has been a recent revival of the two-stage free flap technique for more complex cases.
- Reporting of complications is evolving as definitions are changing and patients are being followed longer postoperatively. This may lead to increases in complication rates being published.
- With improving functional results the challenge is now to obtain the optimal cosmetic result to provide patients with a penis of normal appearance regardless of the severity of the original abnormality.

FURTHER READING

Baskin LS. Hypospadias. In: Stringer MD, Oldham KT, Mouriquand PDE (eds), Pediatric Surgery and Urology: Long-Term Outcomes. Cambridge: Cambridge University Press, 2006: 611–620.

Bouty A, Ayers KL, Pask A, Heloury Y, Sinclair AH. The genetic and environmental factors underlying hypospadias. Sex Dev. 2015;9(5):239–259.

Bracka A. Hypospadias repair: the two-stage alternative. Br J Urol. 1995;76 (Suppl 3):31–41.

Mouriquand PDE, Persad R, Sharma S. Hypospadias repair: current principles and procedures. Br J Urol. 1995;76(Suppl 3):9–22.

Rynja SP, de Jong TP, Bosch JL, de Kort LM. Functional, cosmetic, and psychosexual results in adult men who underwent hypospadias correction in childhood. J Pediatr Urol. 2011;7(5):504–515.

Van der Horst HJR, de Wall LL. Hypospadias, all there is to know. Eur J Pediatr. 2017;176(4):435–441.

Wilcox D, Snodgrass W. Long-term outcome following hypospadias repair. World J Urol. 2006;24(3):240–243.

The Prepuce

KIM A R HUTTON

Topics covered

Development and function of the prepuce
Preputial disorders and abnormalities
Pathological phimosis (BXO)
Balanoposthitis
Paraphimosis, preputial cysts, congenital
   megaprepuce

Circumcision
   Ritual or non-therapeutic
   Medical
Alternatives to circumcision
Topical steroid
Preputioplasty

INTRODUCTION

Circumcision was practised during the Sixth Dynasty of Ancient Egypt (2345–2181BC) and has been a feature of many cultures across the world up to modern times. It is currently estimated that approximately one-third of the world's adult male population have been circumcised. In the United Kingdom (UK), circumcision for non-medical reasons is now virtually confined to ritual circumcision in accordance with religious or cultural beliefs. By contrast, routine neonatal circumcision is still widely performed in the United States (US). The number of "medical" circumcisions in children performed in the UK has declined steadily in recent decades as a consequence of adult surgeons performing fewer unnecessary circumcisions.

DEVELOPMENT AND FUNCTION OF THE PREPUCE

The prepuce first appears as an epithelial ridge at 8 weeks' gestation and then advances over the developing glans. By 16 weeks, the prepuce is fully formed but there is no plane of separation at the epithelial interface between the prepuce and glans. 'Preputial adhesions' are, therefore, a feature of normal development and not a pathological entity.

The prepuce is almost invariably non-retractable at birth and remains so for a variable period thereafter. Attempted retraction of the foreskin during this period creates the appearance of a blanched and apparently tight ring of skin proximal to the preputial opening. Viewed end-on, the preputial orifice is supple and unscarred, with an opening likened to a flower when the foreskin is pulled back (Figure 17.1).

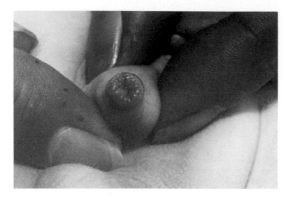

Figure 17.1 Developmentally non-retractile foreskin: attempted retraction reveals an apparent constriction ring a few millimetres proximal to the preputial orifice.

The term phimosis is often applied to the finding of a non-retractable prepuce. However, this is potentially misleading since it creates the impression of a pathological condition when this is, in fact, the normal state. 'Non-rectractile foreskin' or 'physiological phimosis' are therefore, more appropriate terms.

The natural history of non-retractile foreskin and preputial adhesions was documented in younger boys by Gairdner in 1949 and in older boys by Øster in 1968. These authors convincingly demonstrated that without intervention the prepuce spontaneously progresses to become fully and easily retractable by late childhood in the overwhelming majority of boys.

"Ballooning" of the foreskin during micturition is common during early childhood (typically between 2 and 4 years of age) and occurs at a time when the foreskin in not yet fully retractile but a substantial degree of separation from the glans has taken place. It is a transient self-limiting phenomenon, which does not require any intervention and resolves spontaneously when the prepuce becomes more fully retractable. Parents can be reassured that the appearance of ballooning does not signify obstructed voiding because non-invasive studies have established that urine flow rates, post-void residual bladder volumes and bladder-wall thickness are all unaffected by physiological phimosis (Figure 17.2).

Preputial Function

The foreskin typically remains non-retractable before the age of toilet training and this may serve a protective function by preventing exposure of the glans and meatus to the damp ammoniacal environment within the nappy.

The other function relates to sexual satisfaction. The prepuce has a rich somatosensory innervation, which constitutes an important component of the normal complement of

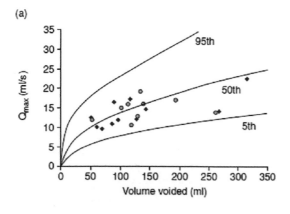

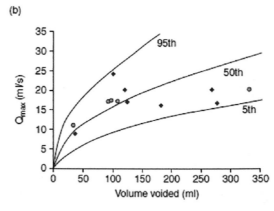

Figure 17.2 Uroflow age-related nomograms plotted with the Q_{max} and voided volume data in 32 boys with physiological phimosis. (a) nomogram for 3–7-year-old boys; (b) nomogram for boys aged 8–12 years. The blue diamonds represent flow data from patients with, and pink circles from boys without, ballooning of the foreskin. The two groups have a similar distribution of flow rate values and all points are within the normal range.

penile erogenous tissue. Circumcision removes around 30% of this innervated penile skin and results in exposure and superficial keratinisation of the surface of the glans. However, because of the highly subjective nature of sexual pleasure it is impossible to draw meaningful comparisons between the circumcised and uncircumcised state other than on a purely anecdotal basis.

DISORDERS OF THE PREPUCE

Balanitis Xerotica Obliterans

True pathological phimosis with scarring of the preputial orifice (Figures 17.3 and 17.4) is caused by the chronic cicatrising skin condition **balanitis xerotica obliterans** (BXO). This also affects the prepuce, glans and occasionally the urethra. The histological features are the same as lichen sclerosis et atrophicus of the vulva including; hyperkeratosis, lymphoedema, hyalinosis and chronic inflammatory infiltrate. BXO typically presents with irritation, local infection, dysuria, bleeding, secondary non-retractability of the foreskin or a deteriorating urinary stream. Advanced cases can sometimes present with acute urinary retention or secondary diurnal or nocturnal enuresis resulting from chronic outflow obstruction. Ultrasonography may reveal thickening of the

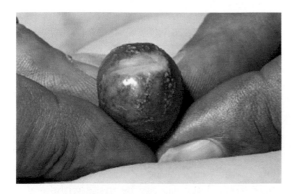

Figure 17.3 Pathological phimosis due to balanitis xerotica obliterans. Characteristic pallor, scarring and stenosis of the prepuce.

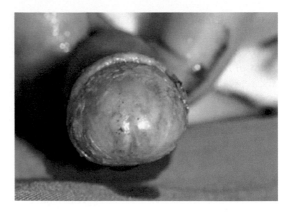

Figure 17.4 BXO, extensive glandular involvement and meatal stenosis.

bladder wall and/or significant residual urine, which may very occasionally be accompanied by upper tract dilatation.

BXO is rare under the age of 5, with a peak incidence between 9 and 11 years. It is estimated that approximately 0.5% of boys will develop BXO before the age of 16. Glandular involvement occurs in around a half the cases, although the meatus is affected in only a small proportion.

The aetiology is unknown with no familial predisposition or identifiable infective basis. Recurrent episodes of balanoposthitis do not predispose to BXO.

The preferred treatment is circumcision and indeed, pathological phimosis due to BXO constitutes the only absolute indication for circumcision in childhood. Although mild forms may respond to potent topical steroid application (e.g. 0.05% mometasone furoate, 0.05% clobetasol propionate or 0.05% betamethasone cream) this is not usually curative and rarely avoids the eventual requirement for circumcision. Preputioplasty alone is not a worthwhile option because the ongoing inflammatory process leads to recurrent stenosis of the preputial opening. However, the combination of preputioplasty and intralesional injection of a potent steroid has been claimed to be curative in milder cases. In approximately 5% of cases, meatal stenosis necessitates meatotomy or meatoplasty at the time of circumcision. The risk of recurrent meatal stenosis can be significantly reduced by postoperative application of topical steroid creams. In adults,

BXO is strongly linked to the development of penile cancer although the nature of this causal relationship is unclear. The longer term implications of BXO in childhood are unknown because the relevant prospective studies have never been undertaken.

Acute Balanoposthitis

In its most severe form acute balanoposthitis consists of purulent, pyogenic, infection of the entire preputial space. This is typically accompanied by a purulent discharge and overlying oedema and cellulitis of the prepuce, which may occasionally extend to involve the entire penile shaft. In less severe forms, more correctly termed posthitis, the inflammatory process is limited to the preputial orifice and the outer areas of the lining of the foreskin. The clinical features comprise localised erythema, oedema and discomfort but do not include purulent discharge. Dysuria is a common complaint – as is minor bleeding from the inflamed preputial orifice. The most common causative organisms are *Staphylococcus aureus*, *Escherichia coli* and *Proteus* spp. but the preputial discharge is sterile on culture in a third of cases.

Treatment consists of antibiotic therapy for acute episodes and attention to hygiene. Therapeutic intervention should be limited to boys who have suffered from recurrent episodes. Where appropriate topical steroid creams, preputiolysis or preputioplasty should be considered as alternatives to circumcision.

Schönlein–Henoch purpura involving the penis
The preputial and penile swelling and oedema which may be features of this condition can be confused with balanoposthitis – particularly if these appear before the characteristic purpuric rash on the legs, lower abdomen and buttocks. Likewise, idiopathic scrotal oedema can occasionally extend upwards from the perineum to involve the penile shaft, although this is unlikely to cause diagnostic uncertainty.

Paraphimosis

This is a rare condition in boys which results from manipulation of the foreskin and a failure

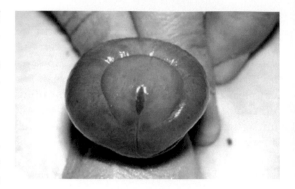

Figure 17.5 Paraphimosis. oedema of the foreskin and glans due to a constriction ring at subcoronal level.

to draw the prepuce forward again following retraction. Sometimes this may be an unforeseen consequence of instructing the boy to retract his foreskin as a treatment for physiological phimosis. After becoming trapped in the region of the coronal sulcus the prepuce becomes increasingly oedematous and difficult to return to its normal position over the glans (Figure 17.5). Treatment consists of reducing the preputial oedema by manual compression, multiple needle puncture or topical cooling before drawing the foreskin forwards over the glans. It should not usually be necessary to resort to urgent surgical intervention such as a dorsal slit. The occurrence of paraphimosis does not signify underlying pathology of the foreskin and a single episode is not an indication for surgery. Recurrent episodes of paraphimosis are relatively unusual but circumcision is a reasonable option in such cases.

Preputial Cysts and Adhesions

Preputial adhesions usually resolve spontaneously during the course of childhood. However, it is not uncommon for collections of smegma to become trapped by surrounding preputial adhesions to create yellowish subcutaneous lumps, which are typically diagnosed (incorrectly) by general practitioners as sebaceous cysts or lipomas of the penile shaft (Figure 17.6). However, the correct diagnosis can be made without difficulty by anyone familiar with this condition. Reassurance is all that is required. In time the trapped smegma will be discharged from under

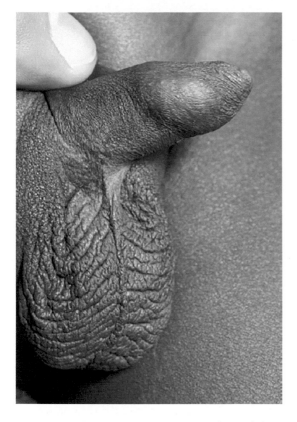

Figure 17.6 Smegma retention 'cyst'. The mobile, subcutaneous, firm lump at coronal level has a yellowish appearance and is often mis-diagnosed in primary care as a dermoid cyst or lipoma.

the prepuce when the surrounding adhesions separate spontaneously. There is only a very limited role for surgical division of preputial adhesions because disruption of the epithelial surface of the glans tends to promote the development of recurrent adhesions. Topical steroid cream, circumcision or preputioplasty (in older boys) are preferable options.

Congenital Megaprepuce

This unusual condition has only recently received recognition as an entity in its own right. On cursory inspection it resembles a buried penis but closer examination reveals an enormously capacious preputial sac, engulfing the whole penile shaft and upper scrotum. Urine dribbles more or less continuously from the preputial orifice

and although the capacious urine-filled sac can be readily emptied by compression there is never a normal urinary stream (Figure 17.7). Despite being termed 'congenital' it is arguable whether this is a genuine congenital anomaly or an acquired condition. Moreover, the natural history is poorly documented because surgery is usually performed when the condition first presents – thus making it impossible to establish whether the potential exists for spontaneous improvement. Surgical correction of congenital megaprepuce can be technically challenging and should be undertaken by an experienced paediatric urologist. Various reconstructive procedures have been described – all of which result in a circumcised penis. Although initial results generally appear promising it is not uncommon for further revision to be required because of redundant penile skin or recurrence of the buried appearance.

MEGAMEATUS INTACT PREPUCE

Although this rare condition is a congenital abnormality of the glans rather than prepuce (indeed the prepuce appears entirely normal) it merits brief consideration because it is often recognised for the first time during the course of a medical circumcision. The management is considered in Chapter 16. On some occasions the abnormality is first recognised shortly after a ritual circumcision – prompting parents and doctors to mistakenly attribute the characteristic cleft-like abnormality of the glans to an iatrogenic circumcision injury. Surprisingly, even experienced paediatric urologists have been known to make the same error and misguidedly endorse unwarranted claims for medical negligence.

CIRCUMCISION

Ritual or Non-Therapeutic Circumcision

In the UK, ritual circumcision is largely confined to the Muslim and Jewish religions but it is

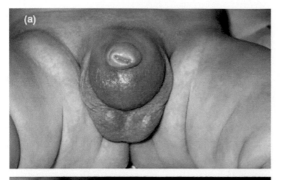

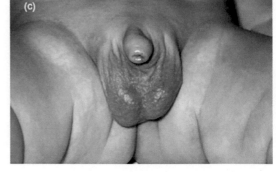

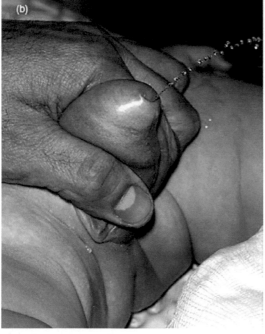

Figure 17.7 Congenital megaprepuce. This series of photographs shows the distended state where the penile shaft is no longer visible, being surrounded by a collection of urine within the dilated subcutaneous preputial sac (a), manual expression of the megaprepuce produces a stream from the retained urine (b) and the decompressed more normal appearance prior to a modified circumcision (c).

also practised within predominantly Christian West African communities. Ritual circumcision is not generally funded within NHS Hospitals but in some cities with a large Muslim population, circumcision services are provided under the auspices of local NHS organisations. In the United States, it is estimated that 70–80% of infants currently undergo non-therapeutic circumcision regardless of religious considerations. However, the prevalence of neonatal circumcision varies considerably between different parts of the USA and between different ethnic and socioeconomic groups. The Circumcision Policy Statement issued by the American Academy of Pediatrics (AAP) endorses the practice of newborn circumcision by stating that the health benefits outweigh the risks and are sufficient to warrant third-party payment for circumcision of male newborns. However, the same Policy Statement later observes that 'the health benefits are not great enough to recommend routine circumcision for all male newborns'. From a European perspective the AAP guidelines appear to be ambiguous, based on a flawed analysis of the evidence and partly influenced by financial rather than scientific considerations. The AAP Policy Statement also contrasts strongly with published guidelines of other developed countries, such as the UK, the Netherlands, Denmark and Canada, which all conclude that the weight of evidence does not support routine neonatal circumcision.

The 'medical' arguments which are usually cited to justify routine neonatal circumcision relate to urinary tract infection (UTI), sexually transmitted infections and penile cancer.

In the first year of life, the incidence of **UTI** is around ten times higher in uncircumcised boys compared with their circumcised peers. Nevertheless, the absolute incidence of urinary infection in boys is low and calculations based on systematic reviews of randomised trials and observational studies indicate that around 110–125 normal male infants would need to be circumcised to prevent one UTI. Neonatal circumcision cannot be regarded as a rational routine prophylactic measure on this basis. By contrast, there is now persuasive evidence that circumcision can be a worthwhile intervention in reducing the risk of UTI in male infants with predisposing urinary pathology, such as vesicoureteric reflux or urinary tract dilatation associated with posterior urethral valves.

Randomised controlled trials in sub-Saharan Africa have demonstrated that circumcision in men and adolescent males confers partial protection against heterosexually acquired HIV infection. But whilst circumcision may be a valid public health intervention in developing countries with a high prevalence of **HIV infection** this is far less relevant to routine circumcision of newborns male infants in countries with a much lower prevalence of HIV. Penile cancer is virtually confined to uncircumcised men but it is a rare malignancy in developed countries. Health education and treatment of phimosis are much more appropriate preventative measures than widescale circumcision of healthy newborn infants.

Circumcision for medical indications

Current estimates indicate that around 3–5% of boys aged 0–16 years undergo circumcision for medical reasons in the UK. The principal indications being 'phimosis' (BXO) and balanoposthitis. Notwithstanding the marked reduction in medical circumcisions over recent decades, unnecessary circumcisions are almost certainly still being performed – particularly for physiological phimosis in boys under 5 years of age.

Contraindications to circumcision

Hypospadias, epispadias or ambiguous genitalia are absolute contraindications to newborn circumcision because removal of the prepuce is highly likely to compromise the outcome of any later genital reconstruction. Special considerations relating to buried penis are outlined below.

Surgical aspects

RITUAL OR NON-THERAPEUTIC CIRCUMCISION

A wide variety of surgical techniques have been used to perform non-therapeutic (ritual) circumcision in infants and children. Of these, the Plastibell technique is the one mostly widely used in the UK (Figure 17.8).

In addition to the general complications of circumcision, complications which are specific to the Plastibell technique include haemorrhage due to slippage of the haemostatic ligature and delayed separation of the ring.

MEDICAL CIRCUMCISION

This should be undertaken as a formal surgical procedure under general anaesthesia, with additional local anaesthesia (caudal or penile block) to provide postoperative analgesia. The technical details are a matter of individual surgical preference, but the following general points should be observed:

- The prepuce must be completely separated from the underlying glans and coronal sulcus prior to circumcision. Failure to do so may result in the formation of persistent skin bridges between the glans and the penile skin.
- To ensure the best cosmetic result the outer and inner layers of preputial skin should be excised separately and trimmed further if necessary. Some surgeons delineate the planned incisions with a marking pen.

a   b   c

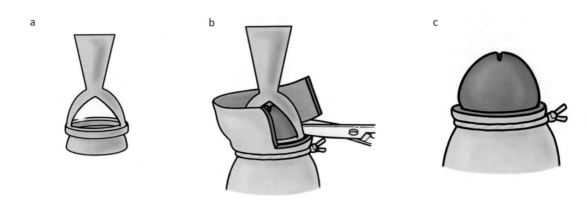

Figure 17.8 **(a)** Plastibell device. **(b)** A dorsal slit is performed to enable a Plastibell device of appropriate size to be introduced between the glans and prepuce. A haemostatic ligature is tied around the base of the prepuce overlying a groove in the Plastibell device. The foreskin distal to the ligature is excised with scissors to complete the circumcision. The handle and section of the Plastibell protecting the glans is then snapped off and discarded. **(c)** The plastic ring remains in place before detaching spontaneously after an interval of 3–7 days.

Failure to excise sufficient of the outer layer of skin may result in unsatisfactory cosmetic outcomes (incomplete circumcision) and a requirement for secondary surgical revision.

- Conversely, removal of too much skin may leave insufficient to cover the penile shaft. This risk is greatest in boys with so-called 'buried penis' in whom even a standard circumcision may result in a denuded penile shaft and a requirement for skin grafting. A modified technique is required in such cases in order to redistribute rather than remove preputial skin.
- Careful attention to haemostasis is important and bipolar diathermy is more effective than ligation of individual vessels.
- Sutures chosen for skin closure (e.g. Vicryl© rapide) should be rapidly absorbed to reduce the incidence of suture tract formation. The use of subcuticular sutures may minimise this risk. The use of tissue glues instead of sutures is well documented and has been claimed to reduce operating times and improve cosmetic outcomes.

The choice of postoperative dressing (if any) is also a matter of individual preference. Many surgeons avoid dressings because of the distress caused on removal.

Complications of Circumcision

Parents should be made aware that circumcision is associated with a significant incidence of postoperative distress and morbidity. Early complications include urinary retention and haemorrhage. The former can be prevented by adequate analgesia or intraoperative local block with levobupivacaine. Haemorrhage of sufficient severity to necessitate early re-operation has been reported to occur in 2–5% of boys. The most common postoperative problems are encrustation, scabbing and infection of the exposed glans. Complications such as buried penis, urethral fistula, injury to the glans and partial penile amputations are virtually confined to religious circumcisions performed in the community (Figure 17.9). Glans ischaemia – a serious but fortunately rare complication, may be related to the dorsal penile nerve block commonly used for postoperative pain relief (Figure 17.10).

ALTERNATIVES TO CIRCUMCISION

These are not appropriate for boys with BXO (in whom circumcision is required) and should not

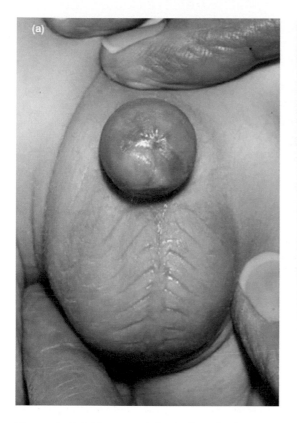
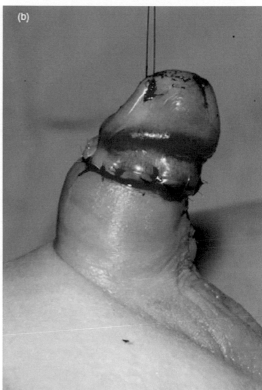

Figure 17.9 **(a)** Iatrogenic buried penis due to scarring and occlusion of the residual skin following ritual circumcision. **(b)** Appearances following surgical release and revision circumcision.

be employed simply because of parental concerns about foreskin non-retractility or 'ballooning'. Reassurance and an explanation of the natural history of the healthy non-retractile foreskin is what is required in these circumstances. However, the combination of topical steroids and regular retraction may be justified for boys who are troubled by localised symptoms or recurrent balanoposthitis.

Topical steroids: There is good evidence from prospective studies that steroid creams are capable of altering the physical characteristics of the foreskin to make it easier to retract. Amongst the preparations that have been used for this purpose are; 0.05% betamethasone cream, 0.05% clobetasol propionate cream and 0.02% triamcinolone acetonide cream. Treatment regimens typically comprise twice daily application of the cream for 4–8 weeks, with a further course if initial results are unsatisfactory. Although 'success rates' of 70–95% have been reported, 'success' is often

loosely (and subjectively) defined – with some authors extending the definition of 'success' to include partial response or retractability deemed 'appropriate for age'. For this approach to be successful it is important that application of the steroid cream is combined with regular attempts at gentle retraction of the prepuce.

Preputioplasty

This alternative to circumcision is particularly suited to older boys with a persistently non-retractile foreskin, which is predicted to cause problems after the onset of sexual activity. Unlike circumcision, preputioplasty enables the boy to retain a normal foreskin. Regular postoperative self-retraction of the foreskin is essential to ensure a satisfactory outcome. For this reason, the procedure is less suitable for use in younger boys and those who are unwilling to comply with the postoperative regimen of regular retraction.

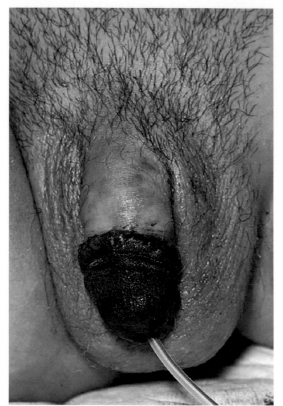

Figure 17.10 Complication of circumcision. Glans ischaemia developing shortly after corrective surgery for phimosis and a buried penis in an adolescent boy. A colour Doppler ultrasound study of the penile vasculature showed normal appearances. This complication resolved completely within a few days following treatment with oral sildenafil, subcutaneous enoxaparin and caudal anaesthesia with levobupivacaine (for its vasodilatory effect). There were no long-term implications.

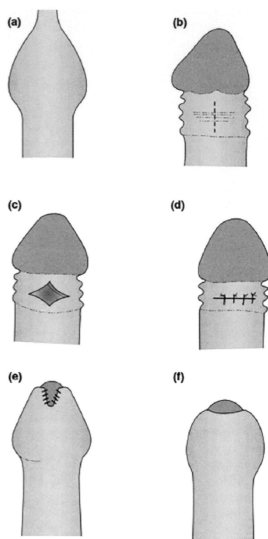

Figure 17.11 Technique of preputioplasty (a) adhesions divided, prepuce retracted. (b) Constricting ring incised and (c,d) incision closed transversely. (e) 'Dorsal slit' appearance on completion of the procedure evolves into normal retractile prepuce (f) if regular retraction is performed postoperatively.

Preputioplasty is performed under general anaesthesia. The procedure consists of incising the 'constriction ring', which is apparent on retracting the foreskin and then closing this incision transversely with interrupted sutures (Figure 17.11). Initially the appearance resembles a limited dorsal slit but with time and regular retraction this evolves to create the appearance of a normal foreskin. Various modifications have been described using multiple incisions or Y–V plasties.

KEY POINTS

- The foreskin is almost invariably unretractable at birth, but becomes fully and easily retractable in approximately 95% of boys by 16 years of age.

- Conservative treatment of the non-retractable foreskin involves advising parents of the natural history of the foreskin and its normal tendency to become retractable when preptutial adhesions resolve spontaneously.
- Effective alternative treatments for the non-retractable foreskin include topical steroid therapy and, where appropriate, preputioplasty.
- Surgical intervention is justifiable in boys experiencing recurrent episodes of balanoposthitis.
- Balanitis xerotica obliterans is the only absolute indication for circumcision but this condition rarely affects boys under the age of 5.

FURTHER READING

American Academy of Pediatrics Task Force on Circumcision. Circumcision policy statement. Paediatrics. 2012;130:585–6.

Babu R, Harrison SK, Hutton KA. Ballooning of the foreskin and physiological phimosis: is there any objective evidence of obstructed voiding? BJU Int. 2004;94:384–7.

Cuckow PM, Rix G, Mouriquand PD. Preputial plasty: a good alternative to circumcision. J Pediatr Surg. 1994;29:561–3.

Singh-Grewal D, Macdessi J, Craig J. Circumcision for the prevention of urinary tract infection in boys: a systematic review of randomised trials and observational studies. Arch Dis Child. 2005;90:853–8.

Sorokan ST, Finlay JC, Jefferies AL. Canadian Paediatric Society, Fetus and Newborn Committee, Infectious Diseases and Immunization Committee. Newborn male circumcision. Paediatr Child Health. 2015;20:311–20.

Yang SS, Tsai YC, Wu CC, Liu SP, Wang CC. Highly potent and moderately potent topical steroids are effective in treating phimosis: a prospective randomised study. J Urol. 2005;173:1361–3.

18

Testis, Hydrocoele and Varicocoele

PRASAD P GODBOLE and NICHOLAS P MADDEN

Topics covered

INTRODUCTION

Hernias, hydroceles and undescended testes are some of the commonest congenital anomalies treated by paediatric urologists and paediatric surgeons. Historically, many children with these conditions were treated by adult surgeons but with changes in training and greater specialisation they are now being managed increasingly by paediatric specialists. This chapter will provide an overview of undescended testis (UDT) (including impalpable testis, retractile testis and ascending testis), hydrocele and varicocele.

UNDESCENDED TESTIS (CRYPTORCHIDISM)

Incidence

Undescended testis (UDT) is the commonest congenital anomaly in males, with a reported incidence of 1.5–3% in term infants and up to 30% in premature infants. Some congenitally undescended testes descend spontaneously in the first few months of life in response to high levels of circulating testosterone. This phenomenon, termed 'mini-puberty' results from stimulation by pituitary gonadotrophins in the early postnatal period. Because some undescended testes descend spontaneously during this period the incidence of UDT falls to 1–2% by 6–12 months of age. Spontaneous descent does not occur after 6 months and hence a 'wait and watch' strategy after this age is not justified.

Pathophysiology

Maintenance of a testicular temperature 2–3 degrees below the core body temperature is essential for normal spermatogenesis. When the testis is located in the inguinal canal or abdomen it is exposed to a higher ambient temperature than in the scrotum and spermatogenesis is consequently impaired.

The onset of spermatogenesis does not commence until puberty but differentiation and maturation of the germ cells which will eventually be responsible for the production of spermatozoa begins in fetal life and continues postnatally. At the time of birth, the seminiferous tubules are populated by fetal stem cells (gonocytes). In response to the surge of gonadotropins and testosterone (mini-puberty) these cells undergo transformation to become adult dark (Ad) spermatogonia between 3 and 9 months of age. After a period of inactivity, Ad spermatogonia proliferate and mature into primary spermatocytes at around 5–6 years of age. The primary spermatocytes remain quiescent until puberty when they are stimulated by gonadotrophins and testosterone to undergo meiotic division to create secondary spermatocytes. These then undergo a further meiotic division to form spermatids and spermatozoa. As a consequence of the two sequential meiotic divisions a single primary spermatocyte eventually gives rise to four spermatozoa. Of the neonatal gonocytes which are present in the testis at the time of birth only a minority transforms into Ad spermatogonia and the remaining gonocytes undergo involution by apoptosis. By 2 years of age there should normally be no undifferentiated gonocytes remaining within the testis.

Gonocyte transformation into Ad spermatogonia is impaired or absent in undescended testes. Moreover, the redundant neonatal gonocytes which would normally be eliminated by apoptosis persist – thus contributing to the increased risk of the later development of malignancy. The impairment of normal germ cell transformation in undescended testes results in a diminished pool of adult stem cells available for spermatogenesis at puberty, with a resulting reduction in sperm density, impairment of semen quality and possible infertility.

The histological appearances of testes which have undergone secondary ascent ('acquired UDT') have been reported to resemble those of congenitally undescended testes which have remained outside the scrotum until orchidopexy in later childhood. There is therefore a substantial body of evidence to indicate that elevated temperature is a major factor in the degenerative changes occurring in undescended testes. Undescended testes are also associated with an appreciable incidence of coexisting congenital abnormalities of the epididymis and vas deferens, which may also contribute to impaired fertility in adult life.

Classification

The most practical distinction lies between palpable and the impalpable testes. Approximately, 10–15% of UDT are impalpable. An impalpable testis may be intra-abdominal – in which case it may be visualised on laparoscopy or, alternatively, it may have atrophied following torsion or some other vascular event in intrauterine life. In addition, a testis lying within the inguinal canal may sometimes be difficult or impossible to palpate if it moves in and out of the internal ring – or is obscured by subcutaneous fat in boys who are overweight.

The anatomical classification of UDT can be further subdivided into maldescended testes, which are located somewhere along the normal line of descent, and ectopic testes lying outside the normal line of descent. Ectopic gonads are most commonly located in the perineum, lateral to the scrotum (Figure 18.1), occasionally in the thigh, and exceptionally, as crossed ectopia, in which the testis is located in the contralateral hemiscrotum. Although undescended testes are often found within a region commonly termed the 'superficial inguinal pouch', this location is no longer considered to be genuinely 'ectopic'.

Presentation

Undescended testes are most frequently diagnosed during routine neonatal examination. If the testis cannot be identified in the scrotum at that stage the infant should be re-examined at 3 months of age (or 52 weeks postconceptual age

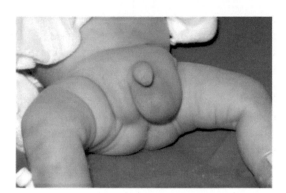

Figure 18.1 **Right ectopic testis. Empty right hemi-scrotum, and a visible swelling (ectopic testis) in the perineum lateral to the scrotum.**

in premature infants). During the first 3 months of life, the cremasteric reflex is absent, so it should be possible to assess the true location of the testis more reliably at this age than in later infancy and childhood. Testicular maldescent may also be identified for the first time during routine developmental assessments at 6–8 months of age, or subsequent school medical examinations.

The right testis is more commonly undescended than the left, and in approximately 20% of cases the condition is bilateral.

Older boys who are referred for an opinion on an 'UDT' more often prove to have a retractile or ascending testis. The term 'retractile testis' should be confined to a testis which, regardless of its initial position can be brought fully to the floor of the scrotum without tension on the spermatic cord. However, the distinction between undescended and retractile testes is not as clear cut as was once thought because incompletely descended testes may also demonstrate 'retractility' due to over-activity of cremasteric muscle surrounding the spermatic cord.

History and Examination

Relevant aspects of the history include ; the antenatal history, duration of pregnancy, information on any medication taken during pregnancy and whether the parents were notified of any abnormal findings following the routine neonatal examination. On inspection, both testes may be visible in the bottom of the scrotum – in which

case the diagnosis is evidently one of retractile testis. Sometimes there is obvious asymmetry of the scrotum or the scrotum may appear small or 'shallow'. The examiner's hands should not be cold and the examination should be conducted in a relaxed, warm environment. Starting laterally to the internal ring, one hand moves down the inguinal canal, 'milking' the testis towards the scrotum. Once this hand reaches the pubic tubercle, the other hand is used to locate the testis and draw it gently downwards towards the scrotum.

A testis which can be readily manipulated to the floor of the scrotum, and remains there, is evidently 'retractile' and essentially normal (Figure 18.2). In other instances, although the testis can be brought to the base of the scrotum, this can only be achieved with some difficulty and is followed by immediate reascent once traction is released. This is commonly termed a 'high retractile testis'.

In infants, thickening of the spermatic cord may denote the presence of a patent

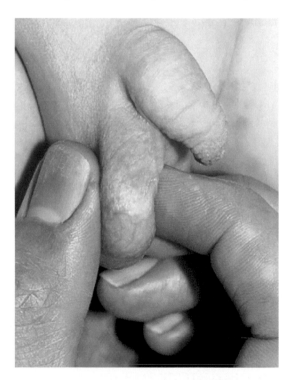

Figure 18.2 **True retractile testis, brought easily to the floor of the scrotum without undue traction.**

processus – raising the possibility of an associated inguinal hernia. It is also important to look for possible ectopic testes – which are most often located in the perineum immediately lateral to the scrotum.

Management

Hormonal treatment

There is a very limited role for hormonal treatment in the management of high retractile testes. However, the findings of a large double-blind placebo cross-over trial conclusively demonstrated that it is ineffective in treating congenitally undescended testes. Hormonal treatment typically consists of intramuscular injections of **human chorionic gonadotrophin (HCG)** once or twice weekly for three weeks. Alternatively, **luteinising hormone-releasing hormone (LHRH)** can be administered via an intranasal route four to six times daily for the same period. Pre-operative hormonal treatment has also been advocated to facilitate a potentially difficult orchidopexy.

Surgery

PALPABLE UNDESCENDED TESTIS

The standard single-stage orchidopexy is usually undertaken as a day-case procedure. Historically, orchidopexy was performed at a much later age – typically at 10–15 years of age in the 1950s. However, the recommended age for orchidopexy was then gradually lowered to 2 years of age by the 1980s and is currently between 6 and 12 months of age. The rationale is based on evidence that relocating the testis to the lower temperature of the scrotum at this age may help to minimise the impairment of gonocyte transformation and thus contribute to an improved outlook for fertility. There is some evidence that early orchidopexy is associated with better testicular growth. Orchidopexy at 6–12 months of age may also help to reduce the risk of germ cell malignancy in later life.

IMPALPABLE TESTIS

Between 10% and 15% of undescended testes are impalpable. Before embarking upon definitive surgery, it is necessary to establish whether the testis is absent (anorchia), whether it is located within the abdomen or is represented by an atrophic nubbin of tissue within the inguinal canal. In approximately 40% of cases, the testis lies intra-abdominally. In 30% the testis has 'vanished', with vas and vessels ending blindly deep to the internal inguinal ring, in 20% the vas and vessels end blindly within the inguinal canal and in 10% of cases, the impalpable testis is present but concealed within the inguinal canal.

Ultrasound is an unreliable diagnostic modality for determining whether a testis is intra-abdominal or absent – yielding both false-positive and false-negative results. Magnetic resonance imaging (MRI) is also unreliable (unless combined with angiography) and usually requires the a general anaesthetic. Ultrasound can occasionally play a useful role, however, by visualizing a testis in the inguinal canal of an overweight boy in whom the testis cannot be identified on clinical examination.

Laparoscopy remains the investigation of first choice in cases of impalpable testis, being both highly reliable and providing positive guidance for further management. The possible findings should be explained to the parents pre-operatively and consent obtained for possible orchidectomy in certain situations. **There are five possible laparoscopic findings:**

- **Testis lying adjacent to the internal inguinal ring**. Such testes are usually amenable to a single-stage orchidopexy using a conventional or a preperitoneal approach. An experienced laparoscopist may be able to manipulate the testis towards the inguinal canal to assess the feasibility of a single-stage procedure.
- **Testis located on the posterior abdominal wall or ectopically within the pelvis**. (Figure 18.3). This finding calls for a decision on whether to remove the testis (either laparoscopically or as an open procedure) or whether to embark upon orchidopexy. For this, the options lie between open or laparoscopically assisted orchidopexy - as either a single or a staged procedure.
- **Failure to visualise blind-ending vessels or testis**. In this rare situation, a limited laparotomy is indicated in view of the high risk

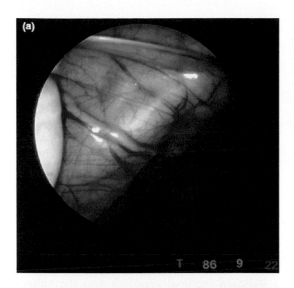
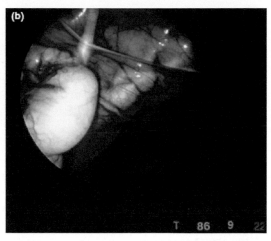
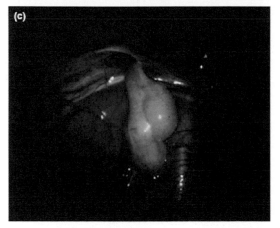

Figure 18.3 **(a, b)** Intra-abdominal testis and vas viewed laparoscopically. **(c)** Intra-abdominal testis lying above the entry to the inguinal canal.

of subsequent malignancy associated with leaving an undetected intra-abdominal testes left in situ.

- **Vas and vessels ending blindly together at or above the internal ring**. This finding ('vanished testis') is usually thought to result from intrauterine torsion and no further exploration is required.
- **Vas and vessels seen entering the inguinal canal**. It impossible to be certain whether the inguinal canal contains a normal testis or an atrophic nubbin of testicular tissue. Opinion varies on whether inguinal exploration is still mandatory in this situation.

Alternatively, it has been suggested that inguinal exploration is unnecessary if a nubbin is palpable and the contralateral testis is hypertrophied (>1.8 cm polar length or 2 ml in volume).

BILATERAL IMPALPABLE TESTES

Further investigation is indicated, including a karyotype (to look for sex chromosome mosaicism or chromosomal abnormalities such as the Prader–Willi syndrome) and an HCG stimulation test to determine whether any functioning testicular tissue is present. However, whilst a positive result from an HCG test is reassuring for the parents, a negative result does not obviate the need for laparoscopy. The combination of bilateral impalpable testes and hypospadias should always raise the possibility of an underlying DSD – notably 46XX DSD due to congenital adrenal hyperplasia (see Chapter 20).

ORCHIDOPEXY – SURGICAL CONSIDERATIONS

For a palpable congenitally undescended testis the crucial step consists of isolating the processus vaginalis from the cord structures to enable them to be completely mobilised back to the internal inguinal ring. This manoeuvre can be extended retroperitoneally above the internal ring if necessary (Figure 18.4). If there is no patent processus vaginalis, orchidopexy is usually more straightforward and the testis can be brought down to the scrotum without undue difficulty following separation of the cremasteric coverings from the cord structures.

Even an experienced surgeon may occasionally operate for what is thought to be a palpable testis, only to be confronted by an empty inguinal canal. If a patent processus vaginalis is present, this should be opened. Frequently an 'emergent' testis will enter the mouth of the processus through the internal ring. Careful dissection is then required to mobilise the vessels and vas, which are usually covered by the friable peritoneal wall of the sac. Nevertheless, a standard single-stage orchidopexy is usually achievable in such cases.

PREPERITONEAL APPROACH (JONES)

This is a useful technique for high inguinal testes. The skin incision is slightly higher than for a standard inguinal approach and the oblique abdominal muscles are split to gain access to the peritoneum above the inguinal canal. Thereafter, the testis is mobilised extraperitoneally (or transperitoneally) and is brought down to the scrotum either via the inguinal canal or more directly

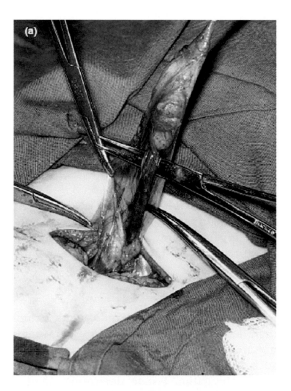
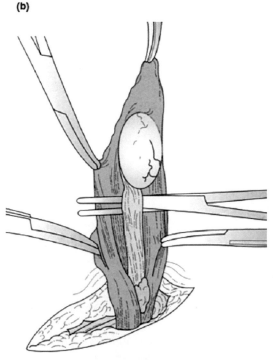

Figure 18.4 Conventional inguinal orchidopexy. (a) Intraoperative photograph. (b) Diagrammatic representation illustrating mobilisation of cord structures from the processus vaginalis.

through the posterior wall of the canal medial to the inferior epigastric vessels.

The following specialised techniques are required for testes lying high within the inguinal canal or within the abdomen.

FOWLER–STEPHENS PROCEDURE (FIGURE 18.5)

The difficulty in bringing an intra-abdominal testis to the scrotum usually arises from the inadequate length of the testicular blood vessels rather than the vas deferens. Following ligation or clipping of the testicular vessels performed

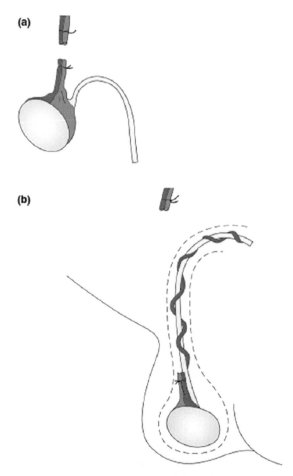

Figure 18.5 Fowler–Stephens orchidopexy. (a) Stage I, testicular vessels ligated or clipped in continuity. (b) Stage II, collateral vascularisation of the testis via the artery to the vas. After 6 months the testis is mobilised on the vas and a strip of surrounding peritoneum and brought to the scrotum by the most direct route.

during the Fowler Stephens procedure the blood supply to the testis is provided by the collateral vessels surrounding the vas. Better results are achieved with a two stage procedure. During the first stage (which can be performed by either an open or laparoscopic approach), the testicular vessels are divided or clipped, taking care not to disturb the vas and its important collateral vessels. The second stage is undertaken 6 months later – by which time a more substantial collateral supply has developed in response to occlusion of the testicular vessels. The testis and vas are mobilised, together with a broad strip of overlying peritoneum, and are then brought to the scrotum through the posterior wall of the canal medial to the inferior epigastric vessels. The second stage may be undertaken as an entirely open procedure or with laparoscopic assistance.

MICROVASCULAR ORCHIDOPEXY

This procedure can be used for intra-abdominal testes, especially if the vas is too short to permit a Fowler–Stephens procedure. The testicular vessels are mobilised and divided as high as possible. The testis and vas are then brought to the scrotum and the testicular vessels are anastomosed to the inferior epigastric vessels in the inguinal canal (Figure 18.6).

LAPAROSCOPICALLY ASSISTED ORCHIDOPEXY (FIGURE 18.7)

The intraperitoneal pedicle of testicular vessels is extensively mobilised laparoscopically. Once sufficient length of vessels has been obtained, the testis is placed in the scrotum by either an open inguinal approach or an entirely laparoscopic procedure.

Management of retractile testis

If the testis meets the criteria of being genuinely retractile the parents can be reassured that this is a relatively common phenomenon, particularly between the ages of 3 and 7 years. Although surgical intervention is not usually required it has become apparent that some retractile testes progress to become ascending testes by adopting a fixed position in the groin or upper scrotum. For this reason it is now recommended that all boys with retractile testes should be seen for annual

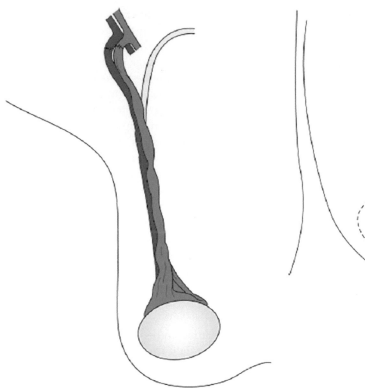

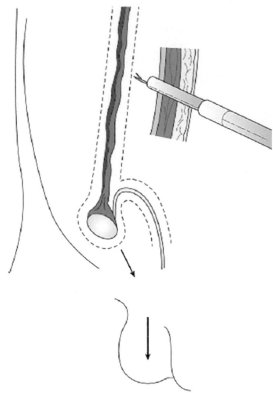

Figure 18.6 Microvascular orchidopexy. Testicular artery and single vein anastomosed to inferior epigastric vessels (or branches).

Figure 18.7 Laparoscopic or laparoscopically assisted orchidopexy. Extensive intraperitoneal mobilisation of testicular vessels enables the testis to be brought down to the scrotum with its vascular pedicle intact.

review until such time as it can confirmed that the testis is no longer retractile and has reverted permanently to a normal position at the floor of the scrotum.

Although hormonal treatment may be considered, orchidopexy is generally regarded as the treatment of choice for a 'high retractile' testis which cannot be brought to the bottom without tension on the spermatic cord or which appears to be becoming an ascending testis. In such cases it is usually possible to perform a satisfactory orchidopexy using a scrotal approach. However, it is not sufficient to simply anchor the testis in the scrotum. The cord structures should be adequately mobilised and the overlying cremasteric coverings completely divided to enable the testis to be positioned in the scrotum without any residual tension on the cord structures.

Ascending testis

This phenomenon, also termed acquired UDT, is now well documented and is thought to account for a relatively high percentage of boys undergoing orchidopexy in later childhood.

The distance between the internal inguinal ring and the scrotum increases from 4 to 5 cm in infancy to around 8–10 cm at puberty – with the corresponding requirement for the spermatic cord to double in length. Failure of this elongation of the spermatic cord is one possible explanation for secondary testicular ascent, another being tethering of the testis by the remnant of a processus vaginalis. In 10–30% of cases, the ascending testis has passed through a retractile phase. Conservative management has been advocated by a group in the Netherlands who reported that >80% of ascending testes reverted spontaneously to the scrotum at the time of puberty. However, this approach has not gained wider acceptance because of concerns that even if the testis does revert to the scrotum at puberty it will nevertheless have sustained thermal damage during the time spent outside the scrotum. Indeed, histological studies have shown that ascending testes demonstrate similar degenerative changes to those found in congenitally undescended testes. For this reason it is current practice to advise orchidopexy for any ascending testis which is lying in a fixed elevated position in the groin or upper scrotum – regardless of the boy's age and previous history.

Surgical results and complications

Success is usually defined in terms of the postoperative position and viability of the testis. The published outcome data indicate that single stage open inguinal orchidopexy has a success rate in excess of 95% whereas the success rates of orchidopexy for intra-abdominal testes (by single stage or staged approach – open or laparoscopic) are in the range of 85–90%.

The principal complications are postoperative atrophy, injury to the vas and re ascent of the testis. The incidence of complications is strongly influenced by the preoperative position of the testis, with one large review identifying a complication rate of 8% for testes located beyond the external inguinal ring, 13% for testes within the inguinal canal, and in the case of intra-abdominal testes 16% for microvascular procedures and 27% for two-stage Fowler–Stephens procedures.

Concerns that the presumed benefits for fertility of orchidopexy at 6–12 month may be offset by a higher incidence of testicular atrophy appear to be unfounded. One comparative study found that the atrophy rate was the same (5%) in boys who had undergone orchidopexy under 2 years of age and those in whom orchidopexy had been performed from 2 years upwards. Another study reported an atrophy rate of 1.4% in a series of boys who had undergone orchidopexy at a mean age of 9 months. A figure of 1–2% is sometimes cited for the incidence of vasal injury but the true incidence is probably higher since intraoperative damage to the vas or its blood supply may go unrecognised or unreported.

Long-term Outcomes of Orchidopexy

Fertility

Virtually all the published long-term outcome data have been derived from retrospective studies - with the inherent limitations of such methodology. In addition, assessment of fertility by paternity (the actual ability to father children) does not correlate closely with the assessment of fertility by semen analysis. Outcomes for fertility are consistently better when assessed by paternity. The published data consistently demonstrate that men with a history of unilateral UDT have a significantly better outcome for fertility (judged by both semen analysis and paternity) than those with a history of bilateral undescended testes (Table 18.1). Studies have generally shown that paternity rates of men with a history of unilateral UDT are only marginally lower than those of the normal population. However, the time taken to achieve conception is longer than controls. The published data have been mainly derived from men who underwent orchidopexy at a later stage in childhood than is current practice. Although there is evidence to indicate the recent trend towards earlier orchidopexy (currently 6–12 months) will probably lead to improved long-term results for fertility it will be some time before this can be reliably confirmed by long-term studies.

The published data do not distinguish adequately (if at all) between men with congenitally undescended testes and men whose testes underwent secondary ascent. Ascending testes could be expected to have a better potential for spermatogenesis because normal gonocyte transformation should have occurred while the testis was still in the scrotum in the first 2 years of life. However, once they are no longer in the scrotum, ascending testes are likely to be at a similar risk of acquired temperature-related degenerative changes as congenitally undescended testes.

Table 18.1 Fertility (paternity) of men with a previous history of undescended testis (UDT)

Authors	Number of patients	Paternity rate of unilateral UDT (%)	Paternity rate of bilateral UDT (%)
Gilhooly et al	145	80	48
Kumar et al	56	84	60
Lee	467	88	59
Lee and Coughlin	408	90	65

Source: Hutson JM. Undescended testes. In: Stringer MD, Oldham KT, Mouriquand PDE (eds), Paediatric Surgery and Urology: Long-term Outcomes, 2nd Edition. Cambridge: Cambridge University Press, 2006: 652–663.

The published evidence can be summarised briefly as follows:

- The long-term prognosis for fertility is better when judged by paternity than semen analysis.
- Published series report **paternity rates in the range 80–90%** for men with a history of **unilateral UDT** (percentage of men with normal semen analysis 55–95%).
- Published series report **paternity rates in the range 45–65%** for men with a history of **bilateral undescended testes** (percentage of men with normal semen analysis 25–30%).
- The evidence of biopsy studies supported by limited clinical data indicate that the prospects of fertility are likely to be improved by early orchidopexy (6–12 months of age).
- Testes arrested in a higher position of maldescent have a poorer prognosis for fertility.
- Fertility may be potentially better in ascending testes because normal gonocyte transformation should have occurred while the testis was still in the scrotum. However, ascending testes have similar histological features to congenitally undescended testes and the impact on fertility may be comparable.

Malignancy

Men with a history of UDT are at a greater increased risk of developing testicular malignancy. However, the magnitude of this risk was overstated in the past. A large case–control study in the UK found that the relative risk was 3.8 times greater than the normal population when orchidopexy had been performed after 9 years of age but was not significantly higher in men who had undergone orchidopexy before the age of 9. In a study reported from Sweden, men who had undergone orchidopexy after 13 years of age had a risk of testicular cancer which was 5.4 times higher than the normal male population whereas the risk was 2.3 times higher in those who had undergone orchidopexy under this age. It is difficult to translate relative risk into a figure for the life time risk of developing testicular cancer in an individual with a history of UDT but current data suggest that this is probably of the order of 1 in 100. The available evidence suggests that the current policy of performing orchidopexy in the first year of life may reduce this risk further by facilitating the elimination of residual gonocytes which have not undergone transformation into Ad spermatogonia.

Regardless of the age when it was performed men who have undergone orchidopexy should be advised to practise testicular self-examination.

Testicular microcalcification (TM)

This disorder is characterised by the presence of multiple small echogenic foci of calcification throughout the testis (Figure 18.8).

The prevalence of testicular microcalcification in adults has been variously reported to be between 0.6% and 9.0% in men with symptoms

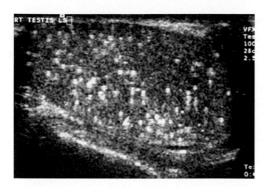

Figure 18.8 Testicular microcalcification. Ultrasound image demonstrating characteristic appearances.

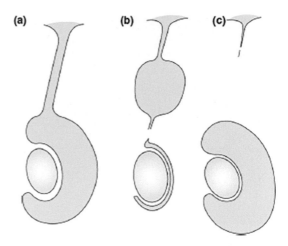

Figure 18.9 Anatomical classification of hydrocoele. (a) Communicating hydrocoele. (b) Hydrocoele of the cord ('encysted hydrocoele'). (c) Non-communicating hydrocoele.

and 2.4–5.6% in asymptomatic men. The frequency of TM is significantly higher in men with Klinefelter syndrome and Down syndrome (17.5% and 36%, respectively).

Although testicular ultrasound is performed far less frequently in children and adolescents than in adults, the presence of testicular microcalcification is being identified by ultrasound in this age group. It has been suggested that TM is a potential marker of premalignancy but this is probably only of relevance when it is associated with other recognised risk factors such as cryptorchidism, infertility, testicular asymmetry or atrophy. The weight of evidence indicates that asymptomatic microcalcification is an incidental finding in the majority of individuals and that prolonged ultrasound surveillance is not required unless other risk factors are present. In adolescents and young adults there is certainly no evidence to support testicular biopsy.

HYDROCOELE

With few exceptions, hydrocoeles in infants and children share a common underlying aetiology with indirect inguinal hernias: namely, failure of closure of the patent processus vaginalis following descent of the testis – see Chapter 1 (Figure 18.9). The two conditions differ mainly in the diameter of the processus, which in communicating hydrocoeles is narrow and will only permit the passage of intraperitoneal fluid

(Figure 18.10). Non-communicating hydrocoeles are rare in boys and occur mainly around or after puberty (Figure 18.11). Communicating hydrocoeles are common in newborn males, with an incidence of 2–5%. More than 90% of communicating hydroceles in infants resolve without intervention following spontaneous closure of the processus vaginalis. However, for reasons which

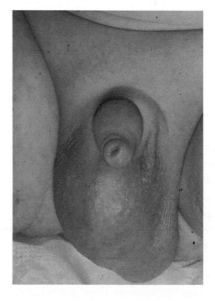

Figure 18.10 Congenital (communicating) hydrocoele.

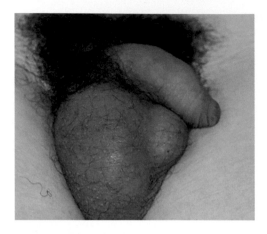

Figure 18.11 **A 14-year-old boy presenting with 1-year history of increasing scrotal swelling. Non-communicating 'adult type' hydrocoele managed by scrotal approach and plication of the hydrocoele sac.**

are often unclear, communicating hydroceles sometimes present for the first time in later childhood – although this is rare after the age of 5 years.

Presentation

Hydrocoeles usually present as a painless scrotal swelling. The size may vary over the course of the day, being comparatively small in the morning and enlarging later in the day. Hydroceles sometimes develop following the insertion of a ventriculoperitoneal shunt for hydrocephalus and may also present acutely in association with a viral illness. Although rare, a hydrocele may sometimes develop in response to the presence of omentum incarcerated in a hernial sac or an underlying testicular tumour. Encysted hydrocoeles of the cord sometimes present as a painless 'irreducible' swelling in the groin, which can be confused with an incarcerated inguinal hernia.

Examination

The principal differential diagnosis lies between hydrocoele and inguinoscrotal hernia, but whereas hernias are reducible, hydrocoeles are not. Transillumination does not reliably distinguish between a hernia and hydrocele in infants because a hernia will also transilluminate in

bright light. The diagnosis can usually be made reliably on purely clinical grounds but an ultrasound scan should be performed if there is any suspicion of an underlying testicular tumour or incarcerated hernia. It may also be helpful in elucidating an encysted hydrocele.

Management

Congenital hydrocoeles should be managed conservatively, as the majority resolve spontaneously during the first 2 years of life.

Surgical intervention is indicated for congenital hydrocoeles which persists beyond 2 years of age, and for hydroceles presenting for the first time in later childhood. Surgery is also justified for occasional cases in which a communicating hydrocele changes to resemble an enlarging, tense non-communicating hydrocele (possibly because of a valve-like effect in the involuting patent processus). Hydrocoeles of the cord are rarely present at birth but can acutely in a way that mimics an irreducible hernia. If the diagnosis is uncertain the combination of clinical examination and ultrasound should avoid an unnecessary emergency operation.

Operative Technique

The operation for communicating hydrocoeles is similar to that for an indirect inguinal hernia and is performed via a small skin-crease incision in the groin. It is not usually necessary to open the entire inguinal canal because the cord can be delivered through a 'window' incision in the external oblique aponeurosis forming the anterior wall of the canal. Once the patent processus has been identified it is isolated from the other cord structures, traced back to its junction with the peritoneal cavity at the internal ring and transfixed, ligated and divided at this point. The hydrocoele sac is then drained by incising the distal portion of the processus, or by percutaneous needle aspiration of the sac.

If the processus is very narrow or of doubtful patency (suggesting a non-communicating hydrocele) the groin procedure should be combined with a scrotal procedure to open, drain and evert the hydrocoele sac rather than risk recurrence.

VARICOCOELE

The significance of varicocoeles lies principally in their association with subfertility. However, there is considerable individual variation in both the clinical characteristics of varicocoeles and their impact, if any, upon fertility. Opinion remains divided on the indications for surgical intervention in childhood or adolescence. There is also debate regarding the optimal surgical technique.

Incidence

One large, population-based study identified a prevalence of 0.8% in boys aged 2–6 years, 1.0% at 7–10 years, 7.8% at 11–14 years and 14.1% at 15–19 years. Numerous studies have shown that varicocoeles occur more commonly in taller individuals and those with a lower body mass indices (BMIs). Among the male partners of infertile couples, the incidence of varicocoele is 30%.

Aetiology

The tortuosity and dilatation of the veins of the pampiniform plexus is the result of incompetence of the valvular mechanism which normally protects the spermatic veins from the hydrostatic pressure of the column of venous blood transmitted from the great veins. The fact that more than 90% of varicocoeles are left-sided is due to differences in venous anatomy, with the left testicular vein draining into the renal vein, whereas the right testicular vein drains into the vena cava. Several patterns of abnormal venous anatomy predisposing to varicocoele formation have been described:

- Absence of valves within an otherwise normal single testicular vein
- Anomalous venous drainage, for example between testicular and retroperitoneal veins
- Bifurcation of the left renal vein, with an abnormal point of entry of the spermatic veins.

Although venous obstruction by a renal tumour accounts for less than 1% of varicocoeles during childhood, this possibility should never be overlooked.

Pathology

Studies involving the use of heat-sensitive strips have confirmed that the presence of a varicocoele causes an increase in the temperature of the scrotal contents, leading to reduction in the normal temperature differential which is necessary for spermatogenesis. The role, if any, of venous pressure-related damage to the testis is more difficult to assess. Histological features observed in testicular biopsies include; reduced spermatogonia, seminiferous tubal atrophy, endothelial cell proliferation and Leydig cell abnormalities. When these histological changes are present in patients under the age of 18 years they are potentially reversible, but the more extensive histological changes found in older adults are not. This observation has been cited as argument for treating varicocoeles during adolescence rather than later.

Classification

The classification devised by Dubin and Amelar is widely employed:

- Subclinical: neither palpable nor visible, but demonstrable by Doppler ultrasound.
- Grade I: palpable only on Valsalva manoeuvre.
- Grade II: palpable at rest but not visible. Visible only with Valsalva
- Grade III: visible and palpable at rest.

Presentation

Varicocoeles may be detected during the course of routine medical examination or may present symptomatically, either as a scrotal swelling, classically likened to a 'bag of worms', or by a dragging sensation within the scrotum, which is often worse during hot weather (Figure 18.12).

Diagnosis and Investigation

The patient should be examined both lying and, more importantly, standing. During the examination the patient should be asked to perform

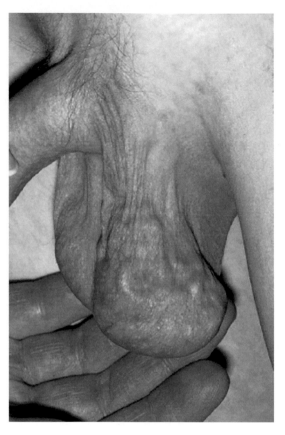

Figure 18.12 Grade III varicocoele. Visibly distended cremasteric veins ('bag of worms').

a Valsalva manoeuvre. In addition to clinical examination a scrotal ultrasound scan should be performed assess the varicocoele and measure testicular volume. This should be combined with an abdominal scan to exclude a renal tumour.

Indications for Treatment

The criteria which warrant **consideration of surgical intervention in adults** include.

- Persistently abnormal semen quality
- Altered sperm function tests
- Infertility
- Pain or significant discomfort
- Differences in testicular volume between the two testes exceeding 15–20%
- Peak retrograde flow on Doppler ultrasound >38 cm/s

- '20/38 harbinger' – combination of difference in testicular volume of > 20% and peak retrograde flow on Doppler ultrasound.

Of these, impaired testicular growth and significant differential in testicular volumes are indications for possible intervention which are also applicable to boys and adolescents. However, semen quality and infertility are far less relevant – particularly in younger adolescents with asymptomatic varicoceles. In these patients the issues surrounding 'prophylactic' treatment remain controversial. The **arguments in favour of surgical intervention in adolescents** can be summarised as follows:

- Persistence of an untreated varicocoele into adult life leads to a demonstrable reduction in testicular volume and there is evidence that surgical correction may partly reverse this process, leading to some degree of subsequent 'catch-up growth'.
- The incidence of varicocoele among men investigated for infertility is higher than in the male population at large.
- Some studies have found an improvement in semen quality and pregnancy rates following treatment of varicocoele in subfertile men.

Arguments against prophylactic surgical intervention in adolescents are:

- Varicocoeles exist in some 15% of adult males, most of whom, as judged by paternity, have normal fertility.
- Although a link exists between varicocoele and infertility or subfertility there is no consistent correlation between the presence or size of the lesion and semen quality or fertility.

Opinion remains divided but the present tendency is to advise 'prophylactic' intervention for larger, grade III lesions, particularly if there is testicular asymmetry with a discrepancy in testicular volume of >20%. From the mid teens onwards the decision on whether to proceed to surgical correction of grade III varicoceles can also be guided by semen analysis.

Treatment Options (Figure 18.13)

Embolisation

Embolisation may be carried out under sedation, although a general anaesthetic is usually used in prepubertal boys. A catheter introduced via the right femoral or internal jugular vein is screened into the left renal vein and thence into the spermatic vein. Venography is performed to identify collaterals. Embolisation is undertaken using

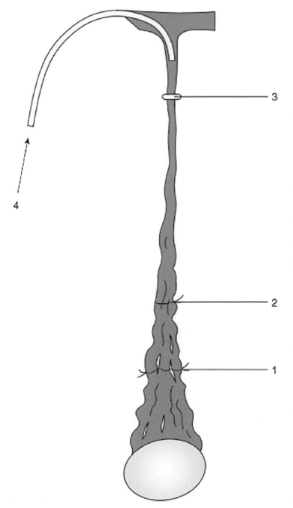

Figure 18.13 Varicocoele treatment options. (1) Surgical ligation of individual veins, inguinal approach. (2) Surgical ligation of veins and artery, high approach. (3) Laparoscopic clipping, all vessels or selective 'artery sparing'. (4) Embolisation.

coils inserted into the testicular vein or, less often, by the injection of a sclerosant.

Surgical ligation

Using the inguinal approach (Ivanissevich), the internal inguinal ring is exposed via the inguinal canal; the spermatic veins are exposed deep to the transversalis fascia and divided at this level.

In the high approach (Palomo), a short transverse incision is performed lateral to the internal inguinal ring. The testicular vessels are identified extraperitoneally above the point they diverge from the vas deferens. In Palomo's original description, the testicular artery, vein and lymphatics are all ligated and divided together but many surgeons ligate only the veins.

Microvascular ligation of the veins can be performed beyond the external inguinal ring or within it. Magnification is employed and intraoperative ultrasound may be helpful in identifying and preserving the arteries. Care is taken to preserve the testicular and cremasteric arteries, the vas deferens and its artery. The lymphatics should also be preserved as this is believed to minimise the incidence of postoperative hydrocoele.

With laparoscopic ligation, three ports are placed and the testicular vessels identified. The veins can either be dissected and divided alone or clipped and ligated en bloc, along with the artery - as in the Palomo technique. This approach also allows easy identification and division of any abnormal veins and is also especially applicable to the rare case of bilateral varicocoele. As with open techniques, lymphatic vessels should be preserved as far as possible in order to reduce the risk of postoperative hydrocele. This can be facilitated by injecting methylene blue into the scrotum preoperatively to demonstrate the lymphatics more clearly at operation.

Complications and Outcome

The fact that several surgical techniques continue to be employed for treating varicocoeles indicates that no single technique gives consistently satisfactory results. High success rates have been claimed for laparoscopic ligation and the Paloma technique (100% and 93%, respectively). Recent data in adults suggest that the best surgical results are typically obtained with the inguinal or subinguinal microscopic techniques – with low recurrence rates (2%) and low incidence of hydrocele formation (0.75%). However, these results in adults have not yet been replicated in the paediatric age group.

Improvement in fertility has been reported in subfertile men following varicocoele ligation, although subfertile men represent only a minority of all men with varicocoeles. Whether prophylactic treatment of asymptomatic varicocoeles in adolescents is beneficial for fertility has yet to be ascertained.

KEY POINTS

- The optimal age for orchidopexy remains uncertain. Paediatric urologists and paediatric surgeons favour the first year of life any time after 6 months of age.
- The risk of testicular atrophy should be specifically discussed with parents when obtaining consent for orchidopexy.
- Laparoscopy is the investigation of choice for impalpable testes.
- In infants a clear diagnostic distinction must be made between an inguinal hernia (which requires prompt surgical intervention in this age group) and a communicating hydrocoele (which generally resolves as a result of spontaneous closure of the patent processus vaginalis within the first 2 years of life).

- The available evidence suggests that treatment of varicocoeles in adolescence should be limited to boys with grade III varicocoeles, symptoms and/or evidence of impaired testicular growth.

FURTHER READING

Balawender K, Orkisz S, Wisz P. Testicular microlithiasis: what urologists should know. A review of the current literature. *Cent European J Urol.* 2018;71(3):310–314.

Esposito C, Escolino M, Turrà F, et al. Current concepts in the management of inguinal hernia and hydrocele in paediatric patients in laparoscopic era. *Semin Pediatr Surg.* 2016;25(4):232–240.

Macey MR, Owen RC, Ross SS, Coward RM. Best practice in the diagnosis and treatment of varicocele in children and adolescents. *Ther Adv Urol.* 2018;10(9):273–282.

Niedzielski JK, Oszukowska E, Słowikowska-Hilczer J. Undescended testis – current trends and guidelines: a review of the literature. *Arch Med Sci.* 2016;12(3):667–677.

Hutson JM. Journal of paediatric surgery-sponsored Fred McLoed lecture. Undescended testis: the underlying mechanisms and the effects on germ cells that cause infertility and cancer. *J Pediatr Surg.* 2013;48(5):903–908.

The Acute Scrotum

DAVID F M THOMAS

Topics covered

Overview of clinical aspects and investigation	Epididymo-orchitis
Torsion of the testis	Idiopathic scrotal oedema
Torsion of testicular appendage	Other acute scrotal pathology

OVERVIEW OF CLINICAL ASPECTS

Acute scrotal pathology constitutes one of the few real emergencies in paediatric urology because of the risk to the testis posed by testicular torsion.

Testicular torsion accounts for 80–90% of cases of acute scrotal symptoms in pubertal boys and adolescents. Urgent surgical exploration is mandatory unless there is compelling evidence of an alternative diagnosis. The differential diagnosis is more varied in prepubertal boys. Although torsion of a testicular appendage (hydatid of Morgagni) is the commonest diagnosis in this age range testicular torsion nevertheless accounts for approximately one-third of cases. Other causes of acute scrotal symptoms in prepubertal boys include; epididymo-orchitis, idiopathic scrotal oedema, acute hydrocoele and Henoch–Schonlein vasculitis (Figure 19.1).

INVESTIGATION

The definitive "investigation" in children and adolescents presenting with acute scrotal symptoms is urgent surgical exploration. A negative exploration is preferable to the loss of a potentially viable testis because of the failure to explore the scrotum.

The role of diagnostic imaging, notably colour Doppler ultrasonography, is largely confined to prepubertal boys in whom testicular torsion has been effectively excluded on clinical grounds. Doppler ultrasonography provides information on blood flow in addition to real-time anatomical imaging of the scrotal contents (Figure 19.2). Drawbacks include operator dependency, limited out-of-hours availability, false negative or false positive results and additional delay in restoring blood supply to the testis in cases of torsion.

Radionuclide testicular scanning (RTS) is now of largely historical interest.

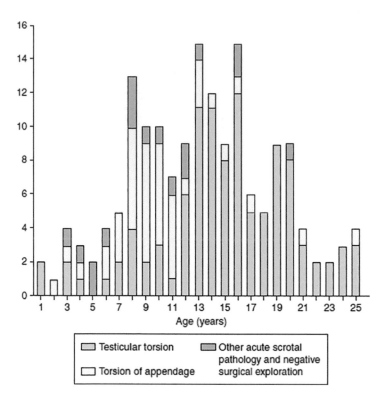

Figure 19.1 The relative frequency of different causes of acute scrotal pathology at different ages in childhood and early adult life. (From Ben-Chaim J, Leibovitch I, Ramon J, et al. Etiology of acute scrotum at surgical exploration in children, adolescents and adults. Eur Urol. 1992;21:45–47.)

TESTICULAR TORSION

The reported incidence is around 1:3,000–1:4,000 with the estimated incidence of neonatal torsion being 1:17,000. Testicular torsion occurs most frequently between the ages of 14 and 16 but can occur into late adulthood. Sporting activity and trauma may be implicated as precipitating factors but most cases occur without any obvious reason and, indeed, torsion can occur during sleep. Torsion in maldescended testes accounts for 2–5% of cases.

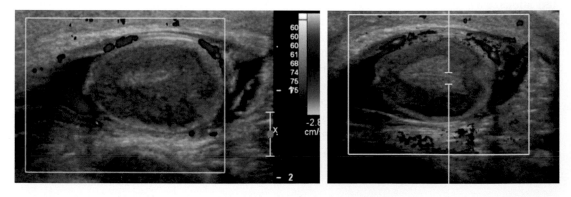

Figure 19.2 Scrotal ultrasound. Colour Doppler signals denote blood flow in the tissues surrounding the testis but absence of perfusion (ischemia) in the testis itself.

Aetiology

In the majority of cases, the testis twists within its coverings in the scrotum (Figure 19.3). This is described as intravaginal torsion – as opposed to extravaginal torsion in which the testis and its coverings twist in their entirety. The extravaginal form is virtually confined to neonatal torsion. Intravaginal torsion is conventionally attributed to a predisposing abnormality ("bell-clapper testis") in which the testis is suspended within the tunica by an abnormally long leash of spermatic vessels. However, autopsy studies suggest that "bell clapper testis" simply represents one end of the normal anatomical spectrum, rather than being a distinct entity.

Pathophysiology

In experimentally induced torsion in animal models, 720° torsion consistently leads to complete cessation of blood flow to and from the testis. This is rapidly followed by the onset of irreversible ischaemic damage to the seminiferous tissue. The correlation between duration of torsion and the timescale of ischaemic damage in experimentally induced 360° torsion is less precise. The majority of published clinical studies are retrospective and are of poor scientific quality. In particular, assessment of potential viability of the testis is often based solely on the subjective judgement of the surgeon (often a relatively junior surgeon) at the time of surgery. Without the inclusion of longer term follow-up data, the "viability" or "salvage" rates reported in such studies are largely meaningless. Where clinical and ultrasound follow-up studies have been undertaken these have consistently found that a high proportion of testes which had been judged to be potentially viable at the time of surgery nevertheless underwent total (or severe partial) atrophy.

The weight of published evidence indicates that the best prospect of conserving a viable testis of normal size lies in restoring its blood supply within 4–6 hours. Complete or partial atrophy

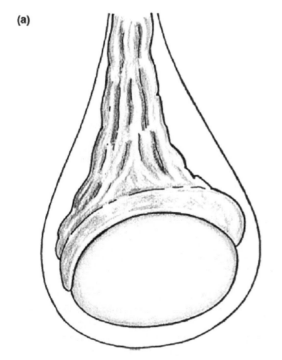
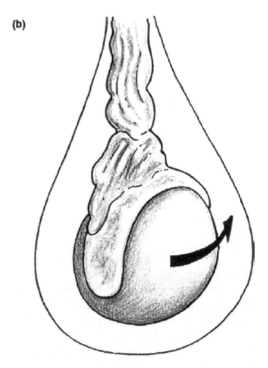

(a)

(b)

Figure 19.3 **(a)** Intravaginal torsion. "Bell-clapper" testis suspended on an abnormally long leash of vessels (mesorchium) within the tunica vaginalis. **(b)** Undue mobility of the testis predisposes to torsion around the axis of the spermatic cord.

is virtually inevitable if the blood supply is not restored within 6–8 hours and atrophy is the rule after 8–10 hours. The "6-hour rule" cited in the context of litigation is broadly supported by the scientific evidence.

Presentation

Testicular torsion is characterised by an acute onset of unilateral scrotal pain and swelling which is accompanied by vomiting in around 40% of cases. However, the clinical presentation can be variable and the "full house" of classic features is probably present in less than 50% of cases. Testicular torsion is often accompanied by referred pain in the groin and/or lower abdominal quadrant which may be perceived as being more severe than the pain arising in the testis itself. In such cases there is a risk of right sided torsion being misdiagnosed as appendicitis and left sided torsion being misdiagnosed as gastroenteritis. Testicular torsion in infants and small children is often relatively painless in the early stages – only coming to light when obvious scrotal swelling and discolouration become apparent (Figure 19.4). Clinical examination may reveal that the affected testis is located in an elevated position within the scrotum as a consequence of contraction of the cremasteric muscle. The testis is usually acutely tender on direct palpation – although this is not always the case in prepubertal boys.

When the torsion has been established for a few hours, oedema and inflammatory changes develop in the overlying scrotal tissues. The features of a more advanced torsion may be misinterpreted as epididymo orchitis – which is a much rarer condition in this age group.

Management

Urgent surgical exploration is the keystone of management. To avoid unnecessary delay (and increased risk to the potential viability of the testis) urgent surgical exploration should usually be performed in the hospital where the child or young person first presents. The Royal College

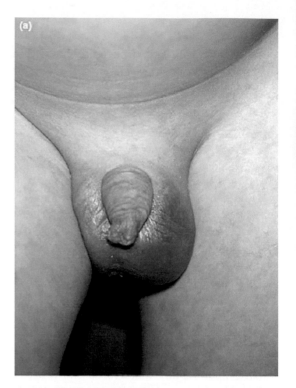

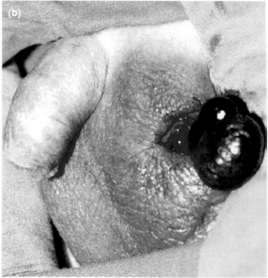

Figure 19.4 (a) Deceptively painless presentation of testicular torsion in an infant with a 3-day history of minimal symptoms. Discolouration of the scrotum prompted his parents to seek medical advice. (b) Prompt surgical exploration nevertheless revealed a necrotic testis.

of Surgeons of England states that *"Transfer of a boy with a suspicion of torsion from a secondary institution to a tertiary care centre should be an exceptional occurrence (e.g. medical comorbidities".)* Following exposure of the testis via a scrotal incision, the spermatic cord is untwisted and testicular viability assessed. Factors influencing the decision to conserve or remove the testis include the duration of the history, the appearance of the testis and arterial bleeding on incising the tunica albuginea (Figure 19.5). Unless the testis is clearly viable it is preferable to err in favour of orchidectomy. If the history is short and the testis is judged to be viable it should be fixed to prevent recurrent torsion. Regardless of the procedure on the affected side, prophylactic fixation of the contralateral testis should always be performed because of the bilateral nature of the predisposing anatomy.

Technical Aspects of Fixation

This is probably best achieved by inserting three non-absorbable sutures (e.g. 4/0 prolene) between the scrotal wall and tunica albuginea of the upper and lower poles and mid zone of the testis. Concerns that puncture of the tunica albuginea by fixation sutures might provoke the production of anti-sperm antibodies have been shown to be unfounded.

No fixation technique offers a total guarantee against further torsion, but three point fixation with a non-absorbable suture material is widely regarded as being the most reliable.

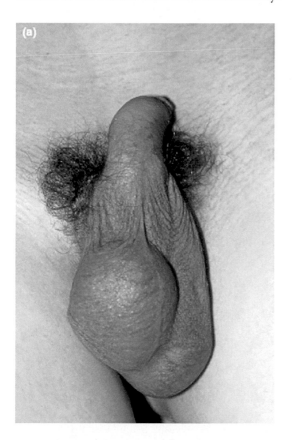 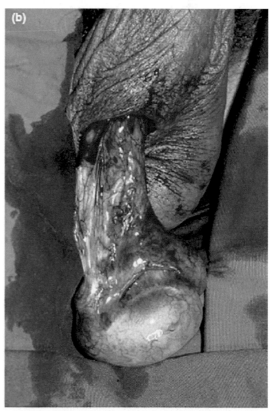

Figure 19.5 **(a)** Characteristic appearances of early torsion (3-hour history). The right testis is tender, mildly swollen, and lies in an elevated position within the scrotum. **(b)** This testis was judged to be viable in view of the short history and operative findings indicating good return of perfusion following detorsion.

Prognosis

Fertility

Men with a history of testicular torsion in adolescence or early adulthood are at increased risk of impaired semen quality. The percentage of men whose semen quality is reduced varies considerably between different studies but is typically in the range 20–50%. Most studies do not differentiate between men in whom the testis was removed and those in whom it was conserved. A number of possible mechanisms have been suggested to account for the reduction in sperm density (sperm count) but the simplest explanation is the quantitative reduction in seminiferous tissue arising from the loss of one testis.

By contrast to the literature on semen quality, there is surprisingly little published evidence on paternity (the actual ability to father children) in men with a previous history of torsion. However, two recent studies have reported that their paternity rates are no different to those in normal age matched controls. In addition, these studies found no difference in the time taken to achieve conception and no difference in paternity between those men who had undergone detorsion and preservation of the testis and those in whom the testis had been removed. One of these studies also looked at quality of life and sexual function and found no differences in self-reported parameters between men with a history of torsion and age matched controls.

Endocrine function: Published studies have consistently reported that plasma testosterone levels are within the normal range in men with a history of torsion – regardless of whether the affected testis was conserved or removed. Levels of gonadotrophin hormones- (Follicle Stimulating Hormone (FSH) and Luteinizing Hormone (LH) are also unaffected – although levels of Inhibin B (a marker of Sertoli cell function) are sometimes reduced.

Testicular prosthesis: The elective implantation of a testicular prosthesis should be offered to young patients who have previously undergone orchidectomy or in whom the testis has undergone severe atrophy. The decision should be deferred until the mid-teens (or later) to ensure that the patient is competent to make a fully informed decision and to enable the surgeon to implant an adult-sized prosthesis of comparable size to the contralateral testis (Figure 19.6).

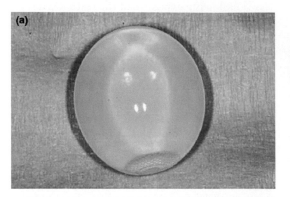

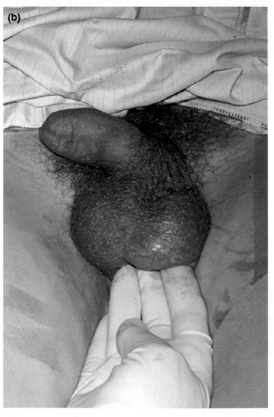

Figure 19.6 (a) Silicone gel testicular prosthesis. This is inserted via an inguinal incision and positioned in the most dependent part of the scrotum by inverting the scrotum and placing an anchoring suture in the reinforced disc at the lower pole of the prosthesis. (b) Postoperative appearances.

RECURRENT TESTICULAR PAIN

The possible risk of impending torsion should always be considered in any boy who is referred with a history of unexplained symptoms of intermittent testicular discomfort or swelling. In practice it is very difficult to assess whether such a history is genuinely indicative of episodes of mild, self-limiting torsion or, alternatively, unrelated symptoms of testicular discomfort, which are not uncommon in this age group. The parents and (depending on his age) the boy himself should be counselled appropriately and offered prophylactic fixation. If they decline this course of action they should nevertheless be strongly advised of the importance of attending the nearest emergency department without delay in the event of a sudden onset of more severe testicular pain.

PREPUBERTAL TORSION

Although testicular torsion is a less frequent cause of acute scrotal symptoms in this age group it nevertheless accounts for around one-third of cases of acute scrotal pathology. The presentation is less distinctive than in older boys and adolescents. The torsion may be relatively (or completely) painless in the early stages and the parents may be unaware of its occurrence until scrotal swelling, erythema and discolouration have supervened. For this reason the opportunities to operate in time to conserve a viable testis are far more limited in this age group.

NEONATAL TORSION

With very rare exceptions, testicular torsion which is diagnosed in the first few days after birth has occurred during intrauterine life rather than the early neonatal period. Indeed, cases of intrauterine testicular torsion have been documented on prenatal ultrasound. "Neonatal" torsion is usually of the extra vaginal rather than intravaginal pattern.

Presentation

Clinical examination typically reveals marked scrotal discolouration and a hard, indurated testis. On ultrasonography the testis and epididymis are enlarged and surrounded by haemorrhagic fluid and oedema of the scrotal tissues. Perfusion is absent on colour Doppler ultrasonography.

Unsurprisingly, the prospects of salvaging a viable testis in these circumstances are effectively zero.

Historically "neonatal" torsion was managed by urgent surgical exploration and fixation of the contralateral testis. In the 1990s, however, a more conservative approach was adopted, which was based on the use of ultrasound to confirm the diagnosis and then monitor the subsequent involution and atrophy of the testis.

However, the rationale for the conservative approach is now being questioned by a growing number of case reports of bilateral synchronous and asynchronous "neonatal" torsion. This appears to occur more frequently than would be expected by chance – indicating that extra vaginal torsion may be associated with higher risk of torsion in the contralateral testis than was previously believed. In addition, there are rare case reports of torsion which appears to have genuinely occurred in the neonatal period. Opinion remains divided: whilst some paediatric urologists continue to favour conservative management of neonatal torsion others favour surgical exploration and prophylactic fixation of the contralateral testis.

No studies have been reported which have looked specifically at long-term outcomes in men with a history of unilateral "neonatal" torsion. However, it can be reasonably assumed that their endocrine function is normal and despite some possible reduction in semen quality (notably sperm density) their overall prospects of achieving paternity are likely to be normal or only marginally reduced.

Any decision regarding implantation of a testicular prosthesis should be deferred until adolescence.

TORSION OF TESTICULAR APPENDAGE (HYDATID OF MORGAGNI)

The appendix testis is a small vestigial remnant of paramesonephric (Müllerian) origin attached to the upper pole of the testis. Torsion of the appendix testis can occur at any age in childhood but the peak incidence is between 10 and 12 years.

Presentation

The condition typically presents with pain, which is usually less severe and more insidious in onset than testicular torsion. However, the two conditions cannot be reliably differentiated on clinical grounds alone. Haemorrhagic infarction of the appendix testis is sometimes visible through the scrotal tissues as a localised area of discolouration at the upper pole of the testis ("blue dot sign"). Whilst this finding is diagnostic of the condition it is only apparent in a minority of cases. Examination may reveal tenderness localised to an indurated nodule but tenderness is often more generalised and accompanied by thickening and erythema of the hemi scrotum.

Diagnosis

The clinical features may be sufficiently distinctive to enable an experienced clinician to make a firm diagnosis. Colour Doppler ultrasound can provide additional confirmation.

Management

The condition can be managed conservatively if the diagnosis can be established with confidence and the pain is mild or resolving. Surgical intervention is indicated when testicular torsion cannot be excluded or when discomfort is more severe. Treatment consists of simple excision of the infarcted hydatid of Morgagni. Prophylactic excision of the contralateral testicular appendage is not necessary nor is prophylactic fixation of the testis.

EPIDIDYMO-ORCHITIS

Aetiology

In children and young people, epididymo-orchitis usually occurs as a consequence of bacterial infection transmitted via the ejaculatory ducts and vas deferens from the posterior urethra. Epididymo-orchitis (particularly when recurrent) may be linked to an underlying urological condition such as neuropathic bladder, persistent Müllerian remnant ("prostatic utricle", "vagina masculina") or ectopic ureter. However, the condition can also occur in infants with urinary infection who have no identifiable anatomical abnormality of their lower urinary tract. Epididymo-orchitis in infants is not always accompanied by demonstrable evidence of urinary tract infection. Such cases are thought to result from the irritant effect of sterile urine transmitted from the lower urinary tract to the testis via the vas (vasal reflux). Epididymitis in sexually active adolescents and young adults may be secondary to sexually transmitted infection – notably chlamydia. As a result of vaccination policy mumps orchitis is now a very rare cause of orchitis in this age group.

Presentation

Scrotal pain and swelling may be accompanied by clinical features of urinary infection such as dysuria or offensive urine. Examination typically reveals marked scrotal erythema and tenderness with induration of the testis. Epididymo-orchitis is often accompanied by fever and some degree of generalised ill health.

Diagnosis

In boys of all ages, testicular torsion is considerably more common than epididymo-orchitis and this diagnosis should therefore be viewed with suspicion. Moreover, epididymo-orchitis cannot always be reliably distinguished from testicular torsion on clinical grounds alone. For these reasons surgical exploration is advisable unless there is a known history of a predisposing urological abnormality or the clinical features are strongly indicative of epidiymo-orchitis. Confirmatory investigations include:

> Urine microscopy – pyuria, bacteriuria and positive urine culture
> Doppler ultrasound – hyperaemia and increased vascularity

Management

Non-operative management comprises analgesia (epididymo-orchitis is an acutely painful condition) and an intravenous antibiotic, e.g. gentamicin or ciprofloxacin, pending the result of urine culture. Antibiotic treatment should be instituted postoperatively when the condition is discovered at exploration.

Surgical intervention may be indicated to resolve any diagnostic uncertainty and to drain a scrotal or testicular abscess.

In cases of recurrent symptomatic epididymo-orchitis it may be necessary to consider vasectomy to prevent retrograde transmission of infecting bacteria to the testis via the vas deferens or surgical correction of an underlying anatomical abnormality, such as a large Müllerian remnant. Excision of this structure can be performed laparoscopically or by an open trans vesical, trans trigonal approach. The late outcome for fertility following these procedures is poorly documented but they undoubtedly carry a significant risk of causing vasal injury.

Prognosis

The fate of the testis cannot be reliably assessed until all the induration has resolved, which is generally a matter of several months. Following an isolated episode in a child without underlying urological abnormalities the prognosis is generally good. However, varying degrees of testicular atrophy can ensue after recurrent attacks of epididymo-orchitis.

IDIOPATHIC SCROTAL OEDEMA

This condition is virtually confined to the prepubertal age group, with a peak incidence between the ages of 5 and 6 years.

Aetiology

Although the aetiology is unknown its association with anal pathology and the occasional finding of erythema extending from the perineum has been interpreted as evidence of reactive oedema secondary to localised lymphangitis.

Presentation

The clinical picture is characterised by marked oedema of the scrotum, which may be unilateral or may affect the entire scrotum – sometimes extending upwards to involve the subcutaneous tissues of the inguinal region (Figure 19.7). Pain is minimal or absent. The diagnosis presents few problems to those clinicians who are acquainted with this distinctive condition.

Management

The scrotal swelling settles spontaneously, usually within 24–48 hours. The use of antihistamines and antibiotics has been described but there is no evidence they are beneficial. As a rule, no specific treatment is required.

OTHER ACUTE SCROTAL CONDITIONS

Incarcerated Hernia

In infancy, scrotal swelling may be the most striking visible manifestation of an inguinoscrotal hernia. On careful palpation it should be possible

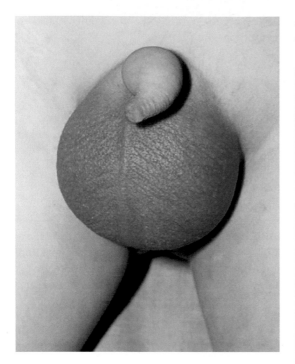

Figure 19.7 Idiopathic scrotal oedema.

to differentiate between an inguinoscrotal hernia (which extends downwards from the inguinal region to the scrotum) and genuine intrascrotal pathology.

Acute Hydrocoele

A tense, rapidly developing hydrocoele can occasionally give rise to diagnostic uncertainty. However, acute hydrocoeles are rarely painful (unless associated with underlying pathology of the testis). Transillumination confirms the diagnosis.

Henoch–Schonlein Vasculitis

Involvement of the testis, giving rise to tenderness, swelling and scrotal discolouration, is a well-documented complication of Henoch–Schonlein vasculitis. The presence of a purpuric rash should give the clue to the diagnosis and thus avert unnecessary surgical intervention. However, testicular torsion can very rarely occur in conjunction with Henoch–Schonlein vasculitis

and it is advisable to obtain an ultrasound scan to assess the underlying testis.

KEY POINTS

- Torsion of the testis accounts for 90% of acutely presenting scrotal symptoms in pubertal boys and adolescents. However, the clinical picture is sometimes dominated by pain referred to the ipsilateral lower abdominal quadrant or groin. The testes should always be examined in any boy or adolescent presenting with a sudden onset of lower abdominal pain.
- Urgent surgical exploration is mandatory unless there is compelling evidence of an alternative diagnosis.
- Prophylactic suture fixation of the contralateral testis should always be performed.
- "Neonatal" torsion is a misnomer since the torsion is usually an intrauterine event and the testis is almost invariably non-viable.
- Torsion of a testicular appendage (hydatid of Morgagni) in a prepubertal boy can be managed conservatively provided a confident diagnosis has been made by an experienced clinician.
- Epididymo-orchitis is uncommon in childhood and, if proven, always merits investigation of the urinary tract.

FURTHER READING

Baglaj M, Carachi R. Neonatal bilateral testicular torsion: a plea for emergency exploration. J Urol. 2007;177(6):2296–2299.

Colliver DW, Thomas DFM. Testicular torsion. In Ledbetter D J, Johnson PRV (eds), Endocrine Surgery in Children. Berlin: Springer, 2017: 293–304.

Drlík M, Kočvara R. Torsion of spermatic cord in children: a review. J Pediatr Urol. 2013;9(3):259–266.

Gielchinsky I, Suraqui E, Hidas G, Zuaiter M, Landau EH, Simon A, Duvdevani M, Gofrit ON, Pode D, Rosenberg S. Pregnancy rates after testicular torsion. J Urol. 2016;196(3):852–855.

Makela EP, Roine RP, Taskinen S. Paternity, erectile function, and health-related quality of life in patients operated for paediatric testicular torsion. J Pediatr Urol. 2020;16(1):44.

Disorders of Sex Development

EMILIE K JOHNSON and ELIZABETH B YERKES

Topics covered

Definitions and nomenclature
Classification of DSD
Evaluation of a child with suspected DSD

Gender assignment/sex designation
Surgical management

INTRODUCTION

This chapter provides a detailed account of the biology and treatment options for the range of conditions classified as differences/disorders of sex development (DSD). The controversial aspects of the medical care of children with DSDs will be briefly addressed although they lie largely outside the scope of this chapter.

DEFINITION AND NOMENCLATURE

The term DSD describes individuals with atypical or discordant chromosomal, gonadal, or phenotypic sex. Historically, DSDs have been broadly classified according to atypical or ambiguous appearances of the genitalia but the current definition encompasses a much wider range of disorders. Until recently, DSDs were typically diagnosed with atypical genitalia in the neonate or with primary amenorrhea in adolescence. However, DSDs are increasingly being diagnosed prenatally or during evaluation of children with conditions such as short stature or hypertension.

MULTIDISCIPLINARY CARE MODEL

In 2006, an international panel proposed a new nomenclature for DSD (Table 20.1) and recommended that all children with DSDs should receive multidisciplinary care provided by a team which, at a minimum should include: pediatric urologists (or pediatric surgeons), pediatric endocrinologists, and appropriate mental health professionals. Wherever possible, the multidisciplinary team should also include specialists in gynecology, social

Table 20.1 Revised nomenclature

Previous	Proposed
Intersex	DSD
Male pseudohermaphrodite	46XY DSD
Female pseudohermaphrodite	46XX DSD
True hermaphrodite	Ovotesticular DSD
Mixed gonadal dysgenesis	Mixed gonadal dysgenesis (unchanged)
XX male or XX sex reversal	46XX testicular DSD
XY sex reversal	46XY complete gonadal dysgenesis

Source: Lee PA, et al. (see Further Reading).

work, nursing, neonatology, fertility medicine, and the provision of peer support.

CONTROVERSIES SURROUNDING NOMENCLATURE

Although the revised nomenclature has generally been embraced by the medical community and is more acceptable for patients and families than the traditional terminology, it nevertheless remains controversial. Some individuals prefer the older term "intersex" while others prefer a named diagnosis, e.g. congenital adrenal hyperplasia (CAH). Indeed, many individuals living with CAH and do not consider themselves to have a DSD but regard themselves as having an endocrine condition. Additionally, while some patients with proximal hypospadias will have a definable DSD diagnosis, others have no clearly defined genetic or endocrinologic condition which would classify them as having a DSD which might benefit from multidisciplinary follow-up. Patients and parents should be asked which terminology they prefer to use. For the purposes of this chapter the medically accepted DSD nomenclature will be used.

EMBRYOLOGY

Knowledge of the normal embryological development of the genital tract provides the key to understanding the etiology and clinical features of the different forms of DSD (see Chapter 1).

DSDs can originate at different stages in the complex pathways of normal development. These can be briefly categorized as follows:

CHROMOSOMAL

Genetically determined defects of gonadal development include mixed gonadal dysgenesis (MGD) and ovotesticular DSD (previously termed true hermaphroditism).

GENE MUTATIONS

DSDs may result from gene mutations which are not apparent on a conventional karyotype examination. For example, mutations of genes on the Y chromosome may result in impaired differentiation, development and function of the testes despite a 46XY karyotype. X-linked mutations occurring in individuals with a 46XY karyotype may be associated with androgen receptor defects.

ENDOCRINE

DSDs may result from defects in endocrine biosynthetic pathways and may also result from defects in the receptors responsible for mediating the effects of sex hormones in the target tissues. Prime examples of the former are CAH and 5-alpha reductase deficiency. Examples of DSDs due to receptor defects include complete and partial androgen insensitivity (CAIS/PAIS).

The severity of the defect in hormonal synthesis or receptor activity can be very variable. Consequently, the genital phenotype and/or functional deficiency can vary considerably even among individuals sharing the same underlying diagnosis.

external genitalia high to androgen levels during intrauterine development. The atypical features of the external genitalia may include enlargement of the clitoro-phallic structure, varying degrees of labioscrotal fusion, and rugated (scrotal like) appearance of the labia. The internal genitalia usually retain a female phenotype with normal uterus, fallopian tubes, and ovaries.

CLASSIFICATION

46XX DSD

This is characterized by masculinization of the genitalia in individuals with a female (46XX) karyotype. It results from exposure of the

CONGENITAL ADRENAL HYPERPLASIA (CAH)

CAH is the commonest form of 46XX DSD and the most frequent cause of ambiguous genitalia in Western countries. It is an autosomal recessive condition linked to mutations in genes encoding for one of three enzymes in the biosynthetic pathways for steroid hormones in the adrenals (Figure 20.1). Enzyme deficiencies give rise to a

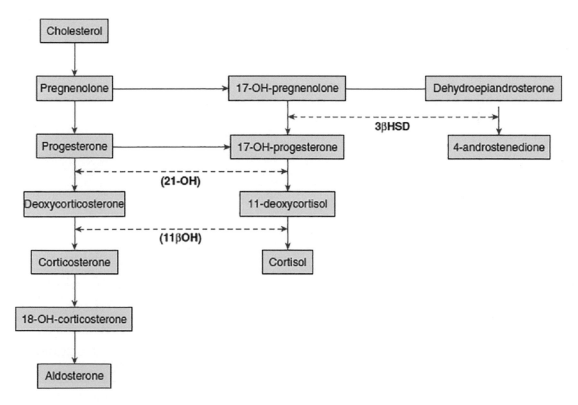

Figure 20.1 Adrenal steroid pathway. Sites of enzyme blockage in congenital adrenal hyperplasia are noted.

block in the biosynthetic pathway of adrenal hormones and consequent accumulation of steroid precursors which are diverted down an androgen synthesis pathway. The pituitary gland responds to the reduced levels of cortisol and aldosterone by increased secretion of adrenocorticotropic hormone (ACTH). In turn, this drives the adrenal biosynthetic pathway to produce even more androgens.

The degree of masculinization of the external genitalia varies according to the specific enzyme deficiency and the severity of the block it causes. Figure 20.2 Further masculinization can also occur postnatally if replacement of adrenal hormones is not sufficient to suppress the ACTH drive. Severe forms of CAH can lead to a life-threatening salt wasting (hyponatremic) condition in neonates. For this reason, any infant born with apparent hypospadias and bilateral non-palpable gonads should be investigated for CAH before being discharged from the hospital.

21-Hydroxylase Deficiency

This is the commonest form of CAH, accounting for >95% of cases. Estimates of the incidence range from 1:10,000 to 1:20,000 live births. The gene encoding for 21-hydroxylase (CYP21A2) is located on chromosome 6. Deficiency of 21-hydroxylase results in increased levels of aldosterone and cortisol precursors, most notably 17-hydroxyprogesterone (17-OHP). This form of CAH can sometimes be diagnosed prenatally, particularly when another family member is affected. Prenatal treatment with dexamethasone to suppress the fetal pituitary adrenal axis and minimize masculinization of the genitalia has been reported but has not been widely adopted.

Approximately 75% of individuals with classical 21-hydroxylase deficiency have the salt-wasting variant which can present with a life-threatening adrenal crisis in the first 2 weeks of life.

11β-Hydroxylase Deficiency

This form of CAH is associated with salt-retention mediated hypertension (via precursors of aldosterone) in addition to masculinization of the external genitalia.

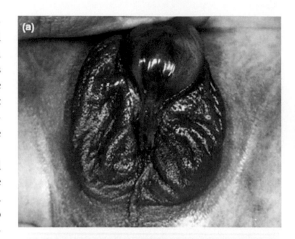
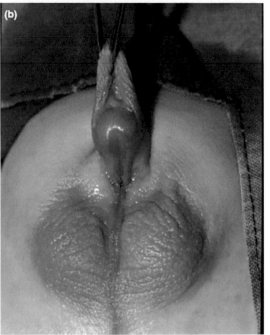

Figure 20.2 Two examples of genital appearance in newborn infants with 46XX congenital adrenal hyperplasia. Note clitoro-phallic structure and a single opening for urogenital sinus. Labioscrotal folds are fused and rugated with no palpable gonads.

3β-Hydroxysteroid Dehydrogenase Deficiency (Figure 20.3)

This is the rarest form of CAH and is the only form which may be associated with an atypical genital phenotype in a 46XY child. In its classic

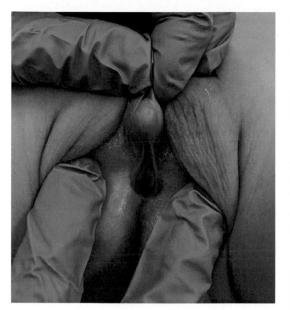

Figure 20.3 Genital appearance in an infant with 46XY 3β-hydroxysteroid dehydrogenase deficiency. Note clitoro-phallic structure with opening at the base and urethral plate "fins", rugated labioscrotal folds with lack of posterior fusion. Gonads were palpable but undescended.

form, 3β-hydroxysteroid deficiency presents with a neonatal salt-wasting adrenal crisis.

MANAGEMENT

The primary management of CAH centers on modulating the effects of the enzymatic defect. As nearly all patients will require corticosteroid replacement, additional dosages of steroid replacement will be needed to cover surgical procedures and at time of illnesses.

Historically, most families have elected for a female sex of rearing and individuals with 46XX CAH usually express a female gender identity. Nevertheless, there is evidence that gender dysphoria and non-binary gender identity are more common than was previously recognized. Males with 21-hydroxylase deficiency generally have typical male external and internal genitalia, and male gender identity. However, they may experience premature onset of puberty due to elevated androgen levels and may also be at greater risk of impaired fertility.

AROMATASE DEFICIENCY

This rare cause of 46XX DSD, is an autosomal recessive condition caused by deficiency of the enzyme responsible for converting testosterone to estrogen. Aromatase deficiency leads to the accumulation of androgens and masculinization of the external genitalia.

MATERNAL ANDROGEN EXPOSURE

Intrauterine exposure to maternal androgens (produced by androgen secreting tumors or due to treatment with androgenic progestins) is a rare cause of masculinization of female external genitalia. This possibility should always be explored by taking a detailed prenatal history.

46XX TESTICULAR DSD

Individuals with a 46XX karyotype may express a typical male genital phenotype if there has been a translocation of genetic material from the sex determining region on Y chromosome (SRY) gene onto an X chromosome and consequent differentiation down a male pathway. The external genitalia are usually unambiguously male. Depending on the nature of the translocation defect, however, some individuals may have undescended testes, hypospadias, and occasionally ambiguous genitalia. Affected individuals are usually infertile.

46XX GONADAL DYSGENESIS

Turner syndrome (45X) is considered below. However, rare individuals with a 46XX karyotype can also experience primary ovarian failure resembling Turner syndrome without displaying the other features of the syndrome. Typically, these patients present with primary amenorrhea and lack of pubertal development. Their ovaries are dysgenetic ("streak") but their external genitalia are female and they usually have a normal uterus. Treatment consists of hormonal replacement.

46XY DSD

This group of DSDs are characterized by variable degrees of masculinization and a spectrum of atypical genital development that commonly includes hypospadias and undescended testes. However, 46XY DSDs that result from a complete failure of testosterone synthesis or androgen receptor function may be associated with unambiguously female appearance of the external genitalia.

In > 50% of individuals with 46XY DSD, the underlying cause cannot be identified by laboratory investigations. This may change with the introduction of advanced genetic testing.

COMPLETE GONADAL DYSGENESIS

In this form of 46XY DSD (Swyer syndrome) the testes are severely dysgenetic and non-functional. Because the external genitalia have not been exposed to the masculinizing effects of testosterone, they exhibit a typical female appearance. Similarly, without exposure to Anti-Müllerian hormone (AMH), a uterus is present. Gonadectomy is usually recommended because the presence of a Y chromosome carries an increased risk of malignancy. Treatment otherwise consists of hormone replacement for sex characteristics and bone health.

PARTIAL GONADAL DYSGENESIS

Incomplete or partial gonadal dysgenesis results in varying degrees of impaired testicular function – which is reflected in highly variable anatomy in affected individuals. The external genitalia are usually ambiguous. Rudimentary or completely formed persistent Müllerian structures may be present, depending on the amount of AMH. Treatment is individualized, and may include hormone replacement, gonadectomy, orchidopexy, and/or genitoplasty.

GONADAL (TESTICULAR) REGRESSION

This condition results from the absence of one or both testes and a corresponding reduction or absence of functioning testicular tissue. Depending on the amount of testicular tissue which is present and the stage in intrauterine life when the testicular regression occurred, the external genitalia exhibit a phenotypic spectrum ranging from a typical male phenotype to a male with a micropenis or a male with a typical female genital phenotype.

ANDROGEN BIOSYNTHESIS DEFECTS

Enzymatic defects in the biosynthetic pathway for testosterone production such as 17β-Hydroxysteroid dehydrogenase 3 deficiency result in incomplete or absent masculinization of the external genitalia and consequently an ambiguous or typical female appearance. Virilization at puberty (notably accompanied by changes in the genitalia and voice) leads to the diagnosis in 46XY individuals who have been raised as girls. In 5-α-reductase deficiency the synthesis of testosterone occurs normally but there is a deficiency of the enzyme responsible for converting testosterone to its more active derivative dihydrotestosterone (DHT). Virilization occurs at puberty in response to the direct effect of exposure to high levels of testosterone. A high percentage of these 46XY individuals who have been raised as girls experience gender dysphoria. Conversion to male gender after puberty is accepted as normal in some societies with a high prevalence of this condition.

DEFECT IN ANDROGEN ACTIVITY

This is an X-linked recessive disorder affecting the androgen receptors. In complete androgen insensitivity syndrome (CAIS) the receptors are incapable of mediating the effects of androgens. This results in failure of masculinization of the external genitalia and correspondingly female appearances. There is a short blind-ending vagina (originating from the urogenital sinus) but no uterus is present because this has undergone regression in response to AMH secreted by the fetal testes. The testes are located in the abdomen or inguinal regions, and Wolffian (mesonephric) duct structures are also present but are typically less well developed than in a normal male. Gender identity is usually female.

CAIS is typically diagnosed either during an inguinal hernia operation in child with a female external phenotype or during the investigation of primary amenorrhea. Some female pubertal changes due to peripheral conversion of testosterone to estrogen (breast development but sparse pubic hair) may occur if the testes are retained through puberty. The risk of testicular malignancy is increased and is of the order of 2–10%. Historically, early gonadectomy was recommended but practice has changed and it is now advised that gonads are retained to permit some degree of endogenous pubertal development and to enable patients to make an informed decision when they reach the appropriate age.

Partial androgen insensitivity syndrome (PAIS) occurs when the androgen receptors demonstrate a partial response to androgens. Individual variability in the extent of the defect of the androgen receptors causes a wide spectrum of genital phenotypes ranging from normal male to normal female with varying degrees of genital ambiguity in between. Gender identity is very difficult to predict in individuals with PAIS. The risk of gonadal tumors is higher than in CAIS, particularly for intra-abdominal gonads.

LUTEINIZING HORMONE RECEPTOR DEFECTS

This receptor defect results in Leydig cell hypoplasia and a broad spectrum of incomplete masculinization related to impaired LH-mediated testosterone production.

ABNORMALITIES OF ANTI-MÜLLERIAN HORMONE (AMH)/ MÜLLERIAN INHIBITORY SUBSTANCE (MIS)

Individuals with AMH/MIS deficiency (persistent Müllerian duct syndrome [PMDS]) have bilateral undescended testes and persistent Müllerian (paramesonephric) duct structures including a uterus and fallopian tubes. In addition to genuine AMH deficiency, a proportion of cases are caused by AMH receptor defects. With the exception of bilateral undescended testes, the external genital phenotype is normal because androgen production by the testes and androgen receptor function are both normal.

SEX CHROMOSOME DSD

Turner Syndrome and Variants

The characteristic karyotype of Turner syndrome is 45XO, but mosaic karyotypes (45X0/46XX, 45X0/46XY) are common and may also be associated with other structural abnormalities of the X or Y chromosome. The external genitalia have a typical female appearance but the ovaries are dysgenetic "streak" gonads with infrequent germ cells (Figure 20.4). Other features include short stature and renal and cardiac abnormalities.

Individuals with Turner syndrome whose karyotype includes Y chromosomal material have a 30–40% risk of developing gonadal malignancy and gonadectomy has been traditionally recommended at the time of diagnosis.

Mixed Gonadal Dysgenesis (MGD)

The 45, XO/46XY karyotype just described for Turner mosaicism may also be associated with ambiguous genitalia. This is the condition of mixed gonadal dysgenesis (MGD). These

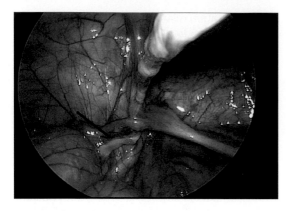

Figure 20.4 Laparoscopic appearance of a streak gonad (black arrow) from a patient with 45X/46XY mosaic Turner syndrome.

consists mainly of ovarian stroma. The ipsilateral ductal system is typically Müllerian with a Fallopian tube, infantile hemiuterus, and a vaginal type structure entering the posterior urethra. The contralateral testis, which may be descended or undescended is typically dysgenetic and the ipsilateral Wolffian (mesonephric) ductal anatomy is variable. The potential for typical male pubertal development or fertility, and the future tumor risk, is determined by the severity of the testicular dysgenesis. Decisions regarding sex of rearing and management are highly individualized but may be informed by extent of testosterone production after the first week of life as an indicator of prenatal exposure to androgens.

individuals do not have Turner syndrome but can demonstrate some of its extragenital manifestations.

MGD classically consists of one streak gonad and a contralateral dysgenetic testis (Figure 20.5). There is a high degree of variability of the genital anatomy but it commonly includes hypospadias. The internal anatomy is determined by the levels of androgen and AMH produced by the dysgenetic testis. The streak gonad is impalpable and

Klinefelter Syndrome (47XXY)

Physical and cognitive development are affected in these individuals. Although their external genitalia are usually typical male, the testes are generally small and soft. Testosterone production is reduced, and infertility is common. Other physical manifestations include a gynecoid body habitus and gynecomastia, which carries an increased risk of breast cancer.

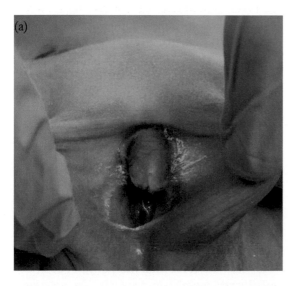

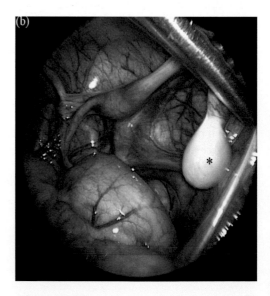

Figure 20.5 External appearance of a patient with mixed gonadal dysgenesis. Note hypospadias, flat right labioscrotal fold, and full, rugated left labioscrotal fold with palpable gonad.

OVOTESTICULAR DSD (HERMAPHRODITISM)

This is defined by the presence of both testicular and ovarian tissue in the same individual. Karyotypes vary considerably, with 46XX being the most common. Prenatal and neonatal masculinization occur to variable extent, but typical male phenotype can occur.

The ovarian and testicular tissue may be distributed as an ovary on one side and a contralateral testis or an ovotestis (one gonad containing both ovarian and testicular tissue) occurring unilaterally or bilaterally. In an ovotestis, the ovarian and testicular tissue may be localized in the poles of the gonad or intermingled throughout it (Figure 20.6). The demarcation between the ovarian and testicular components becomes less well defined after infancy but there is a tendency for

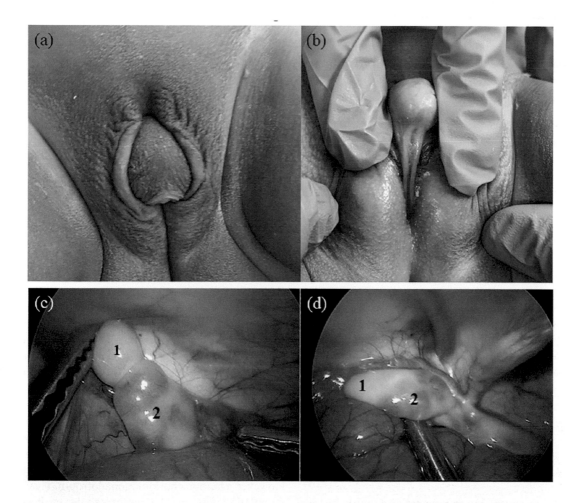

Figure 20.6 Infant with ovotesticular DSD. (a) and (b) External exam shows clitoro-phallic structure with single opening at the base, non-palpable gonads, rugated labioscrotal folds with lack of posterior fusion. (c) Ovotestis during minipuberty (4 months old). (d) Ovotestis after minipuberty (13 months) – the demarcation between the ovarian and testicular components became less distinct. 1, dysgenetic testis; 2, well-developed ovarian parenchyma. ([c] and [d] Reprinted with permission from Johnson EK, Finlayson C, Finney EL, Harris CJ, Tan SY, Laronda MM, et al. Gonadal tissue cryopreservation for children with differences of sex development. Horm Res Paediatr. 2019;92(2):84–91.)

the ovarian tissue to better developed, whereas the testicular tissue tends to be dysgenetic and thus at increased risk for loss of function and for tumor formation. As in other DSDs with variable genital and gonadal phenotypes, decisions relating to sex assignment and treatment are highly individualized.

Other conditions included in the DSD classification are defects of organogenesis and early development which involve the genitalia. These include aphallia, vaginal agenesis (Mayer-Rokitansky-Kuster-Hauser syndrome [MKRH]), vaginal duplication, and cloacal anomalies, including cloacal exstrophy. Given their complex medical needs, these individuals are often managed in the context of a multidisciplinary DSD clinic.

EVALUATION OF A CHILD WITH SUSPECTED DSD

In the initial evaluation of a newborn with a suspected DSD it is most important to reassure the parents that these are rarely life-threatening conditions. Even in CAH, life-threatening complications are mitigated by medical management and surveillance. If there is any uncertainty about possible sex of rearing, it is important to use gender-neutral terminology such as "your baby". Congratulating the parents on the birth of their baby before focusing on the medical aspects can help to make their early medical experience somewhat less bewildering.

EVALUATION OF NEONATES AND OLDER CHILDREN IS SIMILAR

History: A thorough prenatal and family history should include information on maternal symptoms and medications. It is also important to enquire about any history of urogenital abnormalities, infertility, infant death, precocious puberty, and consanguinity.

Physical examination: The following should be recorded: anatomical features of the clitoro-phallic structure, description of labioscrotal folds, the number of perineal orifices, whether the gonads are palpable and, if so, their size and characteristics. A complete examination of the infant/child should also be performed to identify and document any other dysmorphic features.

Genetic evaluation: All patients with a suspected DSD should be evaluated with a karyotype, including examination of a minimum of 40–50 cells to identify low-level mosaicism. If there is evidence of masculinization (suggesting the presence of testicular tissue) but no Y chromosomal material has been identified on the peripheral blood karyotype, a gonadal biopsy with histologic and karyotype analysis of the gonadal tissue may be required to elucidate the diagnosis. The requirement for further, more detailed genetic testing is guided by patient phenotype, hormonal profile, and karyotype results (Table 20.2).

Endocrine Evaluation (Table 20.3)

The recommended protocol for endocrine investigation of a newborn infant with a suspected DSD includes: 17-OHP, androstenedione, Dihydroepiandrosterone – Sulphate (DHEAS), testosterone, AMH/MIS, and gonadotropins (LH and, follicular-stimulating hormone, FSH). Further endocrine investigation may be indicated, depending on the initial results.

Serum electrolytes are measured to detect a hyponatremic salt-wasting state, although clinically relevant electrolyte abnormalities may not present until after 1 week of age.

The protocol for investigating an adolescent with a suspected DSD is similar, although endocrine testing is more targeted. Endocrine function is difficult to assess in the interval between the "mini-puberty" of infancy and onset of puberty. However, a human chorionic gonadotropin (HCG) stimulation test can be performed to evaluate gonadal (testicular) function during this period.

Imaging/Diagnostic Procedures

Ultrasound can help to determine whether gonads are present and assess their location, size, and quality. Müllerian structures can be assessed by

Table 20.2 Adjunctive genetic testing options

Genetic test name	Indication
FISH or SRY	Evaluation of individuals with genitalia/karyotype discrepancy (e.g. 46XX with masculinized genitalia)
Single gene testing	To confirm a diagnosis highly suspected based on history and clinical findings
DSD slice (targeted DSD gene panel)	Evaluate for gene mutations known to be associated with DSD
Microarray	Rapidly scan for multiple mutations (including possible new candidate genes) where diagnosis is unclear, and/or multiple congenital anomalies present
Whole exome sequencing	Indications similar to microarray; broader analysis may yield a diagnosis when other testing is not diagnostic

FISH, fluorescence in situ hybridization; SRY, sex determining region on Y chromosome.

ultrasound. Magnetic resonance imaging provides valuable additional information on gonadal and/or internal genital anatomy. In selected cases a genitogram (x-ray with contrast) can be used to assess the length and configuration of a urogenital sinus.

Endoscopic examination (cystoscopy/vaginoscopy) is valuable for assessing urogenital sinus anatomy. Diagnostic laparoscopy (with or without gonadal biopsy) can be informative in cases where the DSD diagnosis is unclear.

GENDER ASSIGNMENT/SEX DESIGNATION

Although the traditional paradigm advocated raising children with DSDs as either male or female, the option of assigning a third (non-binary) gender has become more acceptable in some cultures. This is increasingly available on official documents such as birth certificates, and driver's licenses.

Table 20.3 Endocrine testing for DSD evaluation

Endocrine test	Result interpretation
17-hydroxyprogesterone	Elevated in congenital adrenal hyperplasia
Anti-Müllerian hormone	Normal levels suggest functional Sertoli cells (testis) and granulosa cells (ovary). Also a measure of ovarian reserve
Gonadotropins – luteinizing hormone and follicle stimulating hormone	Elevation indicates poor gonadal function
Testosterone/Estrogen	Indicate whether functional gonadal tissue is testicular or ovarian
Androstenedione	Elevated in 21-hydroxylase deficiency and 17β-hydroxysteroid dehydrogenase deficiencies
DHEA sulfate	Elevated in 21-hydroxylase deficiency and 3β-hydroxysteroid dehydrogenase deficiency
Testosterone to dihydrotestosterone ratio	Ratio of approximately >30:1 indicates 5α-reductase deficiency
Human chorionic gonadotropin stimulation test	Non-response (lack of testosterone increase) suggests testicular dysfunction (no testicular tissue, no Leydig cells, or luteinizing hormone receptor defect)

The role of the multidisciplinary team is to provide the family with all the available diagnostic information needed to help them reach an informed decision on the sex of rearing. In addition to information on genetic and hormonal status, anatomy, and potential fertility, the family should be provided with a specific diagnosis (when possible) to help guide their decision-making.

Families should be counseled that the assigned sex of rearing is informed by neonatal observations and data but may not accurately predict future gender identity.

SURGICAL MANAGEMENT

For many years, infants with ambiguous genitalia had a sex assigned soon after birth and surgery was recommended to match the genitalia with sex of rearing. Parents were generally accepting of this approach without necessarily understanding the reasons for surgical intervention sufficiently to explain them to the affected individual when they were older.

This approach has, however, evolved into a multidisciplinary model that emphasizes psychosocial support and provides parents with broader understanding of their child's diagnosis and its long-term implications (including tumor risk, potential for fertility, projected likelihood of gender dysphoria). A balanced review of all the treatment options, should enable the team and parents to arrive at shared decisions on future management.

In some countries this model is being challenged by some human rights groups who oppose genital surgery being performed in children who are unable to participate in decisions on their treatment. This has led to calls for a moratorium on surgery before affected individuals reach the age when they can provide informed consent. As a consequence, multidisciplinary surgical decision-making is constantly evolving. Long-term follow-up and psychosocial support for patients and families will be more important than ever if we are to understand the consequences of changes in patterns of care over time.

The following section is intended to provide a general overview of genital reconstruction and to describe the various procedures which are currently available. It is not the authors' intention to advocate for surgical intervention or to suggest which DSDs require intervention. These are shared decisions which should rightly belong to individual patients and/or parents with the benefit of guidance and support from their expert multidisciplinary team.

FEMINIZING RECONSTRUCTIVE PROCEDURES AND FEMALE GENITAL RESTORATION SURGERY

These procedures may be considered for individuals with 46XX DSD (CAH), 45XO/46XY MGD, ovotesticular DSD, and also individuals with 46XY DSD with varied degrees of masculinization of the genitalia.

One or more of the following procedures may be considered;

Clitoroplasty – nerve-sparing clitoral reduction with creation of a cosmetically typical clitoral hood.

This is intended to reduce the size of the clitoral bodies (and possibly the glans clitoris) whilst safeguarding the vascularity and sensory innervation of the clitoral glans for future sexual function. The dorsal neurovascular bundles supplying the glans are isolated and protected while the hypertrophied erectile tissue of the clitoral bodies is removed. The glans is then re-seated onto the base of the clitoral bodies, with the neurovascular bundle preserved.

A clitoral disassembly technique has been described in which the clitoral bodies are separated and buried in the labia majora. The intention is that the clitoro-phallus could be reconstructed in the future, if desired. No data are yet available on the long-term outcome for sexual function or the feasibility of reconstructing a functional clitoro-phallus following this procedure.

Urogenital sinus mobilization – externalization of the urogenital sinus into separate urethral and vaginal orifices.

The anatomy of a urogenital sinus is designated as "low confluence" or "high confluence" according to the distance between the perineal opening of the urogenital sinus and the level at which the vagina joins the urethra.

In low confluence variants it may be possible to separate the vagina from the urethra and exteriorize the opening of the vagina solely by the use of a perineal-based flap. For intermediate or high-confluence variants the urethra and vagina can be mobilized toward the perineum as a unit ("en bloc") by either total urogenital mobilization (TUM) or partial urogenital mobilization (PUM) techniques. Even after successful vaginoplasty in early childhood subsequent surgical revision of the introitus and/or vaginal dilatation is usually required prior to the onset of sexual activity.

Labioplasty: A clitoral hood is created from the skin of the inner layer of the clitoral prepuce and redundant skin covering the clitoral bodies. The remaining clitoral skin is used to construct labia minora, which are usually absent in infants with urogenital sinus anomalies. The skin of the fused labia/labioscrotal folds is redistributed to create labia majora, with excess rugated (scrotal-like) skin being excised.

MASCULINIZING GENITOPLASTY

This is mainly considered when a male gender identity is predicted for the child - notably in cases of partial androgen insensitivity syndrome (PAIS) and androgen biosynthetic defects.

Hypospadias of varying severity is a common feature of these 46XY DSDs and some forms of MGD and ovotesticular DSD. The technical aspects of surgical correction are similar to those of hypospadias in non-DSD patients (Chapter 16).

GONADAL SURGERY

The presence of Y-chromosome material and any degree of gonadal dysgenesis pose a significant risk of tumor formation. The commonest of these is gonadoblastoma, which is typically benign and slow growing, but malignant dysgerminomas may also develop in dysgenetic gonads. Although dysgerminomas are malignant, they are usually curable with surgery and/or multimodal therapy.

Currently, there are no accepted surveillance protocols for the early detection of tumors arising in dysgenetic gonads and ultrasound may not always be a reliable modality for this purpose. Decisions regarding gonadectomy should be reached with the family (and, where feasible, the affected individual) based on patient age, diagnosis, and potential for endocrine function and/or fertility (Figure 20.7). Experimental gonadal tissue cryopreservation can be considered at the time of gonadectomy in the hope that technology will be developed to enable the individual to use assisted reproductive techniques in adulthood. Orchidopexy for undescended testes (dysgenetic or otherwise) is recommended for all young DSD patients who are being raised as male.

Historically, gonadal tissue and Müllerian structures discordant with the sex of rearing were surgically removed. However, current opinion favors their retention unless there is a high risk of malignancy or monitoring is difficult.

In young patients with 46XY DSD due to complete androgen insensitivity there may be benefits in leaving the discordant gonads in situ until the completion of puberty. This may aid breast development through the aromatization of testosterone Although the tumor risk is relatively low, surveillance is important and it may be appropriate to facilitate this by relocating intrabdominal testes to the groin. However, the presence of palpable gonads in the groin or labia may be unacceptable to the young patient.

Ovotesticular DSD presents an additional dilemma in view of the difficulty in identifying and separating the ovarian and testicular components of a gonad. Parents should be counseled about this difficulty and advised on any potential options to cryopreserve excised gonadal tissue for future fertility.

In some forms of DSD it may be difficult to reliably predict the individual's future gender identity and their preferences in terms of anatomy and function. In these circumstances the most appropriate option may be to preserve the existing anatomy, when safe to do so. Parents may not initially understand the reasons for recommending retention of seemingly discordant gonadal tissue and it is important to explain why this might preserve a greater choice of options for their child in the future.

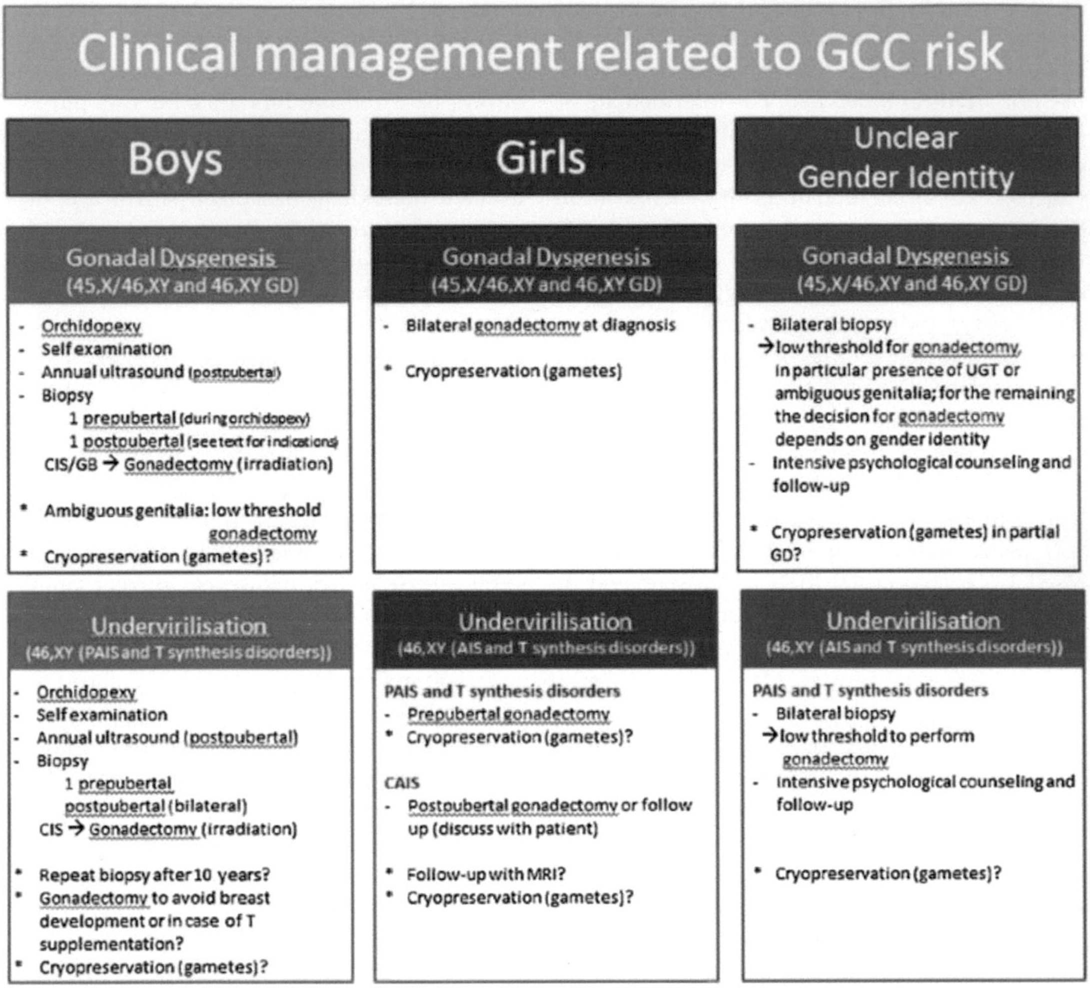

Clinical management related to GCC risk

Boys	Girls	Unclear Gender Identity
Gonadal Dysgenesis (45,X/46,XY and 46,XY GD)	**Gonadal Dysgenesis** (45,X/46,XY and 46,XY GD)	**Gonadal Dysgenesis** (45,X/46,XY and 46,XY GD)

- Orchidopexy
- Self examination
- Annual ultrasound (postpubertal)
- Biopsy
   1 prepubertal (during orchidopexy)
   1 postpubertal (see text for indications)
   CIS/GB → Gonadectomy (irradiation)
 	
* Ambiguous genitalia: low threshold
             gonadectomy
* Cryopreservation (gametes)?
	- Bilateral gonadectomy at diagnosis
	
	* Cryopreservation (gametes)
		- Bilateral biopsy
		→low threshold for gonadectomy, in particular presence of UGT or ambiguous genitalia; for the remaining the decision for gonadectomy depends on gender identity
		- Intensive psychological counseling and follow-up
		
		* Cryopreservation (gametes) in partial GD?

Undervirilisation (46,XY (PAIS and T synthesis disorders))	**Undervirilisation** (46,XY (AIS and T synthesis disorders))	**Undervirilisation** (46,XY (AIS and T synthesis disorders))

- Orchidopexy
- Self examination
- Annual ultrasound (postpubertal)
- Biopsy
   1 prepubertal
   postpubertal (bilateral)
   CIS → Gonadectomy (irradiation)
 	
* Repeat biopsy after 10 years?
* Gonadectomy to avoid breast development or in case of T supplementation?
* Cryopreservation (gametes)?
	PAIS and T synthesis disorders
	- Prepubertal gonadectomy
	* Cryopreservation (gametes)?
	
	CAIS
	- Postpubertal gonadectomy or follow up (discuss with patient)
	
	* Follow-up with MRI?
	* Cryopreservation (gametes)?
		PAIS and T synthesis disorders
		- Bilateral biopsy
		→low threshold to perform gonadectomy
		- Intensive psychological counseling and follow-up
		
		* Cryopreservation (gametes)?

Figure 20.7 One suggested gonadal management paradigm: schematic representation of a risk stratification model and recommendations for clinical follow-up. CIS, carcinoma in situ; GB, gonadoblastoma; GD, gonadal dysgenesis; MRI, magnetic resonance imaging; PAIS, partial androgen insensitivity syndrome; T-synthesis disorders, testosterone-synthesis disorders; UGT, unclear gender identity. (Reprinted with permission from van der Zwan et al.)

KEY POINTS

- A multidisciplinary team approach is the standard model of care for children with DSDs.
- Patients and families should be asked which DSD terminology they prefer.
- Although the karyotype and specific diagnosis represent a useful framework for management they may not always provide a reliable prediction of gonadal function, phenotype or gender identity.

- The degree of masculinization is determined by the extent of intrauterine exposure to circulating androgens. Paracrine factors also play a critical role in determining the anatomical features of DSD, which explains why genital asymmetry is relatively common.
- Congratulating the family on the birth of their child is a simple but important human touch that is valued by the family.
- Routine evaluation of any infant or child with a suspected DSD includes taking a thorough history, a careful physical examination and performing a karyotype and endocrine investigations. More detailed genetic and anatomical evaluation may be indicated on an individualized basis.
- The initial evaluation of an infant with a suspected DSD should include investigations for possible salt-wasting CAH since this can be life threatening.
- The surgical management of DSD is evolving and controversial. Decisions regarding surgical intervention should be individualized and made in the context of a multidisciplinary team. Parents (and where appropriate, the affected individuals) should be closely involved in the decision-making process.

Donohue PA, Migeon CJ. Congenital adrenal hyperplasia. In: Scriver CR, Sly WS, Valle D (eds), The Metabolic and Molecular Basis of Inherited Disease, 7th Edition. New York: McGraw-Hill, 1995: 2929–2966.

Jacobson DL, Yerkes EB. Ambiguous genitalia. In: Chung KC, Disa JJ, Gosain A, Gordon Lee G, Mehrara B, Thorne CH and van Aalst J (eds), Operative Techniques in Plastic Surgery. Philadelphia: Wolters Kluwer.

Johnson EK, Rosoklija I, Finlayson C, Chen D, Yerkes EB, Madonna MB, et al. Attitudes towards "disorders of sex development" nomenclature among affected individuals. J Pediatr Urol. 2017;13(6):608 e1–e8.

Lee PA, Houk CP, Ahmed SF, Hughes IA. Consensus statement on management of intersex disorders. International consensus conference on intersex. Pediatrics. 2006;118(2):e488–500.

Mouriquand PD, Gorduza DB, Gay CL, Meyer-Bahlburg HF, Baker L, Baskin LS, et al. Surgery in disorders of sex development (DSD) with a gender issue: if (why), when, and how? J Pediatr Urol. 2016;12(3):139–149.

van der Zwan YG, Biermann K, Wolffenbuttel KP, Cools M, Looijenga LH. Gonadal maldevelopment as risk factor for germ cell cancer: towards a clinical decision model. Eur Urol. 2015;67(4):692–701.

FURTHER READING

Bouvattier C. Disorders of sex development: endocrine aspects. In: Gearhart JG, Rink RC, Mouriquand PDE (eds), Pediatric Urology, 2nd Edition. Philadelphia: Saunders Elsevier, 2010.

Genitourinary Malignancies

JONATHAN WALKER and NICHOLAS G COST

Topics covered

Pediatric renal tumors
  Wilms tumor
  Renal cell carcinoma
  Congenital mesoblastic nephroma

Genitourinary rhabdomyosarcoma
Prepubertal primary testicular tumors

PEDIATRIC RENAL TUMORS

Introduction

Renal tumors account for approximately 5–10% of all pediatric cancers, with the most common malignant renal tumor in children being Wilms tumor (WT). Other renal tumors, such as congenital mesoblastic nephroma (CMN) and renal cell carcinoma (RCC) are more likely to be diagnosed in patients younger than 6 months and older than 12 years, respectively. Regardless of the final pathologic diagnosis, any newly diagnosed renal tumor in a child should be approached in a standardized fashion based on the assumption that it is a malignant.

Presentation and Differential Diagnosis

The clinical presentation of a renal tumor in childhood can vary depending on the child's age and the tumor burden at the time of diagnosis. The most common presenting symptom is a palpable abdominal mass. Other symptoms may include hematuria (10%), hypertension, lower extremity edema, or the features associated with a related condition or syndrome which predisposes the child to develop renal malignancy. There is a broad differential diagnosis for a childhood renal mass but key points in the history and physical examination findings can help to narrow the diagnostic possibilities. Specifically, age at presentation, the presence of a known predisposing syndrome or medical condition and the characteristics of the tumor on imaging may all help the clinician to identify the most likely etiology of the renal mass.

Initial Evaluation

Diagnostic evaluation of a palpable abdominal mass in children should always begin with an abdominal ultrasound (Figure 21.1A). This will help to establish the anatomical location of the mass and provide a guide to further imaging. In the case of a newly diagnosed solid renal mass, the ultrasound scan should ideally be followed by a single-setting computed tomography (CT) of the chest, abdomen, and pelvis with intravenous contrast. In addition to the renal mass itself, the key findings which may be demonstrated on CT include: possible presence of a tumor in the contralateral kidney (Figure 21.1B), local or regional lymphadenopathy, tumor thrombus in the renal vein and inferior vena cava (Figure 21.1C), and metastatic disease, particularly in the lung fields. In children presenting with gross hematuria, intraoperative retrograde pyelography of the renal collecting system can help to identify tumor involvement of the renal pelvis or ureter, which may be present in up to 2% of cases. Laboratory evaluation should include a complete blood count (CBC), urinalysis and metabolic screen. Coagulation screening should also be performed in view of the 4–8% risk of acquired Von Willebrand disease associated with WT. Although not typically of renal origin, if a paraganglioma or neuroblastoma is part of the differential diagnosis, urinary vanillylmandelic acid, homovanillic acid, and plasma free metanephrine levels can be checked to rule out these common retroperitoneal tumors (Table 21.1).

Wilms Tumor

Etiology and epidemiology

Wilms tumor, also known as nephroblastoma, is the most common primary renal malignancy in children with an incidence of 7–10 per million children. There are approximately 600 new cases a year in the United States (US) alone. Since WT accounts for more than 90% of renal malignancies in childhood this is the presumed diagnosis in most children presenting with a renal mass. The peak age of diagnosis is 3–5 years. Approximately, 5–7% of WTs are bilateral at the time of presentation and 10% are associated with a predisposing syndrome (Table 21.2). These syndromes are typically categorized by their association with the WT1 or WT2 genes on the short arm of chromosome 11. Because of the known association with certain syndromes, it is recommended that children with these syndromes should

be monitored with an abdominal ultrasound scan at 3–4 monthly intervals until 8–10 years of age. Although routine surveillance has not been shown to confer increased survival from WT it may help to minimize treatment morbidity by facilitating earlier intervention.

Histopathology and molecular biology

Classically, WT is described as having a triphasic appearance on microscopy with stromal, blastemal, and epithelial components present (Figure 21.2). The blastemal portion gives rise to the nomenclature of "small round blue cell" tumor. These cells are highly aggressive but typically more chemo-sensitive. The most common stromal components seen in WTs include smooth and skeletal muscle, bone, fat, or cartilage. Immature renal tubules, glomeruli, or papillary structures are classified as epithelial elements. Of note, there is not always equal distribution of these components, and not all of these components are always present in every WT.

The designation of *favorable* vs *unfavorable* histology was an important milestone in the treatment of WT, as it provided one of the first sources of risk stratification. Unfavorable histology, such as anaplasia, is associated with a poorer prognosis and resistance to chemotherapy. WTs with unfavorable histology only represent approximately 10% of all WTs but are responsible for the majority of deaths.

Recent advances in molecular biology have enabled further risk stratification for patients with favorable histology (FH) Wilms tumors. Studies undertaken by the children's oncology group (COG) have demonstrated that abnormalities identified on chromosomes 1 and 16 are predictive of worse overall survival. Loss of heterozygosity (LOH) of chromosomes 1p and 16q is also associated with a poorer outcome and a requirement for additional and more prolonged chemotherapy.

Staging

The children's oncology group (COG), Société Internationale d'Oncologie Pédiatrique (SIOP),

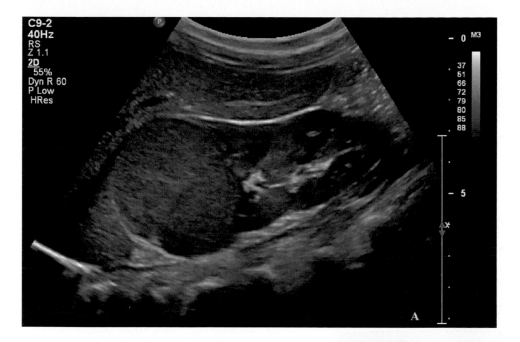

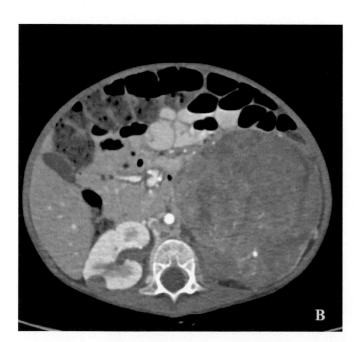

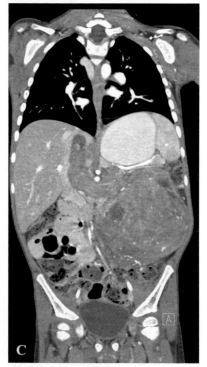

Figure 21.1 (A) Renal ultrasound of the right kidney performed during the initial evaluation of a suspected intra-abdominal mass confirming the presence of a heterogeneous renal mass. (B) Axial computed tomography (CT) with IV contrast images of a patient with a large, left-sided renal mass and a second, smaller lesion in the right kidney. (C) Coronal CT images from the same patient reveal an associated tumor thrombus extending from the left renal vein into the intra-hepatic inferior vena cava.

Table 21.1 Investigational tools for a new renal mass

Test	Purpose
Ultrasound	Primary investigation; helps direct additional imaging work-up
CT chest, abdomen, pelvis with contrast	Ideal imaging for solid renal mass; aids in surgical planning and staging
Complete metabolic panel	Renal and liver function assessment
Complete blood count	Assess for anemia or infectious etiology
Urinalysis or urine studies	Identifies hematuria, proteinuria, or VMA if indicated
Coagulation panel	Assess for the presence of bleeding disorder
Brain imaging and bone scan	Reserved for patients with concerning central nervous system symptoms or evidence of bone metastasis on standard imaging; Not typically included in initial evaluation

VMA, vanillylmandelic acid.

Table 21.2 Wilms tumor predisposition syndromes and associated features

Syndrome	Genetics	WT risk (%)	Features
Denys-Drash	WT1	50–90	XY DSD, hypospadias, UDT, renal failure
WAGR	11p13, WT1	30–50	WT, aniridia, GU anomalies, mental retardation
Perlman	WT2	20–60	Prenatal overgrowth, high infant mortality
Frasier	WT1	5–20	XY DSD, renal failure
Beckwith-Weideman	11p15, WT2	5–10	Hemihypertrophy, Macroglossia
Simpson-Golabi-Behmel	X-linked, GPC3	5–10	Skeletal and cardiac abnormalities, accessory nipples

DSD, difference in sexual development; GU, genitourinary; UDT, undescended testicle.

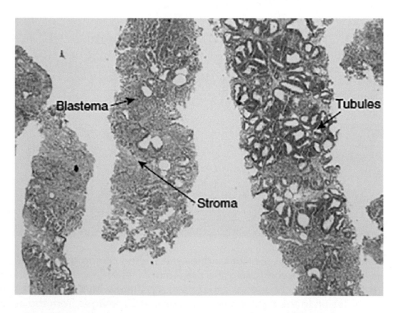

Figure 21.2 Triphasic nephroblastoma. Photomicrograph of a core-biopsy from a 3-year-old child with a unilateral renal mass showing the characteristic triphasic histological features of Wilms tumor.

and the UK National Wilms Tumor Study Group (NWTSG) are independently engaged in multicenter studies of various aspects of treatment of WTs. The staging protocol adopted by the COG is as follows; (Figure 21.3):

- Stage I (40–45%): Tumor confined to the kidney, completely resected, with no evidence of local or distant spread
- Stage II (20%): Tumor spread beyond the kidney, completely resected, with no evidence of local or distant spread
- Stage III (20–25%): Preoperative chemotherapy or biopsy, tumor incompletely resected, or positive nodal involvement
- Stage IV (10%): Distant tumor spread (metastasis)
- Stage V (5%): Bilateral disease

Management and treatment

- Surgery
- Chemotherapy
- Radiation

In North America, the definitive treatment of WT typically involves a combination of surgery and chemotherapy, with the possible addition of radiation therapy. The children's oncology group recommends that most renal tumors are managed by primary radical nephrectomy and lymph node sampling. Staging is performed after nephrectomy, with recommendations on further treatment being based on the surgical findings and tumor histology prior to any chemotherapy. Exceptions to this protocol include bilateral tumors (stage V), tumors which appear to be too locally advanced for initial surgical resection (locally invasive into solid organs) or tumors which are accompanied by thrombus in the inferior vena cava (IVC) extending above the hepatic veins. Another exception relates to children suffering from syndromes which predispose them to developing Wilms tumor. In these different scenarios chemotherapy is given prior to surgical resection in order to minimize morbidity during nephrectomy or permit a nephron-sparing approach where appropriate.

The backbone of chemotherapy is dual-agent vincristine and actinomycin (VA). Patients who

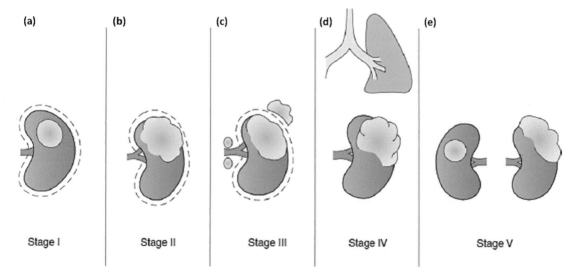

Figure 21.3 Children's oncology group staging of Wilms tumor. Stage I: tumor confined to the kidney and completely excised macro- and micro-scopically. Stage II: tumor extending beyond the kidney but completely excised macro- and micro-scopically. Stage III: tumor (a) biopsied preoperatively or those patients receiving preoperative chemotherapy; (b) incompletely resected; (c) intraoperative tumor spillage; (d) positive lymph nodes. Stage IV: metastatic disease (usually pulmonary). (e) Stage V: bilateral Wilms tumors.

meet stage III or IV criteria receive additional doxorubicin chemotherapy as well as radiation. Those with unfavorable histology may also receive cyclophosphamide, etoposide, and carboplatin in addition to VA.

A different approach is adopted in the UK and in majority of European countries, which follow the SIOP protocols. This approach consists of upfront chemotherapy prior to a delayed nephrectomy. Historically, specialist practice in the UK favored initial biopsy to determine next steps in management- either chemotherapy or upfront surgery depending on the histology. However, recently published data indicates that for patients aged 6 months to 10 years, such biopsy adds little information to change management. Thus, the UK group now follows the general SIOP practice of upfront chemotherapy for routine cases.

The rationale for upfront chemotherapy is to down-stage tumors prior to surgery, facilitate easier surgical resection and decrease the risk of intraoperative tumor spillage. The indications for radiation therapy or additional chemotherapy are determined by a number of factors including tumor response to primary chemotherapy, further imaging/staging and the histological findings.

The surgical approach to the resection of Wilms tumors is fairly standardized (Figure 21.4a–e). A wide transverse abdominal incision (a) gives ready access to the retroperitoneum, particularly the affected kidney and great vessels (aorta and vena cava). Once the overlying colon and its mesocolon have been reflected medially (b), the ureter and gonadal vessels are identified, divided, and followed proximally to the renal hilum. Vascular control of the renal artery and vein is obtained (c). Before ligating the renal vein, careful palpation of the vessel should be performed to confirm the absence of tumor thrombus, regardless of whether the findings on preoperative imaging were negative. After the renal artery and vein have been divided (d), the kidney is removed from the retroperitoneum. Care is needed to avoid capsular rupture (e), as this can affect staging and increase the need for local radiotherapy. The adrenal gland can be left in situ if appropriate. Sampling of a minimum of 7–10 retroperitoneal lymph nodes is essential to permit accurate staging and to guide subsequent management (Figure 21.5).

Minimally invasive nephrectomy for WT has been reported but further studies are needed to select the patients for whom this might be safe and appropriate.

Overall survival for patients with WT has improved dramatically over the last half-century, rising from 70% in the 1970s to over 90% today (Table 21.3). This is due in large part the introduction of multi modal therapy and the findings of collaborative studies undertaken by the COG, SIOP, and NWTSG. Despite differences in the approach to treatment, the overall survival rates of children treated on the varying protocols are remarkably similar. Both the COG and SIOP are running studies to identify which children with advanced disease can be effectively treated without recourse to extended chemotherapy and radiation therapy.

Renal Cell Carcinoma

Epidemiology and etiology

Renal cell carcinoma (RCC) accounts for only 5% of renal tumors in children but is the commonest renal tumor in the second decade of life, accounting for >50% of renal malignancies in this age group. It is more common in patients of Afro-Caribbean descent. Since renal cell carcinomas are indistinguishable from Wilms tumors on imaging by CT or MRI they should both be considered in the differential diagnosis of any renal mass in a child, particularly in the older age group. Nodal involvement and/or metastatic spread are more common at the time of presentation in children than in adults with RCC. A number of conditions are known to predispose to RCC including; Von Hippel Lindau syndrome, sickle cell trait or disease (for renal medullary carcinoma), hereditary leiomyomatosis, and tuberous sclerosis.

Histology and molecular biology

In children and adults under the age of 30 years, RCC is associated with histological appearances

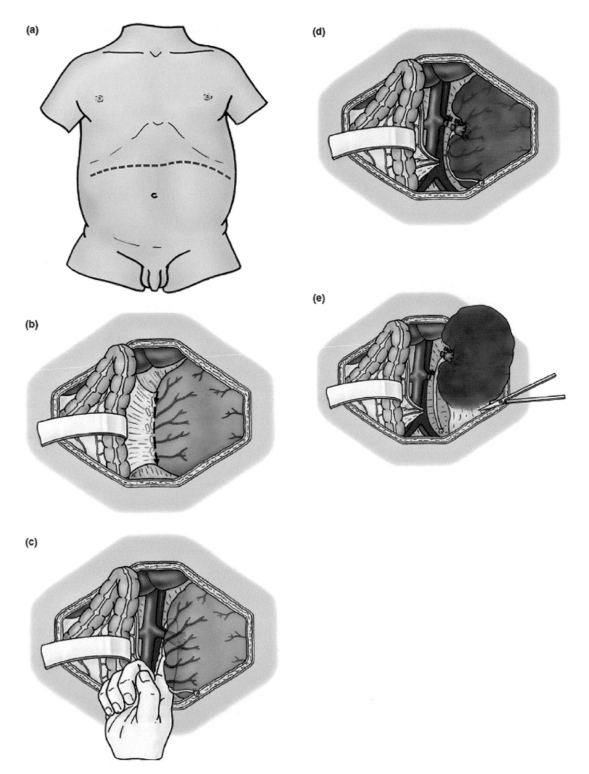

Figure 21.4 Surgical steps of open radical nephrectomy for pediatric renal tumors. See text for expanded description.

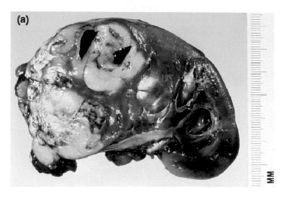

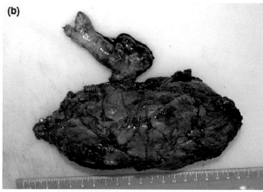

Figure 21.5 (a) Nephrectomy specimen stage II Wilms tumor. Localized penetration of renal capsule with some tumor extension. Full macroscopic and histological clearance achieved. (b) A nephrectomy specimen from a patient with a Wilms tumor. The renal capsule is intact and there was obvious tumor extension into the renal vein and inferior vena cava.

linked to a translocation of the TFE3 gene on the X chromosome in >50% of cases. This variant carries a worse prognosis. Papillary RCC are more common in children than adults and there

Table 21.3 Four-year overall survival (OS) rates for Wilms tumor based on stage and histology

Stage	Favorable histology 4 yr OS (%)	Unfavorable histology 4 yr OS (%)
I	95–100	75–90
II	95–100	80–85
III	95–100	50–90
IV	85–90	30–75
V	95–100	65–100

is a higher incidence of renal medullary carcinoma in patients with sickle cell trait and disease.

Staging

Staging for RCC in children follows the same American Joint Committee on Cancer (AJCC) *tumor, node, metastasis* (TNM) staging that is used for adult patients with RCC.

Management and treatment

- **Surgery**
- **Targeted therapy/clinical trial**

The initial evaluation and surgical approach to RCC is exactly the same as for WT. Unlike WT and other pediatric renal malignancies, RCC is primarily a surgical disease and adjuvant therapy is reserved for advanced tumors with unresectable disease. Metastatic lesions, most often in the lungs, should be surgically removed if possible, as complete surgical resection leads to significantly improved overall survival in adolescents and young adults with RCC. Stage I and II disease have 80–90% 5-year overall survival, decreasing to only 14% for patients with stage IV RCC. Trials of chemotherapy and immunotherapy are in progress to try and improve survival for these patients.

Congenital Mesoblastic Nephroma (CMN)

Epidemiology and etiology

CMN is the most common form of renal tumor in the first 6 months of life but it nevertheless accounts for less than 5% of all pediatric renal tumors. It commonly presents as a palpable abdominal mass in the neonatal period but is detected on prenatal ultrasound in up to 15% cases. The diagnostic evaluation is the same as for WT and RCC, with an initial abdominal ultrasound followed by cross-sectional imaging.

Staging and histology

CMNs are staged by the same criteria as WT, with the vast majority being stage I or II at the time of initial diagnosis. There are three CMN histo-logic subtypes: *classic, cellular,* and *mixed.* Classic and cellular subtypes represent the majority of CMNs, and cellular histology is prone to a more aggressive natural history.

Management and treatment

Despite being commonly regarded as a benign tumor, CMN has the potential to recur locally or give rise to distant metastases after initial therapy. Because most CMNs are localized to the kidney, surgical excision is the primary treatment modality. Even in cases of stage III disease, surgery alone may be curative. Stage III tumors and those with a "cellular" histologic subtype carry a higher risk of recurrence. There is no standardized approach to the management of recurrent or more advanced CMN cases, which often require a combination of surgery, chemotherapy, and radiation therapy.

Overall survival for children with CMN is excellent (96%). Treatment – related complications of surgery or chemotherapy are common causes of death in the small minority who do not survive. The higher mortality rate in children presenting with CMN within the first month of life highlights the need for specialized, multi-disciplinary treatment planning for these extremely young patients.

RHABDOMYOSARCOMA

Introduction

Rhabdomyosarcoma (RMS) is the most common soft-tissue sarcoma in children and arises from undifferentiated skeletal muscle precursors. These tumors are relatively rare in children, with an incidence of approximately 4 in 1 million, of which only 15–25% arise within the genitourinary systems. In the United States, this approximates to 90 new cases of genitourinary RMS a year. There is a bimodal age distribution of presentation with the first peak in the early years of life and a second in adolescence. The location of the tumor,

Table 21.4 Favorable vs unfavorable sites of rhabdomyosarcoma

Favorable	Unfavorable
Biliary tract	Bladder/prostate
Orbit	Urachal
Head and neck (excluding parameningeal)	Retroperitoneal
Paratesticular/penis	Extremity
Vaginal/uterine	Parameningeal

classified as *favorable* vs *unfavorable* (Table 21.4), is an important factor determining plays the treatment and prognosis of genitourinary (GU) RMS. Favorable GU sites include paratesticular, vaginal/vulvar, uterine, and penile. Unfavorable GU sites include bladder/prostate (BP), retroperitoneal and urachal. The most common GU sites are BP and paratesticular. Risk factors for the development of RMS include advanced maternal age, birth weight >4.0 kg, and several syndromic conditions including Li Fraumeni syndrome, DICER-1 and Costello syndromes and neurofibromatosis and multiple endocrine neoplasia Type 2A.

Histology and Molecular Biology

The embryonal type of histology (EMRS) is the commonest, accounting for 60% of all rhabdomyosarcomas in children and up to 90% of genitourinary rhabdomyosarcomas. This histological pattern is associated with higher overall survival (80% 5 years event-free survival) and includes subtypes such as the botryoid variant commonly seen in vaginal RMS. Tumors with the alveolar type of histology (ARMS) are more common in older children, behave more aggressively and have a poorer prognosis (60% 5-years EFS). Tumor genetics, namely the "fusion value" are probably of greater predictive value than the histologic classification. Fusion value refers to the presence or absence of a translocation between the *FOX01* genes and *PAX3 or PAX7* on chromosomes 2 and 13, respectively. Up to 80% of tumors displaying alveolar histology are *PAX/FOX01* fusion positive. Alveolar tumors which are "fusion negative" behave almost identically to tumors with the less aggressive embryonal histology.

Table 21.5 Stage summary for rhabdomyosarcoma

Stage	Site	Size	Node status	Metastasis
1	**Favorable site**	Any	N0 or N1	M0
2	Unfavorable site	**Tumor ≤5 cm**	N0	M0
3	Unfavorable site	Tumor ≤5 cm	**N1**	M0
3	Unfavorable site	**Tumor >5 cm**	N0 or N1	M0
4	Any	Any	Any	**M1**

N0, no positive nodes; N1, nodes positive; M0, no metastatic disease; M1, metastatic disease.

Stratification and Staging

The staging, grouping, and risk stratification of RMS relies on a complex algorithm based on key information on the patient's history and tumor biology. The basics are summarized as follows:

- **Stage**: *Preoperative* determination based on tumor size, location, and clinical node and metastatic status. Of note, bladder/prostate RMS can **never** be stage 1 because of its unfavorable location (Table 21.5).
- **Group**: *Postoperative* classification based on completeness of surgical resection. The assigned group is not static and can be altered prior to the initiation of chemotherapy.
- **Risk group**: This is based on a combination of stage, group, patient age, histology, and fusion status. Risk groups are routinely revised and updated and are used to guide decisions on therapy, to stratify patients in clinical trials, and to counsel parents and patients on prognosis.

Bladder/Prostate Rhabdomyosarcoma

Initial evaluation

The evaluation for a new or suspected bladder/prostate RMS is based on the medical history and physical examination followed by a renal and bladder ultrasound (Figure 21.6A). Information on the age of the child, presence or absence of voiding problems, including gross hematuria or symptoms of outlet obstruction and a possible history of bladder augmentation may help to identify risk factors for less common bladder masses. Basic laboratory biochemical and hematological studies should include a comprehensive metabolic panel, complete blood count, and coagulation panel. Early management of bladder/prostate RMS involves complex decision-making which should be the responsibility of a multi-disciplinary team. These patients will then require complete staging with CT chest, CT/MRI of the abdomen and pelvis, positron emission tomography (PET) CT, and bone marrow biopsies (Figure 21.6B, C).

Treatment

- **Surgery**
- **Chemotherapy**
- **Radiation**

Historically bladder/prostate RMS was initially managed with radical cystoprostatectomy but this approach is now used in less than 10% of cases. The initial diagnosis is most commonly confirmed by endoscopic biopsy. This is then followed by an assessment of the feasibility of an organ-sparing surgical resection. Since most BP RMS are not amenable to complete resection at the time of diagnosis, initial treatment consists of chemotherapy – typically comprising vincristine, actinomycin, and cyclophosphamide (VAC). Numerous alternative chemotherapeutic agents have been evaluated but none have so far been shown to offer superior survival to VAC – which is approximately 80%. Radiation therapy is used primarily for local disease control in cases where the primary tumor is not completely removed. The concept of "pre-treatment re-excision" refers to cases where after the initial biopsy, the tumor is re-excised *before*

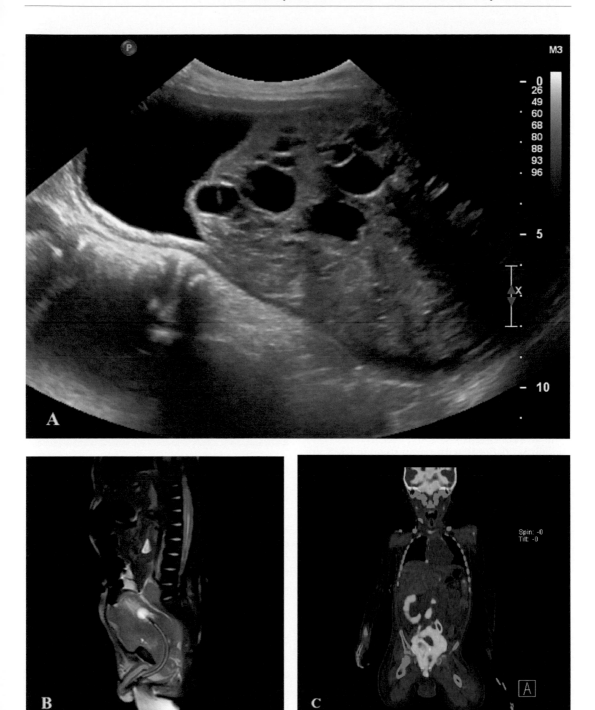

Figure 21.6 **(A)** Bladder ultrasound obtained during the initial evaluation of a suspected pelvic mass revealing a large, heterogeneous mass near the base of the bladder. **(B)** Sagittal T2 weighted magnetic resonance imaging of a patient with a large bladder/prostate rhabdomyosarcoma, which has cranially displaced the Foley catheter. **(C)** Positron emission tomography (PET) computed tomography of the same patient demonstrating PET-avid retroperitoneal lymphadenopathy.

initiating chemotherapy. A number of regimens incorporating different timing of radiation, chemotherapy, and surgery have been described. It is important to note that residual tumor seen on follow-up imaging after chemoradiation therapy may not be malignant tissue but may consist of cells, which have differentiated into mature rhabdomyoblasts which do not require additional treatment.

Paratesticular Rhabdomyosarcoma

Treatment

- **Primary surgery**
- **Chemotherapy**
- **Radiation**

Paratesticular RMS, unlike bladder/prostate RMS, is designated as a favorable site and should therefore be initially managed by radical surgery whenever possible. This includes an ipsilateral radical inguinal orchiectomy with high ligation (at the internal inguinal ring) of the spermatic cord (Figure 21.7A, B). Upon confirmation of the diagnosis, patients with paratesticular RMS are treated with combination VAC chemotherapy. The decision to perform ipsilateral retroperitoneal lymph node dissection (RPLND) is based on the patient's age and imaging findings. In children under 10 years of age this is limited to those with suspicious lymph nodes on staging cross-sectional imaging. Regardless of the presence or absence of lymphadenopathy, ipsilateral retroperitoneal lymph node dissection should be performed in all patients aged 10 and over because of the much higher incidence of occult lymph node involvement in this age range. Radiation therapy is reserved for patients with locally advanced disease, those with confirmed lymph node involvement and those whose orchidectomy had been performed by a transcrotal approach

Vaginal/Uterine

- **Chemotherapy**
- **Radiation**
- **Surgery**

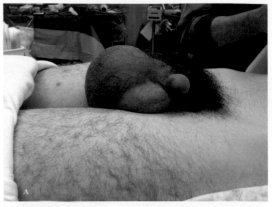

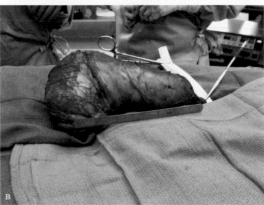

Figure 21.7 **(A)** Paratesticular rhabdomyosarcoma presenting as a solid scrotal swelling. As in adults, exploration and orchidectomy should be performed via an inguinal approach and not by a scrotal incision. **(B)** Specimen delivered through the inguinal incision prior to removal. Penrose drain and clamps proximal to the mass achieve vascular control of the spermatic cord.

Gynecological RMSs are also classified as a favorable site and are usually managed with primary chemotherapy followed by radiation. Surgical intervention is typically limited to the initial diagnostic biopsy, which is then followed by complete staging. Chemotherapy alone is curative in less than 50% of patients but with the addition of radiation therapy, the 5-year survival increases to over 80%. Brachytherapy offers similar survival outcomes to external beam radiation therapy but with fewer short and long-term radiation side effects.

PRE-PUBERTAL PRIMARY TESTICULAR TUMORS

Introduction

Primary testicular tumors comprise approximately 1–2% of all solid tumors in prepubertal children. Although they affect 1 in 100,000 male children, up to 75% of these tumors have little or no malignant potential. The peak age of diagnosis is around 2–4 years of age with a second peak in young adults. Common risk factors include; a previous history of undescended testis, a family history of testicular cancer, and a co-existing disorder of sex development (DSD) particularly one that involves the Y-chromosome.

Initial Evaluation

Key points of the history and physical examination include whether the mass is symptomatic (a painless mass is of greater concern), and pubertal status. Scrotal ultrasound is the initial imaging of choice (Figure 21.8). Careful attention should be made to the appearance of the lesion on ultrasound, its location within or adjacent to the testis (i.e. whether it is a paratesticular mass or a primary testicular mass), and the appearances of contralateral testis. Multifocal tumors are more indicative of malignancy.

Laboratory evaluation should always include the standard serum tumor markers (STM) for testicular tumors, including alpha-fetoprotein (AFP), beta-human chorionic gonadotropin (β-hCG), and lactate dehydrogenase (LDH). However, AFP may not be a reliable tumor market in the first 8 months of life because of a physiological elevation of AFP occurring in this age range. If there is suspicion that the lesion may represent a stromal-type tumor, additional hormonal evaluation is indicated, including serum testosterone, estradiol, and inhibin levels. The differential diagnosis for a newly discovered testicular mass is summarized in Table 21.6.

Because of the relatively low incidence of metastatic disease associated with testicular tumors in children, further evaluation with CT should be used selectively. In asymptomatic children

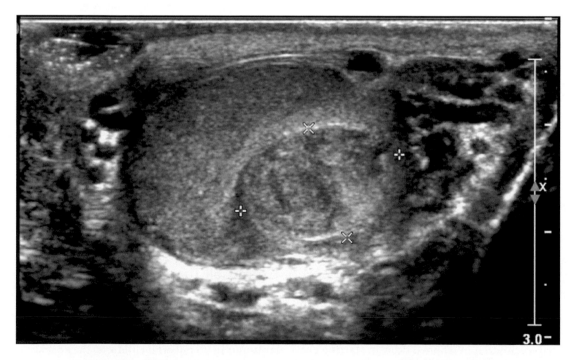

Figure 21.8 Testicular ultrasound demonstrating a heterogeneous intratesticular mass suspicious for a primary testicular malignancy.

Table 21.6 Differential diagnosis for a newly discovered testicular mass

Tumor	Associations
Germ cell tumor	Teratoma and yolk-sac most common
Stromal tumors	Precocious puberty
Epidermoid cyst	Concentric rings on ultrasound
Metastatic lesion	Lymphoma
Gonadoblastoma	Malignant precursor and DSD

DSD, difference in sex development.

Table 21.7 Children's oncology group pediatric testicular tumor staging

Stage	Description
I	Limited to testis, **completely resected** No evidence of disease beyond testis **STM** normal
II	**Microscopic residual disease** **Elevated STM** Tumor rupture or scrotal biopsy prior to orchiectomy
III	Retroperitoneal **lymph node involvement**[a]
IV	Distant **metastasis**

[a] Lymph nodes >4 cm meet imaging criteria, lymph nodes 2–4 cm need pathologic confirmation (i.e. biopsy), and lymph nodes 1–2 cm have unclear significance and may require additional evaluation prior to completing staging.

presenting with a primary testicular tumor it can be deferred until after surgery has been performed and the results of the final pathology evaluation are available. However, a preoperative CT scan to assess the total tumor burden is indicated in children with marked elevation of standard tumor markers or clinical evidence of metastatic disease.

Staging

The staging employed by the children's oncology group differs from the one used for staging testicular tumors in adults (Table 21.7). This reflects the fact that the majority of prepubertal tumors are benign and are confined to the testis. After puberty, however, the staging is the same as for adults with testicular tumors.

Treatment

- **Surgery**
- **Chemotherapy**
- **Radiation**

The initial treatment of testicular tumors in children usually consists of either radical or partial orchiectomy. Preoperative chemotherapy is limited to children in whom a delay in starting chemotherapy could be life threatening because they have a large burden of disease with pulmonary and/

or neurological involvement. An inguinal incision should always be used for surgical exploration of a primary testicular tumor in a pre-pubertal boy because of the possible need to proceed to radical orchiectomy. If the diagnosis is uncertain and preoperative tumor markers are normal, particularly in patients with small (<2 cm), unifocal tumors, partial orchiectomy with intraoperative frozen section is a reasonable approach. In these cases, the use of intraoperative ultrasound can be helpful in locating the margins of the tumor prior to excision. If the frozen section raises suspicion of malignancy the surgeon can proceed to perform a radical orchiectomy, whereas if the pathology is more consistent with a benign process, the affected testis can be spared. The possible requirement for further treatment (surgery, chemotherapy, or radiation therapy) is determined by the pathology and tumor characteristics.

Germ Cell Tumors

Teratoma

Teratomas are the most common benign testicular tumor in prepubertal children. They consist of a combination of the three germ-cell layers: endoderm, ectoderm, and mesoderm. Epidermoid cysts are considered part of this spectrum of tumors but contain only a single germ-cell layer and have the classic appearance of concentric hyperechoic rings on ultrasound. Teratomas are not usually accompanied by elevated serum tumor markers. The definitive treatment is orchiectomy (either radical or partial) performed via an inguinal incision.

Yolk-Sac tumor

Yolk-sac tumors (YST) are the most common malignant testicular tumors in children. They are almost universally associated with elevated levels of AFP and are characterized by the histologic finding of Schiller-Duval bodies on microscopy. Ninety percent of YSTs present as Stage I disease and are managed by radical orchiectomy followed by monitoring serum AFP levels and chest and abdominal imaging at increasing intervals. Patients who present with stage II–IV disease (or stage I patients who experience a recurrence after orchiectomy) are treated with bleomycin, etoposide, and cisplatin chemotherapy. In addition, patients with retroperitoneal lymph node involvement should undergo formal radical lymph node dissection.

Stromal Tumors

Leydig and Sertoli cell tumors

Leydig cell tumors (LCT) are the most common stromal tumor in childhood and are often associated with elevations in serum testosterone, which can lead to precocious puberty. Histologically they are defined by the presence of Reinke crystals, which are pathognomonic for LCTs. In prepubertal patients these tumors are universally benign and complete surgical excision is considered curative. Sertoli cell tumors (SCT), are the second most common testicular stromal tumor and may be may be associated with gynecomastia in the postpubertal age range. They are benign tumors with no reported cases of metastasis in children. A variant of Sertoli cell tumor can occur in patients with Peutz-Jeghers syndrome. Because they are benign tumors, Leydig and Sertoli cell tumors in children can be managed initially by

testicular sparing surgery (partial orchiectomy) with intraoperative frozen section.

Juvenile granulosa cell tumors

Juvenile granulosa cell tumors (JGCT) are almost exclusively seen in the first year of life and can even be present at birth. These tumors are hormonally inactive, benign tumors that are often associated with Y-chromosomal abnormalities. In addition to surgical excision, a karyotype should be performed to rule out a concomitant genetic disorder.

KEY POINTS

- Molecular profiling is likely to play a key role in risk-stratification and the design of targeted therapy for children with renal tumors and genitourinary rhabdomyosarcoma.
- The overall survival of children with genitourinary malignancies is improving dramatically as a result of the introduction of multimodal treatment (surgery, chemotherapy, and radiation therapy). The current challenge is to reduce the burden of treatment – related morbidity without compromising survival rates.
- Prepubertal testicular tumors are not usually as aggressive as testicular tumors in adults. Most cases can be managed with surgery and observation alone.

FURTHER READING

Saltzman, A.F., Cost, N.G., 2018. Childhood kidney tumors. American Urological Association Update Series 37, 187–195.

Husmann, D.A., 2019. Cancer screening in the pediatric cancer patient: a focus on genitourinary malignancies, and why does a urologist need to know about this? Journal of Pediatric Urology 15, 5–11.

Gooskens SL, Houwing ME, Vujanic GM, Dome JS, Diertens T, Coulomb l'Herminé A, et al, 2017. Congenital mesoblastic nephroma 50 years after its recognition: a narrative review. Pediatric Blood & Cancer 64, e26437.

Malempati, S., Hawkins, D.S., 2012. Rhabdomyosarcoma: review of the children's oncology group (cog) soft-tissue sarcoma committee experience and rationale for current COG studies. Pediatric Blood & Cancer 59, 5–10.

Ross, J.H., Kay, R., 2004. Prepubertal testis tumors. Rev Urol 6, 11–18.

Pediatric Genitourinary Trauma

DAVID J CHALMERS

Topics covered

General evaluation	Bladder injuries
Renal trauma	Urethral injuries
Ureteric injuries	Injuries to the external genitalia

INTRODUCTION

Trauma is the leading cause of mortality in children and young people. Management principles generally mirror those of adult trauma, which has the benefit of more evidence-based guidelines. However, there are some key differences. Renal injury is most frequently caused by blunt force – often in conjunction with multisystem organ trauma. With some important exceptions, all but the most severe renal injuries are generally managed non-operatively. Ureteral injuries can occur from penetrating trauma or iatrogenic injury during surgery in the retroperitoneum or pelvis. Bladder and urethral injuries are usually associated with other severe injuries involving pelvic fractures and carry the greatest potential risk of long-term morbidity. Isolated external genital trauma, depending on the history, should always trigger suspicion of possible sexual abuse. While pediatric urologists rarely have prime responsibility for the evaluation and treatment of pediatric trauma patients, they are relied upon heavily as consultants.

GENERAL EVALUATION

History

Evaluation begins by obtaining a comprehensive history from the patient, family or consulting clinician, followed by a physical examination if possible. Information should be sought on the mechanism of injury, associated injuries and any significant comorbidities. It is important to enquire about the presence of hematuria and to look for evidence of abdominal or flank tenderness, rib fractures, and contusions or abrasions to the abdomen, pelvis, or flank. Penetrating injuries to the torso, multisystem trauma and significant hematuria always warrant further investigation. It is important to note, however, that genitourinary injuries associated with multisystem trauma are not always accompanied by hematuria. For this reason, the absence of hematuria should not preclude further investigation if other indications are present.

Physical Examination

Hemodynamic parameters are not reliable indicators of acute shock in children. Tachycardia may be a response to pain or anxiety and the cardiovascular system in children is capable of compensating more effectively for significant blood loss through vasoconstriction and increased cardiac output. Signs of acute blood loss, anemia, and/or hypovolemia are indicators of advanced hemodynamic instability and even if the other vital signs are reassuring the clinician should nevertheless proceed with further evaluation and decisions on management. The physical examination should focus on the abdomen and genitalia. A flank mass or ecchymosis suggests perinephric hematoma – which may also be associated with urinary extravasation. Ecchymosis of the perineum in a butterfly pattern is suggestive of blood tracking within Colles Fasica while scrotal or labial hematoma can result from genital trauma or pelvic injury. The presence of blood at the urethral meatus or urinary retention should raise suspicion of urethral injury or disruption.

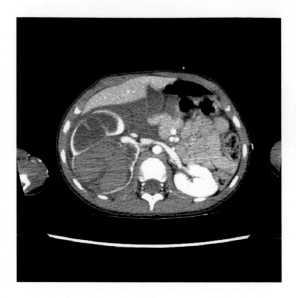

Figure 22.1 Grade 4 renal injury in a kidney with previously undiagnosed ureteropelvic junction obstruction. This occurred following a fall from playground monkey bars. There were no other injuries and the injury failed to improve with conservative management. Ultimately, a nephrectomy was performed.

RENAL TRAUMA

The kidney is the commonest site of injury in the genitourinary system. The majority of renal injuries result from blunt trauma and approximately 80% are accompanied by injuries to other organs. Males outnumber females by almost 2:1, with the commonest causes being motor vehicle collisions, traffic accidents and falls. Contact sports are an uncommon cause of serious renal injury in this age group.

It is thought that the kidney is more susceptible to blunt trauma in children than adults because it is proportionately larger and is less well protected by the ribs. Children also have less retroperitoneal fat and less musculature to buffer and protect the kidneys. Horseshoe kidneys and hydronephrotic kidneys are at particularly high risk of injury even in the absence of associated organ injuries (Figure 22.1).

Evaluation and Investigations

Because hemodynamic signs are a less reliable guide to the severity of injury in children, greater reliance must be placed on the clinical history, physical examination, and the presence of associated injuries.

The indications for radiographic evaluation include;

- Blunt trauma resulting from significant deceleration, such as a high-velocity motor vehicle collision or fall
- Blunt trauma leading to other significant multi-organ injuries
- Penetrating injury to the abdomen or flank
- Gross macroscopic hematuria or significant microscopic hematuria

Haematuria is a much less reliable guide to the severity of renal trauma than in adults and >50% of children who have sustained a renal injury may not have hematuria at the time of presentation.

Ultrasound is a reasonable first-line investigation if the child is clinically stable and the history and findings on examination do not arouse concern. However, the accuracy of ultrasonography in detecting grade III renal lacerations is only 60% and is even lower in the detection of low grade renal injuries. Any evidence of renal injury detected by ultrasonography should then prompt a computerized tomography (CT) scan for a more detailed anatomical and functional assessment.

Contrast-enhanced CT with delayed imaging is the cornerstone of modern staging of blunt renal injuries. The American Association for the Surgery of Trauma (AAST) organ injury scale for renal trauma (Figure 22.2) has been widely adopted to characterize renal injuries and guide their management.

Grade I injuries are defined by decreased uptake of contrast material or subcapsular hematoma. They are essentially renal contusions and account for 80% of renal trauma cases.

Grade II and III injuries are tears in the renal parenchyma. Tears <1 cm are considered grade II and >1 cm as grade III. They are classified as minor if they are limited to the renal parenchyma and do not extend into the collecting system. Grade II and grade III injuries may be associated with extensive perinephric hematomas, but not urinary extravasation.

Grade IV injuries are lacerations, which also involve the collecting system. Grade IV injury may also consist of damage to the hilar vessels – typically as a consequence of rapid deceleration causing shearing damage to the vessel wall, intramural haemorrhage, vascular occlusion, and clot formation. In such cases, renal perfusion in the injured kidney may be compromised even if the parenchyma remains intact.

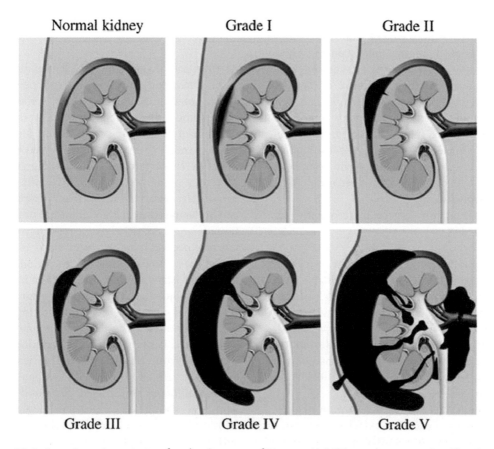

Figure 22.2 American Association for the Surgery of Trauma (AAST) renal trauma classification.

Grade V injury is one in which the renal tissue is separated into multiple renal fragments ("shattered kidney"). It can be difficult to determine which segments of tissue are poorly perfused as a result of severe contusion and which segments have been completely devascularized. Massive bleeding and extravasation within Gerota's fascia is common. Major hilar injury leading to devascularization also constitutes a grade V renal injury.

Management

The goals of care focus on preservation of renal tissue and renal function while minimizing the morbidity and risk of mortality posed by the injury. Most blunt renal injuries can be managed non-operatively, particularly since the majority are low grade (I–III). Conservative management usually involves bed rest until hematocrit measurements have stabilized and hematuria has resolved. Monitoring of vital signs is imperative to assess hemodynamic stability. Although reevaluation with ultrasound can be used to detect any expanding urinoma or hematoma, CT imaging is indicated if there is deterioration in the child's clinical condition or hemodynamic instability which might necessitate surgical intervention. Conservative management is highly successful in preventing long-term complications such as hypertension, loss of renal function and hydronephrosis.

Indications for surgery are frequently relative and include:

- **Hemorrhage**: Intervention may be required to control active hemorrhage which is causing hemodynamic instability (e.g. pulsatile hematoma on CT). Selective angioembolization may be effective in stopping bleeding of minor severity but surgical intervention should be considered if this is unsuccessful or the child is requiring repeated blood transfusions.
- **Urinary extravasation**: A minor degree of contained urinary extravasation may be managed conservatively and monitored whereas larger and/or persistent collections may require percutaneous drainage. Partial disruption of the uretero pelvic junction (UPJ) may be amenable to ureteral stent placement whereas complete disruption may require either percutaneous drainage as a temporizing measure or immediate surgical repair.
- **"Shattered kidney" (grade V injury)**: Even in a hemodynamically stable patient, removal of a non-functioning "shattered" kidney may be justified to hasten recovery and reduce long-term complications. In the presence of other intra-abdominal injuries requiring laparotomy, a "shattered" kidney should be removed concurrently.
- **Hilar injury**: The prospect of successful revascularization is minimal when blood supply is compromised and warm ischemia time exceeds one hour. However, this relatively desperate attempt to conserve the kidney may be justified in very rare circumstances, such as a solitary kidney or bilateral renal injuries.

At the time of operation, the initial priority is to gain vascular control of the renal pedicle and aorta. Once hemostasis has been achieved, the kidney and collecting system can be inspected, devitalized tissue can be debrided and any defects in the parenchyma closed and covered wherever possible. In certain cases partial nephrectomy may be a better way of preserving the remaining viable renal tissue. Urinary extravasation can be managed with a ureteral stent or nephrostomy tube. As stated above, emergency repair of a severe pedicle injury or thrombosis is unlikely to result in preservation of the kidney since the warm ischemic time will already have been exceeded while the child was being evaluated and resuscitated prior to surgery. Penetrating trauma is most commonly the result of gunshot or stab wounds and is, therefore, largely confined to the older age group. Because these injuries tend to be more severe and involve other organs there is usually a greater requirement for blood transfusion and stronger likelihood of nephrectomy. While stab wounds and low-velocity gunshot wounds may cause localized injury, high-velocity gunshot wounds are associated with blast effect tissue damage, which may make it more difficult to determine the true extent of injury on initial evaluation.

Outcomes and Complications

The most serious early complication of renal trauma is acute bleeding, with the highest risk being immediately following the injury. Even if there is a low suspicion for severe injury the child should be admitted for bed rest and serial hemoglobin/hematocrit monitoring. Secondary hematuria is not uncommon within the first few days and weeks of the injury. Although it is rarely of sufficient severity to require active surgical intervention secondary hematuria should be monitored carefully to rule out the development of an arteriovenous malformation or pseudoaneurysm. This risk is highest in patients with higher grade trauma who are managed conservatively. Infection is another potential early complication, particularly if there is a significant urinoma and a substantial amount of devitalized renal tissue. Initially, it may be difficult to distinguish on ultrasound between old blood products, resolving urinoma, and possible abscess formation but serial imaging should enable this distinction to be made. Outcomes following penetrating injuries to the kidney are generally worse than for blunt injury. The most significant late complications of renal trauma are hypertension and loss of renal function. The risk of hypertension is likely to be higher when a significant amount of devascularized renal tissue has been left in place. The true incidence of hypertension is difficult to assess because of the lack of reliable long-term data but the available evidence indicates it is relatively rare with an incidence of 1–2%. Nevertheless, monitoring of blood pressure is generally advisable in view of the small risk of hypertension, which might indicate late complications requiring medical or surgical management.

Full recovery of function can usually be expected following low-grade trauma (grades I–III), whereas grade IV and V injuries are more likely to result in some permanent reduction in renal size and function.

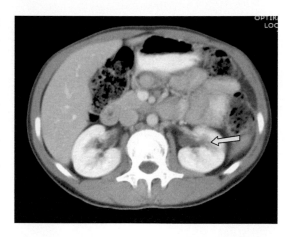

Figure 22.3 A linear scar in the left kidney persisting 3 months following a grade III injury.

Surprisingly, even segments or renal parenchyma in a shattered kidney may sometimes retain their blood supply and viability and become realigned in a functional configuration. However, the prognosis of severe injuries can be adversely affected by the presence of persisting morphological changes including scars, cysts, or segmental hydronephrosis (Figure 22.3). Nuclear medicine studies, such as 99m Tc dimercaptoacetyltriglycine (MAG3) or 99m Tc dimercaptosuccinic acid (DMSA) are helpful in monitoring functional recovery over time and in guiding a decision on whether to perform reconstruction or nephrectomy in the case of an injured kidney, which has been stabilized by nephrostomy drainage (Figure 22.4). If the contralateral kidney is healthy, the risk of post-traumatic renal failure is low. Statistically, the risk of injuring a solitary kidney, even during contact sports, is extremely low so there is little justification for restricting normal activities and sports.

URETERIC INJURY

Injuries to the ureter are rare and usually result from penetrating trauma or iatrogenic damage – for example during ureteroscopy, tumor resection, or laparoscopy.

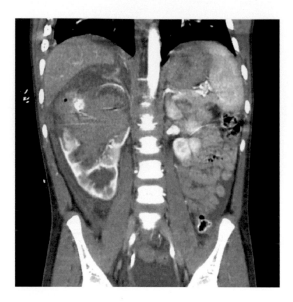

Figure 22.4 A 17-year-old boy experienced a grade IV renal laceration with UPJ disruption following a snowmobile accident. An indwelling ureteral stent could not be placed and a nephrostomy tube was used as a temporizing measure. Delayed MAG-3 test demonstrated only 10% function and an elective laparoscopic nephrectomy was performed.

Evaluation

Gross hematuria is not necessarily present even after a significant ureteral injury. A high index of suspicion must therefore be maintained to avoid missing the diagnosis. Delayed computerized tomography (CT) imaging with use of contrast to visualize the entire collecting system is most helpful in this regard.

Management

Management of ureteral injuries in children generally mirrors the management in adults and should be individualized according the site and nature of the injury. Prompt surgical repair is indicated for injuries which are recognized immediately or shortly after they have occurred. However, a period of temporizing nephrostomy drainage is preferable when the diagnosis is delayed by > 1 week, with definitive repair being delayed for a few months. The key principle of

ureteral repair is the creation of a tension free, spatulated anastomosis. Devitalized segments should be excised to ensure that healthy ureteral tissue is used for the anastomosis. Depending on the level and extent of the injury the options include; spatulation with end-to-end anastomosis, psoas hitch and Boari flap. For more extensive injuries ureteral substitution by ileal interposition may have to be considered.

Outcomes and Complications

If the injury is not recognized or is not correctly managed the primary complication is urinary extravasation into the retroperitoneum resulting in urinoma or abscess formation. Long-term outcomes following repair are generally favorable – although the published data are sparse.

BLADDER INJURY

Traumatic injuries to the bladder are rare in this age group and are usually associated with other severe injuries including pelvic fractures. Motor vehicle accidents are the leading cause of blunt pelvic trauma and bladder injury. By comparison to an adult, the bladder in a child is located in a more vulnerable position which is higher in the abdomen and less protected by the bony pelvis. Penetrating injuries of the bladder are exceedingly rare in children and are usually iatrogenic, for example inadvertent damage to the bladder wall during herniotomy or difficult appendectomy.

Evaluation

The hallmark signs of bladder and urethral injury are suprapubic pain, tenderness, inability to urinate, gross hematuria, and blood at the urethral meatus. Indications for bladder imaging include gross hematuria and/or urinary retention in conjunction with a pelvic fracture.

The initial CT scan may not be adequate to completely characterize bladder injury, although delayed imaging after bladder filling may be helpful when looking for possible extravasation.

Other imaging modalities which may be useful include cystography or intravenous pyelography. CT cystography is sensitive and specific but involves significant radiation exposure and should be used judiciously.

Management

Free leakage of urine into the peritoneum is indicative of an intraperitoneal injury for which surgical intervention is required in the majority of cases. However, non-operative management can be used successfully for small, isolated bladder injuries. Extraperitoneal perforation, with extravasation confined to the perivesical space, can usually be managed by a period of continuous catheter drainage. However, if there are other concurrent injuries requiring surgical intervention this may be an opportunity to close the bladder defect and hasten recovery.

Outcomes and Complications

Early complications include persistent gross hematuria, clot retention, and pelvic abscess. Hematuria is typically self-limiting but may require intermittent or continuous irrigation. Abscess or urinoma can be drained percutaneously. Large intraperitoneal injuries may be complicated by peritonitis, paralytic ileus and metabolic disturbance, such as hyponatremia, hypokalemia, and elevated serum urea and creatinine. Late complications are uncommon but can include urinary fistula, persistent lower urinary tract symptoms or persistent incontinence.

URETHRAL INJURY

These are generally confined to males and can result from either direct blunt trauma to the urethra or injuries associated with pelvic fracture. In adults, the posterior urethra is supported by the prostate but in boys the prostate has not yet developed so that when the pelvic ring is disrupted, shear forces can disrupt the pelvic floor and drag the membranous urethra apart from the bladder

and prostate. Straddle injuries typically result from falls on bicycles, playground equipment and bars, and fences. The mechanism of injury occurs when the urethra and surrounding corpus spongiosum are crushed against the pubic rami.

Evaluation

The signs of urethral injury are an inability to urinate, gross hematuria, and blood at the urethral meatus.

A retrograde urethrogram is widely regarded as the best imaging study for visualizing the urethra. Oblique views are necessary to look for posterior extravasation and demonstrate complete continuity of the urethra.

Management

Initial management of urethral injury involves bladder drainage and radiological evaluation. A Foley catheter may be placed into the bladder under radiographic guidance if the urethra is intact with only a small tear. Alternatively, if the patient has already voided and examination does not suggest urethral injury, a urethral catheter can be placed immediately without a retrograde study. If a catheter has been placed previously, it should not be removed. In such cases, an infant feeding tube can be introduced alongside the catheter in order to facilitate the urethrogram and assess injury.

The management of injuries to the bulbar or anterior urethra is typically straightforward and consists of either observation or urethral catheter drainage alone. The primary risk is the later development of a urethral stricture. The initial management of posterior urethral injuries is more complex. If possible, placement of a urethral catheter will help to align the urethra as well as providing bladder drainage. However, this may not be feasible if there is complete disruption and the urethra is no longer in continuity. As in adults, the management of these severe injuries is controversial. The options include prolonged suprapubic tube drainage followed by delayed urethroplasty or, alternatively, immediate exploration with debridement and primary realignment. If a delayed repair strategy is employed, continuous drainage should be maintained for at least 6–8 weeks before urethroplasty is attempted. Injuries to the urethra which involve the bladder neck and/or prostate require immediate intervention to minimize the risk of long-term complications, such as stricture, incontinence, and fistula. Fortunately, such injuries are very uncommon. Traumatic injuries of female urethra are extremely rare because of the shorter length of the urethra and the more protected location. These injuries typically occur in conjunction with severe pelvic fractures and vaginal injury and may consist of either transverse disruption or a longitudinal tear. Conservative management can be employed if the bladder neck is intact and a urethral catheter can be passed into the bladder. However, immediate surgical repair is indicated if the bladder neck is transected or the vagina is also involved in the injury. In some cases, the preferred management may comprise a period of suprapubic catheterization followed by delayed repair. Long-term outcomes are generally poor because a traumatic force which is of sufficient severity to cause damage to the female urethra usually causes extensive damage to the tissues supporting the urethra as well as causing pelvic fractures.

Outcomes and Complications

Stricture formation is the most significant complication following urethral injuries. Experience with urethral stricture and urethroplasty in children is limited, but the management options are similar to those in adults. Optical urethrotomy may be appropriate for short, well defined strictures. For more extensive strictures the choice usually lies between stricture resection and end to end anastomosis or urethroplasty utilizing onlay grafts of buccal mucosa or other materials. A perineal approach usually provides optimal exposure. Injuries to the posterior urethra which involve the bladder neck, prostatic urethra, and sphincteric complex, carry a high risk of serious long-term complications, notably urinary incontinence and impotence.

INJURIES TO THE EXTERNAL GENITALIA

In the neonatal period, penile injuries are usually iatrogenic and related to circumcision. In older boys, the penis or prepuce may become trapped in a zipper – with resultant contusion or pressure necrosis of the prepuce. Other forms of penile injury include dog bites and high-flow priapism associated with a traumatic arteriovenous fistula secondary to perineal trauma.

The testis may be injured as a result of a bicycle crossbar injury in which the testis is compressed against the pubic ramus, causing disruption of the tunica albuginea. Other causes include kicks to the scrotum during sporting activity or rough play and fights. Traumatic genital injuries are rare in girls and typically result from straddle injuries. Because of the proximity of the urethra and vagina, traumatic injuries of the external genitalia or urethra should prompt an evaluation for associated vaginal injuries. A high index of suspicion of possible sexual abuse is required whenever a girl presents with a genital injury, particularly if the nature of the injury seems discordant with the history.

Evaluation and Management

Excessive removal of penile skin due to neonatal circumcision can be managed conservatively in the majority of cases but later reconstructive surgery (including the use of free skin grafts) may occasionally be required if there has been extensive excision of penile shaft skin. Circumcision injuries involving the glans or urethra are rare but may require complex reconstruction.

Superficial penile contusions and lacerations can typically be managed with topical antibiotic ointments, but may require minor debridement and skin approximation depending on the mechanism and severity of the injury. Zipper injuries usually occur in uncircumcised boys and may be treated using mineral oil to release the trapped skin from the zipper or dividing the zipper with bone cutters. Genital injuries caused by animal bites should be assessed under anesthesia to fully assess the extent of trauma and broad spectrum antibiotics and tetanus prophylaxis should be administered. High-flow priapism may be managed non-operatively because of the likelihood of spontaneous resolution within days to weeks after injury. If conservative measures fail, embolization with autologous clot is the preferred treatment.

In cases of scrotal trauma, ultrasound is an excellent investigation to assess any testicular injury. Early scrotal exploration should be undertaken if there is clinical or ultrasound evidence of testicular rupture or a significant tear in the tunica albuginea (Figure 22.5). In rare cases of penetrating scrotal injury a detailed examination is required to determine the depth of penetration prior to treatment by cleansing and debridement.

Operative management is seldom required for uncomplicated genital trauma in young girls. However, sexual abuse or assault is implicated in up to 25% girls presenting with genital injuries. In these circumstances cystoscopy, vaginoscopy, and rectal examination should be performed to fully evaluate any associated injuries. For more extensive vaginal lacerations, primary repair should be performed if possible to reduce the rate of vaginal stenosis and urethrovaginal fistulae.

Complications

Acute complications of penile trauma include bleeding and infection, particularly in cases of animal bites. Late complications of penile injury include penile entrapment (cicatrix), meatal stenosis, and unsatisfactory cosmetic outcomes. The outcome of circumcision injuries is generally excellent, although a very small proportion will require further surgery to provide adequate skin coverage of the penile shaft. Penetrating scrotal injuries pose a risk of infection but this can be considerably reduced by adequate cleansing, debridement, and the use of broad-spectrum antibiotics. Inadequate surgical management of a significant injury to the testis may lead to a prolonged recovery and convalescence.

The most significant complication following vaginal trauma is stricture – although this is usually confined to severe injuries. Follow-up into puberty is essential to exclude possible stenosis or hematocolpos, especially in patients with extensive urethrovaginal injuries.

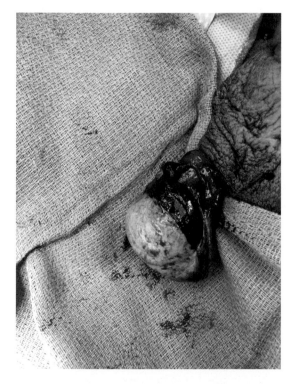

Figure 22.5 **A 12-year-old boy experienced a straddle injury with significant scrotal pain and hematoma. Testicular ultrasound suggested a rupture and exploration is demonstrating a 1 cm tear in the tunica albuginea. 4-0 PDS was used to reapproximate the edges and there was no atrophy on follow-up.**

KEY POINTS

- Potentially serious renal trauma can occur in children after seemingly innocuous injury.
- All children with suspected renal trauma should be admitted for observation, imaging, and evaluation.
- Most cases of renal trauma can be managed conservatively, but grade IV–V injuries are more likely to require intervention.

- After recovery from the acute injury, blood pressure should be monitored.
- The risk of significant injury to a solitary kidney is extremely low and does not usually justify any restrictions on everyday life or sporting activity.
- Extraperitoneal bladder injuries can be managed conservatively with catheter drainage whereas intraperitoneal injury is an indication for surgical repair.
- Surgical management of post-traumatic urethral strictures should only be undertaken by an experienced pediatric or reconstructive urologist.
- The possibility of sexual abuse should always be considered in any child presenting with an injury to the external genitalia.

FURTHER READING

Americal Urological Association Guidelines on UroTrauma. 2017. https://www.auanet.org/guidelines/urotrauma-guideline#x3296

Buckley JC, McAninch JW. Pediatric renal injuries: management guidelines from a 25-year experience. J Urol. 2004;172(2):687–690, discussion 90.

Buckley JC, McAninch JW. The diagnosis, management, and outcomes of pediatric renal injuries. Urol Clin North Am. 2006;33(1):33–40, vi.

McAleer IM, Kaplan GW, LoSasso BE. Congenital urinary tract anomalies in pediatric renal trauma patients. J Urol. 2002;168(4, Pt 2):1808–1810, discussion 10.

Santucci RA, McAninch JW, Safir M, Mario LA, Service S, Segal MR. Validation of the American Association for the Surgery of Trauma Organ Injury Severity Scale for the Kidney. J Trauma. 2001;50(2):195–200.

Laparoscopic Paediatric Urology

KARLY ZAHER, SARA LOBO and IMRAN MUSHTAQ

Topics covered

Overview of benefits and limitations of
    laparoscopic surgery in paediatric urology
Robotic surgery – Benefits and limitations
Patient selection
Fundamentals of technique: Robotic and
    non-robotic
Procedures, indications and outcomes

Nephrectomy
Heminephrectomy
Pyeloplasty (including robotic pyeloplasty)
Adrenalectomy
Reconstructive surgery
Others

INTRODUCTION

The role of laparoscopy in paediatric urology was initially limited to diagnostic indications, such as the investigation of impalpable testes. In 1976, Cortesi was the first to report the use of laparoscopy to perform a therapeutic procedure – in the treatment of crypthorchidism. The well-established benefits of minimally invasive surgery (MIS) have been further enhanced by the introduction of single site surgery. Innovations in robotics have helped to overcome difficulties of working in limited spaces, permitted more effective intracorporeal suturing and provided three-dimensional (3D) visualisation and technology to eliminate manual tremor during operative manoeuvres. These and other developments now enable the surgeon to operate with far greater precision. The advent of MIS and robotics has provided new insights into the anatomy of the urogenital tract and the conditions which affect it. It has also created challenging opportunities for minimally invasive paediatric urologists to develop and introduce innovative techniques for reconstructive surgery of the lower urinary tract.

BENEFITS AND LIMITATIONS

The acknowledged benefits of laparoscopic surgery in children include; reduced postoperative pain, shorter hospital stay, earlier return to normal activities, improved cosmesis and fewer wound complications. The smaller size of the paediatric patient has the great advantage of allowing access to both the upper and lower urinary tract through the same port sites. Laparoscopy also provides superior access to the pelvis when operating, for example, on Müllerian duct remnants, intra-abdominal testes and cloacal anomalies.

Paediatric urology encompasses a wide spectrum of conditions (including a variety of congenital anomalies and benign and malignant tumours) in patients ranging in age and size from neonates to adolescents. In addition, minimally invasive paediatric urologists face the challenge of having to overcome the technical difficulties inherent in operating in relatively confined anatomical spaces (as in the retroperitoneoscopic [RP] approach). However, these have been largely addressed by advances in camera technology and instrumentation. One of the main drawbacks of laparoscopic surgery relates to the high financial costs of the technology and equipment. Although these additional costs may be partially offset by the economic advantage of a reduced duration of hospital stay this consideration is of less importance in children than adults. The complications of laparoscopic surgery in children, however, are broadly similar to those in adults.

Robotic Surgery – Benefits and Limitations

Robotic surgery offers the benefits of a minimally invasive approach whilst overcoming some of the limitations of laparoscopic surgery. Robotic surgery provides better visualisation (with 3D, magnified images), superior ergonomics, tremor filtration and improved dexterity than traditional laparoscopy. However, a major limitation of the Da Vinci robotic system is the lack of tactile feedback – which requires the operating surgeon to rely far more on visual information. Another disadvantage is the large capital outlay for the robot and ongoing costs of consumables. There are also risks which are unique to the robotic system, such as human error in operating the robot and problems arising from mechanical failure and malfunction of the system. Despite recent modifications and upgrades, the bulky equipment still demands a sizeable space for storage.

SCOPE OF MINIMALLY INVASIVE SURGERY IN PAEDIATRIC UROLOGY

MIS now fulfils a key role in paediatric urology and used for a wide range of procedures including;

- Nephrectomy and partial nephrectomy
- Pyeloplasty
- Adrenalectomy
- Excision/marsupialisation of renal cysts
- Pyelolithotomy and ureterolithotomy
- Ureteric surgery including; excision of ureteric stump after partial nephrectomy, ureteroureterostomy, ureterocalicostomy
- Ureteric reimplantation
- Investigation and management of impalpable testis
- Treatment of varicocele
- Investigation and treatment of disorders of sex development (DSD), e.g. gonadal biopsy. Gonadectomy
- Ovarian harvest for cryopreservation
- Excision of Müllerian remnants
- Lower urinary tract reconstruction including; bladder reconstruction (augmentation) Monti/Mitrofanoff procedures, bladder neck reconstruction and Sling procedure

Contraindications

Almost all conditions in paediatric urology are amenable to a minimally invasive approach and there are very few contraindications. The use of MIS has also been extended to the treatment of Wilms tumour. In carefully selected patients the results of laparoscopic total nephrectomy and lymphadenectomy are comparable to those of open surgery. With increasing experience it is likely that large and more complex Wilms tumours may prove to be amenable to MIS. For the time being, however, most oncology centres continue to favour open surgery for Wilms tumour.

Absolute contraindications to the use of MIS include:

- Significant comorbidity (e.g. cardiac, respiratory disease)
- Uncorrectable coagulopathies
- Sepsis

Anaesthesia

Anaesthesia for MIS procedures in children requires endotracheal intubation and the use of volatile and/or intravenous anaesthetic agents. Because respiration in infants and young children is predominantly diaphragmatic, abdominal insufflation during transperitoneal (TP) surgery may compromise diaphragmatic excursion. Insufflation pressures are therefore kept low in infants and children. Younger children absorb proportionately more CO_2 than other age groups during pneumoperitoneum formation and may also experience greater transient elimination of CO_2 postdesufflation. For this reason small children warrant particularly close monitoring during laparoscopy and the immediate postoperative period. Underbody/overbody warming mats are used routinely in children because they are at significant risk of developing hypothermia during laparoscopic surgery, especially with prolonged operating times and a high gas flow.

Instrumentation

Laparoscopic instruments are available in a wide range of sizes (2, 2.5, 3 and 5 mm) – although a 5 mm 30° laparoscope provides optimum visualisation for most procedures. The Hasson cannula, which is used for the initial access, is available in 5 mm and 10 mm sizes. For diagnostic and reconstructive procedures (e.g. pyeloplasty), the 5 mm cannula is sufficient. However, a 10 mm cannula is required when an Endopouch retrieval device is required for specimen extraction. A wide assortment of reusable or disposable instrument trocars are available. Bladeless trocars are generally safer for use in children, in whom the abdominal wall is more compliant and less muscular.

Access

There are two methods of accessing the peritoneum: in the blind technique a Veress needle is inserted into the peritoneal cavity via the skin adjacent to the umbilicus through all layers of the abdominal wall. However, the Hasson technique is the preferred method for establishing a pneumoperitoneum in children. This is an 'open' procedure in which the needle is inserted under direct vision. A stab incision is made in the supraumbilical skin crease, and is enlarged along Langer's line. The underlying linea alba is then grasped and opened transversely with scissors or a scalpel. The peritoneum is opened in a similar manner and the Hasson cannula introduced into the peritoneal cavity and secured in place with a skin suture. Because of the limited working space and relatively large size of the liver, spleen and bladder in children, the insertion of trocars and instrumentation should always be performed under direct vision to avoid iatrogenic complications. For retroperitoneoscopic (RP) procedures a blunt approach is used to access the retroperitoneum (Figure 23.1).

In common with traditional laparoscopic surgery, robotic surgery utilises small incisions and insufflation of the anatomical operative space with CO_2. The robotic camera and instruments are inserted through access ports and are manipulated remotely by the operating surgeon seated at a console. The system has three major components: the robot (mobile tower with three or four arms, including a camera arm and instrument arms), the bedside cart (image processing equipment and light source) and the console (where the surgeon performs the surgery with two handpieces aided by the use of two binocular lenses, which magnify and create a 3D image) (Figure 23.2).

The Da Vinci robotic surgical system is used most widely – with instruments available in

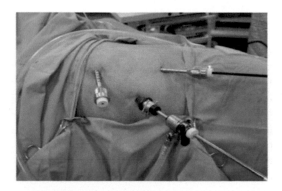

Figure 23.1 Port placement for a transperitoneal laparoscopic nephrectomy.

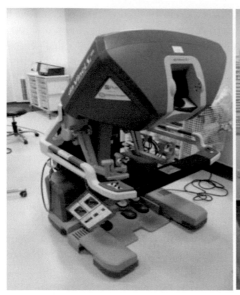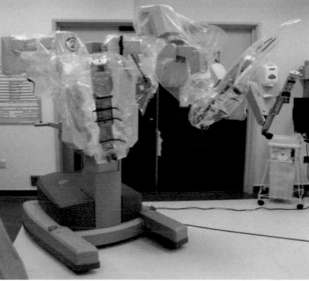

Figure 23.2 Da Vinci system (the console in the left and the robot in the right).

two sizes: 8 and 5 mm. The 8-mm instruments articulate with a pitch-roll-yaw mechanism, whereas the 5-mm instruments articulate in a 'serpentine' manner. The Da Vinci instruments provide seven degrees of freedom in movement. The lack of commercially available 3-mm instruments combined with the minimum 8 cm distance between each port precludes the use of the robot in neonates.

CURRENT INDICATIONS FOR MINIMALLY INVASIVE SURGERY IN PAEDIATRIC UROLOGY

Laparoscopic Nephrectomy

In centres where the expertise is available, minimally invasive surgical techniques have largely replaced open nephrectomy and nephro ureterectomy. The transperitoneal route has the advantage of a larger working space, whereas the retroperitoneoscopic approach obviates the need for colonic mobilisation and avoids the risks of injury to hollow viscera and the potential for adhesion formation. However, the combination of reversed orientation of the kidney and hilum with the patient

in a semiprone or prone position and the comparatively smaller working space make the retroperitoneoscopic approach more difficult to master. Regardless of which approach is adopted, laparoscopic nephrectomy and nephroureterectomy offer undoubted benefits to the child in terms of faster postoperative recovery and improved cosmesis by comparison with open surgery.

Indications

- Congenital dysplastic kidney
- Multicystic dysplastic kidneys (MCDK) – see Chapter 10
- Pelviureteric junction (PUJ) obstruction with severe loss of function
- Reflux-associated nephropathy
- Intractable protein loss associated with congenital nephrotic syndrome
- Native nephrectomy prior to renal transplantation

Operative technique for retroperitoneoscopic nephrectomy

The operating theatre layout for retroperitoneoscopic nephrectomy is shown in Figure 23.3. The patient is positioned prone, with the chest and

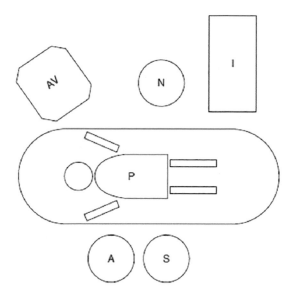

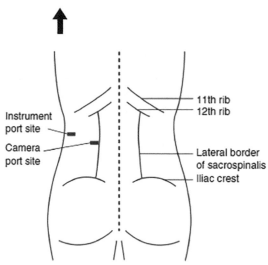

Figure 23.3 Theatre layout for left retroperitoneoscopic nephrectomy, with patient (P) in prone position: monitor and stack system (AV), theatre nurse (N), operating surgeon (S), assistant (A) and instrument table (I).

Figure 23.5 Schematic representation of port position for SIMPL nephrectomy. If required, a second instrument port can also be placed through the sacrospinalis muscle in a position medial to the camera port site.

pelvis raised to allow the abdomen to be dependent (Figure 23.4). Topographic landmarks and anticipated port sites are marked as shown in Figure 23.5.

Through a small incision between the iliac crest and the tip of the 12th rib a small area of the retroperitoneum is dissected bluntly with artery forceps to allow the insertion and inflation of a balloon to create a retroperitoneal working space, which is then insufflated with CO_2 via a Hasson cannula. An instrument port is placed under

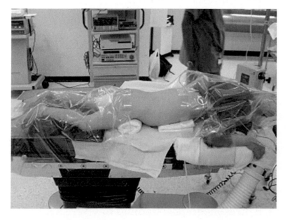

Figure 23.4 Patient positioned for right retroperitoneoscopic nephrectomy.

direct vision below the tip of the 11th/12th ribs and above the iliac crest.

Following incision of Gerota's fascia, the kidney is dissected on its posteromedial aspect to expose the hilar vessels, which are individually identified and divided between haemoclips or with a harmonic scalpel. The ureter is traced inferiorly as far as necessary and is then divided. If there is reflux into the ureter it is ligated before being divided or alternatively the bladder is drained with a urethral catheter for 48 hours. Small kidneys can be removed directly via the camera port, whereas larger kidneys may require entrapment in an Endopouch retrieval device and piecemeal removal.

Results

A systematic review of the literature found that whilst the overall results of transperitoneal (TP) and retroperitoneoscopic (RP) nephrectomy were broadly similar, recovery was faster after RP nephrectomy – which also had a lower conversion rate (<3%) and fewer complications. Because the peritoneum remains intact during RP nephrectomy, this approach is particularly suitable for performing bilateral nephrectomy in children with end-stage renal disease since postoperative peritoneal dialysis can be performed immediately – thus obviating the need for a period of haemodialysis. Unlike transperitoneal nephrectomy the retroperitoneoscopic approach has the advantage of enabling the entire procedure to be performed with a single instrument port. In the authors' institution the single instrument port laparoscopic technique nephrectomy (SIMPL) has been used successfully to perform over 150 nephrectomies in patients ranging from 1 month to 18 years of age (Figure 23.5).

Laparoscopic Heminephrectomy

Minimally invasive surgery has been widely used to perform heminephrectomy and the results are comparable to open surgery, even in small infants. The indications relate mainly to renal duplication anomalies.

Upper pole heminephrectomy. This is the most commonly performed procedure. The anatomy is typically characterised by dilatation of a poorly functioning upper pole renal moiety in conjunction with a dilated upper pole ureter. Laparoscopic heminephrectomy is also used to remove a poorly functioning upper pole, which is accompanied by an ectopic ureter causing incontinence in girls.

Lower pole heminephrectomy. This is mostly performed to remove a poorly functioning lower pole renal moiety in cases of reflux-associated nephropathy or, rarely, lower moiety PUJ obstruction with loss of function.

The laparoscopic dissection may prove difficult in children with a history of recurrent or recent UTI's which have given rise to dense adhesions between the kidney, the ureter and the peritoneum. In such cases, an open approach may be preferable for technical reasons and to avoid excessive excessive blood loss.

Operative technique for retroperitoneoscopic heminephrectomy

The initial steps are the same as for a retroperitoneoscopic nephrectomy. Care is taken to establish the anatomy of the kidney and dupex ureters and

to identify the blood vessels supplying both renal moieties. Following division of the blood vessels supplying the affected moiety, the ureter draining this moiety is carefully mobilised from the ureter which is being preserved before being divided. Pallor of the renal parenchyma following division of the blood vessels to the affected moiety serves to demarcate it from the healthy moiety. The kidney is then transected between the two moieties using monopolar diathermy, ligasure or an endoloop (Figure 23.6). The distal ureteric stump is traced as far as possible down into the pelvis before being removed – with care being taken to visualise and safeguard the remaining ureter.

Results

Conventional transabdominal laparoscopy has become the 'gold standard' technique for heminephrectomy in children. Retroperitoneoscopic heminephrectomy is a challenging procedure with long learning curve, especially for lower pole heminephrectomy. However, it offers the advantages of direct visualization of the duplex kidney, decreased risk of intra-abdominal adhesions and a shorter hospital stay.

Laparoscopic Pyeloplasty

Laparoscopic pyeloplasty was initially introduced for the management of PUJ obstruction in older children but despite being more technically challenging in infants, it has also been adopted in many centres as the modality of choice in young children and infants (including those under 6 months of age).

Indications

- Symptomatic PUJ obstruction
- Worsening hydronephrosis on serial imaging
- Ultrasonographic findings of significant hydronephrosis (pelvic anteroposterior [AP] diameter >20 mm with calyceal dilatation) and reduced differential renal function (<40%)
- Ultrasonographic findings of severe hydronephrosis (pelvic AP diameter >30 mm with calyceal dilatation)

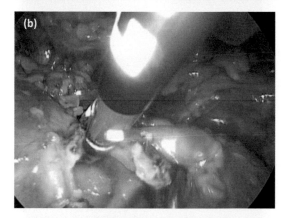

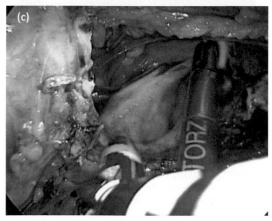

Figure 23.6 Intraoperative images of retroperitoneoscopic heminephrectomy. (a) Upper pole heminephrectomy using endoloop; (b) and (c) lower pole heminephrectomy using ligasure.

Contraindications for laparoscopic pyeloplasty include a small extrarenal pelvis, previous renal surgery and anatomical variants, such as a horseshoe kidney.

Operative technique for laparoscopic pyeloplasty

Laparoscopic pyeloplasty can be performed via the transperitoneal or retroperitoneoscopic route. Although there is no particular advantage of one approach over the other, the authors' preference is for the transperitoneal route since it provides a relatively larger working space for intracorporeal suturing.

The child is positioned in a lateral decubitus position with the affected kidney uppermost. The camera port is placed in the region of the umbilicus and two working ports are inserted: one under the costal margin and the other in the ipsilateral iliac fossa. The kidney is identified either by reflecting the colon medially or through a transmesenteric window. Once the pelvi ureteric junction has been visualised, the renal pelvis is stabilised with a 'hitch stitch' through the abdominal wall. A dismembered pyeloplasty is then performed – with excision of redundant renal pelvis if required. A length of proximal ureter is 'spatulated' and anastomosed to the lower end of the open renal pelvis (Figure 23.7). The posterior wall of the anastomosis is performed with a continuous absorbable suture. A JJ stent is introduced and passed antegradely down to the bladder over a guidewire before completion of the anstomosis

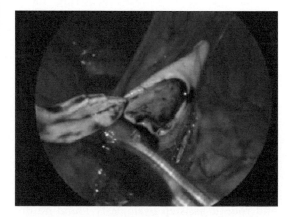

Figure 23.7 Intraoperative view of laparoscopic left pyeloplasty. The renal pelvis is stabilised with a 'hitch stitch' through the lateral abdominal wall (top right corner).

with a further continuous absorbable suture. A urethral catheter is left in situ for a minimum period of 48 hours or until the patient is fully mobile. The stent is removed cystoscopically after a period of 4 weeks. As an alternative to using a JJ stent the authors prefer to protect the anastomosis and drain the kidney post-operatively with a 'nephrostent', which drains externally. This overcomes the complications associated with an indwelling JJ stent and can be removed without the need for a second procedure.

Laparoscopic pyeloplasty is a safe and effective operation in children and numerous studies have found that outcomes are comparable to those achieved by open pyeloplasty.

Robotic Pyeloplasty

Robotic pyeloplasty is based on the same concepts as laparoscopic pyeloplasty. The patient is placed in the lateral decubitus position with the operative side facing up and slightly rotated from the vertical plane. To maximize the range of movement for the robotic arms, the child is positioned as close to the edge of the operating table as possible. The port placements for a robotic pyeloplasty are illustrated in Figure 23.8. Care is taken to ensure that the ports are separated by at least 6–8 cm to maximize robotic arm movements. If necessary, an additional port is used to facilitate passage of sutures, suctioning, and/or retraction of the liver when operating on the right kidney. Following port placement, and 'docking' of the robot, the dilated renal pelvis is identified and the procedure is performed using the same steps as those performed during conventional laparoscopy.

In one large, single centre study, 98% of robotic-assisted laparoscopic pyeloplasty (RALP) were performed by a transperitoneal approach with an operating time averaging 199 minutes. The overall success rate was 96%. A comparative study of open, conventional laparoscopy and robotic-assisted pyeloplasty found no difference in success rates between these three modalities. However, RALP was associated with reduced analgesic requirements and shorter hospital stay.

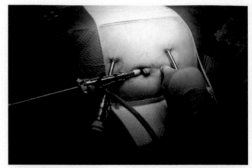
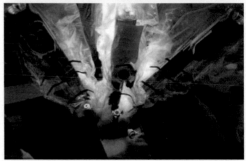
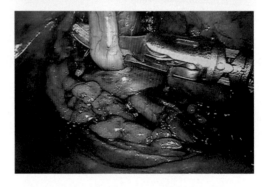

Figure 23.8 Right robotic-assisted laparoscopic pyeloplasty (with crossing vessels at PUJ level).

Laparoscopic 'Vascular Hitch'

Antenatally detected hydronephrosis is usually associated with some form of intrinsic obstruction at the pelvi ureteric junction with lower pole crossing vessels being present in only 6–11% of cases. By contrast, lower pole vessels are found in 50–60% of cases of PUJ obstruction in older children and adults. When the presence of crossing vessels is identified during pyeloplasty, the conventional approach has been perform a dismembered pyeloplasty in which the vessels are re-positioned so they lie posterior to the completed anastomosis. If, however, there is no evidence of intrinsic obstruction at the time of surgery and if the obstruction can be attributed to extrinsic compression of the PUJ by crossing lower vessels, a vascular hitch procedure can be considered as an alternative to dismembered pyeloplasty. In this procedure, the lower pole vessels are relocated away from the PUJ and anchored in more cranial position on the anterior wall of the renal pelvis (Figure 23.9). The principal candidates for this procedure are older children who present with intermittent episodes of pain and who have no preceding history of antenatal hydronephrosis. The vascular hitch procedure avoids the need to transect the pelvis and therefore minimises the risk of any postoperative urinary leak. It is also less technically demanding than laparoscopic pyeloplasty, carries a lower complication rate and results in a shorter hospital stay. A recent multicentre study found that with appropriate patient selection, the vascular hitch procedure offers can excellent long-term outcomes – as evidenced by 100% resolution of symptoms, decreased hydronephrosis grade and improved drainage on MAG3 renogram.

Laparoscopic Adrenalectomy

Laparoscopic adrenalectomy is now widely regarded as the optimal surgical procedure for removing the adrenal gland. Since the initial report of laparoscopic adrenalectomy in 1992, the technique has evolved to become a safe and effective means of removing benign and malignant adrenal tumours in both adults and children. Although the transperitoneal approach is used more widely, the retroperitoneoscopic approach offers distinct advantages particularly for paediatric urologists who already familiar with this approach for renal surgery. Despite developments in technique, however, laparoscopic adrenalectomy remains a challenging surgical undertaking urgery – particularly in view of the paramount importance of avoiding capsular breach and tumour spillage.

Indications

- Phaeochromocytoma
- Adrenal adenoma
- Adrenocorticotrophic hormone (ACTH)-dependent Cushing's syndrome
- Neuroblastoma

Contraindications include; previous renal surgery, large tumours exceeding 8 cm in diameter, evidence of tumour thrombus within the adrenal vein and/or inferior vena cava (IVC) coagulation

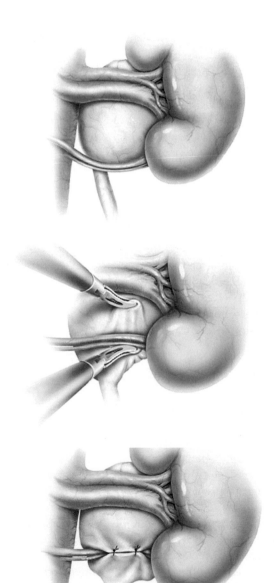

Figure 23.9 **Laparoscopic 'vascular hitch'.**

disorders and a suspected diagnosis of adrenal carcinoma.

Preoperative assessment

A detailed ultrasound scan of the adrenal glands can provide valuable information on the location and size of a mass, and whether it is cystic or solid. In selected cases, the use of Computerised Tomography (CT) and Magnetic Resonance Imaging (MRI) can also be very informative (Figure 23.10). Some conditions affecting the adrenal glands (notably 'central' Cushing's syndrome) are associated with bilateral diffuse enlargement rather than a focal lesion.

Imaging is also valuable in establishing whether there is intravascular extension into the adrenal vein and/or IVC since this information will help to determine the suitability of a laparoscopic approach and the safest approach for specimen retrieval.

Children with hypertension caused by phaeochromocytoma receive 7 days preoperative administration of α-blockers, such as phenoxybenzamine, to which β-blockers, such as propranolol may be added to decrease the risk of tachyarrhythmias.

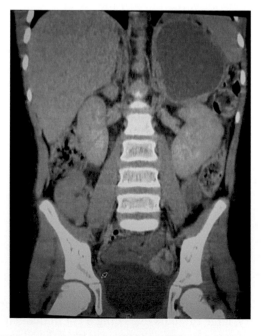

Figure 23.10 CT scan showing left cystic phaeochromocytoma in an 8-year-old male child.

Operative technique for retroperitoneoscopic adrenalectomy

The child is positioned fully prone in a similar manner to a retroperitoneoscopic nephrectomy and the same landmarks and access technique are used to enter the retroperitoneum.

The dissection commences around the kidney and continues until the inferior margin of the adrenal gland is visualised at the superomedial border of the kidney. The arterial blood supply to the adrenal is then identified and divided. To minimise bleeding from the surface of the gland, dissection is performed in a plane within the surrounding adipose tissue. Left adrenalectomy is more difficult than right adrenalectomy due to the smaller size of the gland and adrenal vein and the lack of clear landmarks, such as the inferior vena cava. Once the veins have been divided and adrenal has been fully mobilised it is placed within an endobag and removed through the camera port incision.

Opinion remains divided on whether the transperitoneal or retroperitoneoscopic approach is preferable. There are no reliable comparative data in children and most reports have consisted of small series. The authors' have performed more than 30 RP adrenalectomies, with excellent intraoperative haemodynamic stability and complete excision of lesions in every case.

Other Techniques

Laparoscopic ureteric reimplantation

Although open ureteric reimplantation (with either the intravesical or extravesical approach) remains the most widely performed surgical approach to the correction of vesico ureteral reflux, the use of minimally invasive surgery has also been reported. The techniques which have been deployed include; vesicoscopic ureteral reimplantation using the Cohen technique and laparoscopic or robotic-assisted extravesical ureteral reimplantation using the Lich-Gregoir technique).

In the vesicoscopic technique, the bladder is insufflated with CO_2 to create a pneumovesicum. The refluxing ureter is mobilised in a similar manner to the technique for open reimplantatation and is then reimplanted using a cross-trigonal submucosal tunnel. The limited published data indicate that this is a safe and effective technique, with success rates comparable to conventional open anti-reflux surgery and a lower incidence of postoperative bladder spasms.

Laparoscopic extravesical ureteral reimplantation also has a high success rate and has been reported to offer superior cosmetic outcomes and reduced postoperative morbidity by comparison with open surgery in the older children. As with open extravesical ureteral reimplantation the laparoscopic technique has been reported to carry some risk of damage to pelvic innervation – with consequent bladder dysfunction leading to urinary retention and constipation.

Laparoscopy in disorders of sex development

Laparoscopy plays a valuable role in the investigation and management of children with DSD by permitting direct visualisation of the internal genital anatomy including the uterus, Müllerian duct remnants, gonads and vasa deferentia. Laparoscopy also provides an opportunity to perform gonadal biopsies where indicated and to remove dysgenetic gonads or gonads, which are discordant with the sex of rearing. Symptomatic Müllerian duct remnants can be evaluated and removed with relative ease.

Laparoscopic reconstructive surgery

In addition to the wide range of laparoscopic procedures now available for complex upper tract surgery, the use of minimally invasive surgery has been extended to include lower urinary tract reconstructive procedures, such as bladder augmentation (with or without appendico-vesicostomy) and bladder neck sling procedures.

In a small series of young patients who had undergone robot-assisted laparoscopic augmentation ileocystoplasty and Mitrofanoff procedures

the results were reported to be excellent and comparable to those achieved by open surgery. The operating time was significantly longer but the duration of hospital stay was shorter and the use of epidural anaesthesia was avoided. Diagnostic laparoscopy is performed initially to confirm that the length of the appendix is adequate for use in a Mitrofanoff procedure prior to docking the robot. In other respects, the technical manoeuvres are similar to those employed in the open operation.

The evolution of robotic procedures for use in paediatric urology will increase the availability of alternative approaches to conventional open reconstructive surgery – offering the prospect of advances in patient care and improvements in quality of life. However, the acceptance of robotic reconstructive surgery is currently limited by the paucity of published data and lack of randomized controlled trials.

KEY POINTS

- Minimally invasive alternatives to conventional open urological procedures are now routinely practised in major paediatric urology centres. Indications include nephrectomy, heminephrectomy, pyeloplasty and adrenalectomy.
- The relatively small size of paediatric patients permits access to both the upper and lower urinary tract through the same ports. Both the transperitoneal and retroperitoneoscopic approaches are utilised in children, although the retroperitoneoscopic technique is favoured for renal surgery.
- Laparoscopic pyeloplasty is the gold standard for older children and adolescents. The advent of robotic technology has made intracorporeal suturing more precise and less challenging.
- Minimally invasive techniques have provided new insight into disease processes and can be applied to complex reconstructive surgery of the lower urinary tract.

FURTHER READING

Barashi NS, Rodriguez MV, Packiam VT, Gundeti, MS. Bladder reconstruction with bowel: robot-assisted laparoscopic ileocystoplasty with Mitrofanoff apendicovesicostomy in paediatric patients. J Endourol. 2018;32:119–126.

Cho A, Mushtaq I. Retroperitoneoscopic lower pole heminephrectomy. J Pediatr Urol. 2019;15:89–90.

Esposito C, et al. Retroperitoneoscopic heminephrectomy in duplex kidneys in infants and children: results of a multicentric survey. J Laparoendosc Adv Surg Tech A. 2015;25:864–869.

Garg S, Gundeti M, Mushtaq I. The single instrument port laparoscopic (SIMPL) nephrectomy. J Pediatr Urol. 2006;3:194–196.

Sakoda A, Cherian A, Mushtaq I. Laparoscopic transposition of lower pole crossing vessels ('vascular hitch') in pure extrinsic pelviureteric junction (PUJ) obstruction in children. BJU Int. 2011;108:1364–1368.

Song SH, Lee C, Jung J, Kim SJ, Park S, Park H, Kim KS. A comparative study of paediatric open pyeloplasty, laparoscopy-assisted extracorporeal pyeloplasty and robot laparoscopic pyeloplasty. PLoS One. 2017;20:12.

Upasani A, Paul A, Cherian A. External stent in laparoscopic pyeloplasty: the K-wire technique. J Pediatr Urol. 2018;14:298–299.

Adolescent Urology

CHARLOTTE DUNFORD, CHRISTOPHER R J WOODHOUSE and DAN WOOD

Topics covered

Renal impairment	Posterior urethral valves (including transplantation)
Vesicoureteric reflux	Prune-belly syndrome
Bladder exstrophy	Enterocystoplasty
Female genital reconstruction	Spina bifida
Hypospadias	Fertility

INTRODUCTION

The major anomalies of the genitourinary tract are commonly reconstructed in infancy and from a paediatric point of view the results are generally good. However, they leave a legacy of potential morbidity in adolescence and adult life. Many problems are predominantly medical or psychosocial rather than surgical in nature and it is essential to adopt a holistic approach to long-term care. Close collaboration between paediatric and adolescent or adult urologists is also important to ensure continuity of follow-up and specialist care. Where surgical input is required, particularly for the revision of previous reconstructive procedures, it may be necessary to adopt a multi-disciplinary approach involving gynaecological, colorectal and renal transplant surgeons. Collaboration with a renal physician to optimise preservation of renal function is paramount. The young patient's transition from the care of paediatric specialists to the relevant adult disciplines is of pivotal importance in determining their future engagement with follow-up and lifelong maintenance of their renal function. This chapter reviews the management of complex congenital urological anomalies in the context of their long-term outcomes and the legacy of morbidity in later life.

RENAL FUNCTION

The renal damage associated with many of the congenital urological anomalies dates from fetal life and despite successful correction of the structural anomaly - such as resection of posterior urethral valves (PUV) shortly after birth (or even in utero), hypertension and renal failure may nevertheless supervene in later life. Monitoring of renal function is therefore an integral part of adolescent care.

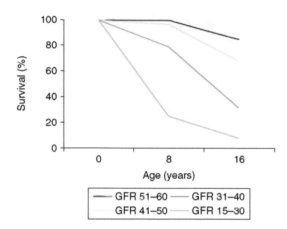

Figure 24.1 Percentage of patients surviving *without* dialysis/transplantation by initial GFR (ml/min) corrected to 1.73 m². Time zero was at entry into adolescent follow-up around puberty.

Historical data suggest that patients who reach adolescence with a glomerular filtration rate (GFR) of less than 40 ml/min/1.73 m² are at substantial risk of progressing to end-stage renal failure within 16 years (Figure 24.1). The downward trajectory can, however, be delayed with rigorous control of proteinuria and blood pressure using angiotensin-conversion enzyme (ACE) inhibitors.

Around 20–40% of patients with PUV have (or will develop) renal impairment and 10–15% will require renal replacement therapy. Prognostic risk scores for patients are based on baseline plasma creatinine level, nadir creatinine level and proteinuria. When stratified according to their level of risk of significant renal impairment (defined as CKD ≥3), those categorised as low risk have 6% incidence of renal impairment whereas those categorised as medium or high risk have a 40% and 70% incidence, respectively. The later decline in renal function is generally attributed to hyperperfusion/hyperfiltration injury to the remaining nephrons but it is important not to overlook the potential additional contribution made by high-pressure bladder dysfunction.

Although measurement of plasma creatinine represents the simplest and most practical means of monitoring renal function it may be potentially misleading in patients with congenital malformations, particularly since a significant loss of GFR can sometimes occur before this is reflected in abnormal plasma creatinine levels (see Chapter 2). What is clear is that all patients transitioning from paediatric to adult care require risk assessment of their renal function and many will then go on to require long-term surveillance in specialist units.

VESICOURETERIC REFLUX

Four groups of adults must be considered:

1. **Adults whose vesicoureteric reflux (VUR) has either ceased or been corrected in childhood**. If their kidneys have not sustained any renal damage no follow-up is necessary for these patients.
2. **Adults whose VUR has ceased or been corrected in childhood but in whom reflux nephropathy is present**. These patients need lifelong follow-up. By the age of 18 years, 11% of those with unilateral scarring and 18% of those with bilateral scars have developed hypertension, a figure rising to 23% at 27 years. If the renal damage is sufficiently severe to reduce the GFR below 40 ml/min/1.73 m², the eventual onset of renal failure may be inevitable.
3. **Reflux persisting from childhood beyond puberty**. There is no consensus on management. However, it is reasonable to recommend either endoscopic treatment or surgical reimplantation in symptomatic females since their kidneys may still be at risk of developing pyelonephritic scarring in pregnancy. However, it has been reported that women who have previously undergone reimplantation are at greater risk of urinary infection in pregnancy than any other group. The reason is unclear. It may be that the women who underwent ureteric reimplantation were those who originally had the most severe forms of reflux and a greater likelihood of reflux nephropathy. Alternatively, it may represent some unexplained consequence of reimplantation. In asymptomatic males there seems to be no indication for

surgery in the absence of bladder outflow obstruction.

4. **Adults presenting for the first time with VUR**. These are mainly women presenting with symptomatic urinary tract infections (UTIs). Medical management with continuous antibiotic prophylaxis (CAP) is appropriate in the first instance but surgical treatment (either endoscopic or open) is indicated if this fails.

The controversies surrounding the management of VUR in children are reviewed in Chapter 6.

BLADDER EXSTROPHY

Most children with exstrophy have an isolated anomaly and their overall development is normal, with many being both intelligent and well-motivated. Despite the excellent results of bladder reconstruction reported from major centres, there remains a perception that early diversion is also an acceptable form of management and one with a lower complication rate. Certainly, reconstruction should only be undertaken by surgeons with the appropriate training and extensive experience. In the United Kingdom, the surgical management of children born with bladder exstrophy is now concentrated in two specialist supra regional centres.

A successful outcome from bladder reconstruction in childhood may not be maintained into adulthood. Historically, only 23% of exstrophy patients who underwent bladder reconstruction in childhood progressed into adult life without the need for urinary diversion. Of those whose bladder reconstruction did endure beyond childhood, 60% nevertheless required further reconstruction in adolescence or early adult life.

In one large study of exstrophy patients who were followed for over 40 years it was found that only 25% of patients were still voiding spontaneously per urethra. The remaining 75% were either reliant on catheterisation or had undergone urinary diversion. Most patients required complex reconstruction and subsequent revisions in order to achieve urinary continence. A continence rate

of 93% was reported in patients who had undergone bladder neck closure combined with formation of a continent catheterisable stoma. Bladder augmentation or subtotal substitution cystoplasty with intestinal (e.g. ileocaecal) segments may be required. Historically the surgical options have also included cystectomy and external urinary diversion or internal diversion by ureterosigmoidostomy. In one long-term follow-up study of ureterosigmoidstomy with follow up of 24 years, 97% of patients were continent by day and 87% had stable renal function. However, 40% of patients had disturbances of acid base balance which required them to take alkaline supplements. Although sexual function was impaired in all patients, 40% of the men achieved achieve paternity and the women in this series gave birth to a total of six healthy children.

Malignancy

Bladder exstrophy is associated with a significantly higher incidence of malignancy. In a study reported from the authors' unit 4 out of 61 patients developed bladder cancer at a mean age of 41 years – an incidence which is 694 times greater than that of the normal population. Most reported cases have occurred in bladders which were defunctioned by urinary diversion in childhood. It is possible that the risk of malignancy will be lower in patients who have retained a functioning bladder following reconstruction in childhood but, as yet, there are no long-term data to confirm this.

Ureterosigmoidostomy is associated with a 15% incidence of malignancy (usually adenocarcinoma) occurring within the bowel reservoir. However, there is typically a latent period of 20–30 years before the malignancy develops.

Genital Reconstruction in Exstrophy

Males

The penis in exstrophy is short but often has an increased girth and is accompanied by a tight dorsal chordee. If uncorrected in infancy the chordee is likely to prevent the adult patient from having penetrative sexual intercourse (Figure 24.2). In adults the extent of the deformity is evaluated by

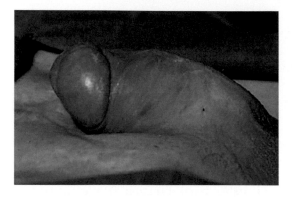

Figure 24.2 Clinical photograph of an epispadiac penis showing dorsal chordee and retraction into the recessed mons area.

an artificial erection test in which saline is injected into the corporal bodies. Minor defects may be corrected by a ventral Nesbit's procedure, whereas severe penile deformity requires more extensive correction which typically involves penile disassembly and inward or outward rotation of the corpora to achieve a more normal configuration.

Females

The vagina is short and lies in a more horizontal plane than normal. The labia are located on the anterior abdominal wall, the introitus is narrowed and the clitoris is bifid (Figure 24.3).

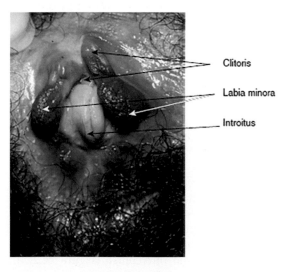

Clitoris

Labia minora

Introitus

Figure 24.3 Female perineum in exstrophy.

Although the labia cannot be repositioned, the overall appearances can be improved by labioplasty and patients can have normal sexual function. Fertility is unaffected, but troublesome uterine prolapse (procidentia) occurs in up to 50% of women. Historical data suggest that when one parent has bladder exstrophy the risk of exstrophy or epispadias in their offspring is approximately 1:70. However data collected in the authors' unit and elsewhere suggest that the risk is far lower than this.

FEMALE GENITAL RECONSTRUCTION OF AMBIGUOUS GENITALIA

The timing and nature of genital reconstruction in females with virilised or ambiguous external genitalia has become a highly controversial topic. Historically, very few studies have attempted to document the long-term functional and psychological outcome of feminising genitoplasty and vaginoplasty performed in childhood. Importantly, there are virtually no published data on long-term outcomes for women with disorders of sex differentiation (DSDs) who were not operated upon in childhood. However, evidence is accumulating which challenges some of the assumptions about female genital reconstruction, particularly the belief that one-stage surgery in childhood will suffice. In 2006, the Chicago Consensus Document noted that clitoral surgery in childhood carries a risk of impaired sensation and advocated a two stage approach – particularly with regard to vaginoplasty. Studies have shown that many young women who underwent vaginoplasty in childhood in the past nevertheless went on to require further vaginal surgery (ranging from simple introital revision to complex vaginoplasty) in order to experience normal comfortable intercourse (Figure 24.4). More recently, published data indicate that although there have been changes with regard to the timing of vaginoplasty, clitoral surgery is still being performed in infancy or early childhood. Further surgical revision is required in around 25% of women after clitoral surgery in childhood but this figure

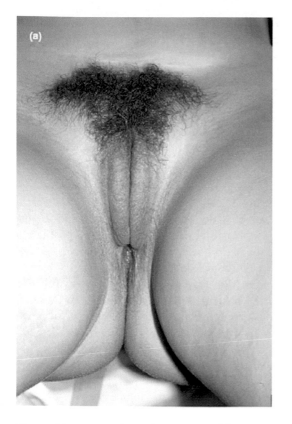
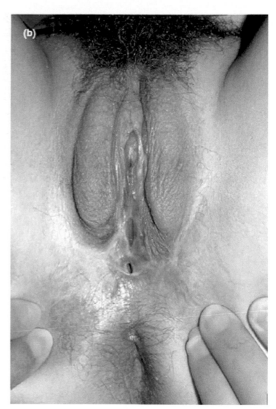

Figure 24.4 Postpubertal outcome of feminising genitoplasty for the correction of virilisation associated with congenital adrenal hyperplasia. Single-stage feminising genitoplasty previously undertaken in the first year of life. (a) External cosmetic outcome satisfactory, with no visible phallic hypertrophy and normal appearance of labia created from 'scrotalised' skin. (b) Retraction of the labia reveals introital scarring, requiring introitoplasty to permit normal, comfortable intercourse.

may be lower in the future because of changes in surgical techniques for feminising genitoplasty. The issues surrounding the management of DSD in childhood are addressed in greater detail in Chapter 20. Continuity of follow-up from childhood into early adulthood is essential, with further care being provided in a centre specialising in adolescent gynaecology to ensure that these patients have access to relevant specialist expertise and appropriate psychological support.

HYPOSPADIAS

Surgeons tend to view their own results more favourably than their patients (and parents). Published reports of excellent results (e.g. 100%

of patients having straight erections and a normal urine stream) should be viewed with considerable scepticism. When viewed more objectively, the late results are less impressive- with up to 50% of men experiencing a poor functional or cosmetic outcome. In general, repair of proximal hypospadias is associated with the worst long-term results.

Patients' dissatisfaction tends to centre on those aspects of hypospadias which are often the most difficult to correct, namely size of the penis and glans, penile curvature, scarring and the absence of a normal prepuce.

There is little consensus on the impact of hypospadias on sexual and psychosexual development. This partly reflects the fact that the majority of adult patients underwent correction of their hypospadias with outdated techniques which yielded

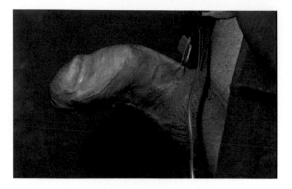

Figure 24.5 Clinical photograph of a patient with persistent chordee following repair of hypospadias in childhood.

inferior results to those in current use. Although an overall sexual satisfaction rate averaging 80% has been reported in different studies, what constitutes sexual satisfaction is not always clearly defined and it has been found that men who have undergone surgical correction of hypospadias are more inhibited in seeking sexual contact.

The presence of gross persistent abnormalities, especially chordee, may preclude normal intercourse (Figure 24.5). With less severe anomalies, particularly of a cosmetic variety, the ages of sexual debut and intercourse may be nearly normal. One study found no differences in the development of standard sexual milestones in patients who had undergone surgical correction of hypospadias in childhood when compared with those who undergone surgery for hernia or phimosis. Reduced semen quality has been reported in up to 50% of men with a history of hypospadias although this does not appear to be accompanied by a corresponding decrease in paternity rates. Intercourse is possible following repair of penoscrotal or perineal hypospadias (which has often presented initially as ambiguous genitalia) but ejaculation is poor and infertility is common. Uroflowmetry studies have demonstrated that reduced flow rates are relatively common following hypospadias surgery. This has been attributed to reduced elasticity/compliance of the reconstructed neo urethra – although some patients may also have varying degrees of fixed stenotic narrowing. There is some evidence that flow rates tend to improve after puberty. Moreover,

reductions in measured flow rate are not usually of clinical significance and rarely give rise to symptoms.

POSTERIOR URETHRAL VALVES (PUV)

Bladder Function

The main long-term consequences of PUV are the result of bladder outflow obstruction and secondary upper tract damage in utero and postnatally in the period before the obstruction was relieved by valve resection. Differing patterns of bladder dysfunction may persist despite successful relief of the obstruction by valve resection. These are considered in more detail in Chapter 9 but can be briefly summarised as poor compliance, detrusor overactivity and reduced functional capacity (the 'valve bladder'). In adults, however the pattern may evolve to one of chronic retention, often with high pressure.

Renal Function

The progressive nature of renal impairment in PUV boys has been recognised for many years. A study published in 1988 reported the incidence of renal failure as 23% at 10 years, 30% at 16 years and 43% at 30 years. In spite of improvements in management and a greater understanding of the pathophysiology of the 'valve bladder' more recent data have shown no real change in recent decades with 10–15% of PUV patients requiring renal replacement therapy and a 20–40% incidence of renal renal impairment. These figures illustrate the importance of congenital renal damage in determining the long-term functional outcome. Increasing muscle mass at the time of puberty places an increased load on the renal reserve, with the result that normal levels of plasma creatinine at the beginning of puberty do not guarantee that the plasma creatinine will still be normal at the end of puberty.

The combination of a poorly compliant 'valve bladder' and polyuria arising from renal tubular concentration defects may result in dangerously high bladder storage pressures – thus creating a vicious cycle of worsening renal damage.

Significant prognostic factors indicating poor long-term outcome include:

- Diagnosis before the age of 1 year (including prenatal diagnosis)
- Diurnal incontinence persisting after 5 years of age
- Persistent bilateral reflux
- Polyuria

There is some evidence that the onset of renal failure can be delayed (or is some cases possibly averted) by aggressive bladder management with anticholinergics, self-catheterisation and clam cystoplasty (see also Chapter 9).

Ejaculation

Like the bladder, the prostate is exposed to the effects of high pressure outflow obstruction before the valves are resected. Damage to the prostatic tissue may cause impaired semen quality and poor ejaculation in up to 50% of patients. The seminal abnormality is characterised by lack of liquefaction, low sperm count, poor motility and high pH (up to 9.5). Dilatation of the posterior urethra may result in inadequate pressure being generated at the beginning of orgasm, resulting in less forceful (or absent) ejaculation. Up to a third of men with a history of PUV encounter difficulty in achieving paternity.

Transplantation

A bladder which has contributed to the destruction of the two native kidneys and caused end-stage renal failure has the potential to do the same to a transplanted kidney unless it is managed appropriately. In the past, the published 5-year graft survival in PUV patients was approximately 50% lower than in all other recipients. However, current 5-year graft survivals figures are comparable, although PUV transplant patients tend to experience more UTIs and have higher levels of plasma creatinine than other transplant patients, especially from 7 years onwards. A large series published

from France reported a 60% graft survival rate at 15 years. When appropriate measures had been taken to ensure that the bladder was 'safe' prior to transplantation, graft survival rates were not significantly different between patients who had undergone enterocystoplasty and those who had not.

PRUNE-BELLY SYNDROME

Prune-belly syndrome is now very rare, at least in the UK. This is probably because the condition is being detected prenatally and affected pregnancies are being terminated. However, there is a cohort of adult patients born this condition from the 1960s onwards who have generally done well.

There are three components to the syndrome (Figure 24.6):

- Bilateral undescended testes
- Absence of the muscle of the anterior abdominal wall
- Variable functional and anatomical anomalies of the urinary tract

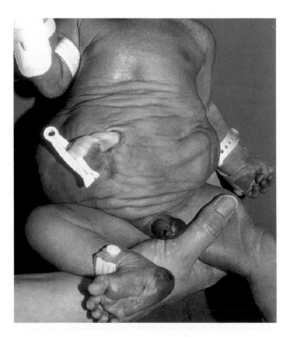

Figure 24.6 Characteristic appearance of the abdominal wall in a newborn infant with prune-belly syndrome.

Although each of these components has the potential to affect long-term development, most prune-belly patients develop to acquire normal stature. Other, associated anomalies, notably skeletal, may be present, but with the exception of kyphoscoliosis (and possible respiratory compromise) these are seldom of great consequence.

Undescended Testes

Historically men with prune-belly syndrome were thought to be sterile, with 'Sertoli cell only' histology on testicular biopsies. Orchdiopexy was therefore delayed to coincide with major reconstructive surgery or until later childhood. However, it has become apparent that testes are not always devoid of germ cells and consequently the outlook for fertility might not be so bleak as was once thought. Although it was once believed that undescended testes in men with prune-belly syndrome did not carry the same increased risk of malignancy there have been three reported cases of germ cell neoplasia.

Serum testosterone levels in adulthood are usually in the normal range and adequate to maintain normal masculinisation but serum luteinising hormone (LH) levels are significantly elevated.

The Abdominal Wall

The literature on the value of abdominal wall reconstruction during childhood is contradictory (Figure 24.7). Although it is certainly possible to improve the 'prune-like' wrinkled appearance of the skin, it is doubtful whether this alone is of any long-term benefit since the abdominal wall lacks the necessary underlying muscular or fascial support.

In adult life the abdomen is protuberant, resembling a premature 'pot-belly'. However, this creates no functional problem other than an inability to sit up directly from the lying position. Patients in the authors' practice are physically fully active.

The Kidneys

The long-term function of the kidneys is dependent on the degree of renal development in utero (and severity of any renal dysplasia) and the

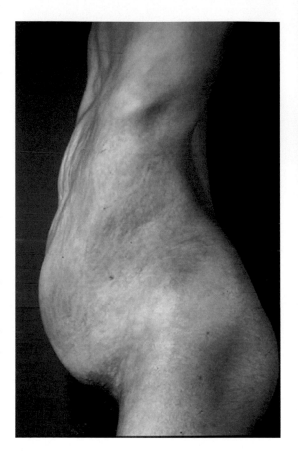

Figure 24.7 Clinical photograph of an adult with prune-belly syndrome. Note the 'pot-belly'. Pectus cavus, a common anomaly in prune-belly syndrome, is also present.

management of urinary tract abnormalities in childhood. In a cohort of 21 adults who had undergone minimal surgery in childhood, 17 had normal renal function, with a mean GFR of 85 ml/min/1.73 m^2 at a mean age of 24 years. Four patients were in end-stage renal failure and another four were hypertensive. However, out of eight patients who had been born with significant renal impairment and undergone major reconstruction in childhood, five were in end-stage renal failure as adults.

Satisfactory bladder function is usually maintained although there may be a risk of UTI due to incomplete bladder emptying and post void residual urine. If this problem is identified, it is most important to look for (and rectify) possible outflow obstruction, either at the level of the urethra or the bladder neck.

ENTEROCYSTOPLASTY

All urinary reservoirs created from intestinal segments share the same basic long-term problems. Because no type of intestine is superior to another, the surgical strategy must be tailored to the individual patient. Hyperchloraemic acidosis occurs in up to 14% of patients – although many more may have a metabolic acidosis with respiratory compensation. Anaemia occurs in 8% and Vitamin B_{12} deficiency is a potential complication after 5 years – especially if terminal ileum has been used. The reported incidence of stone formation in reconstructed urinary reservoirs is at least 15% with risk factors including infection, intermittent catheterisation (CIC) and retained mucus. The commonest complication of continent urinary diversion (Mitrofanoff procedure) is stenosis at the junction between the skin and catheterisable channel (usually appendix). The reported incidence is 40%, with further revision being required in 40% of patients. Nevertheless, overall patient satisfaction with continent urinary diversion is very high.

The interaction of urine and fecal bacteria in the sigmoid is known to result in the formation of nitrosamine and other known carcinogens. Although these agents have been identified in bladders following enterocystoplasty, the overall risk of malignancy is likely to be considerably lower than following ureterosigmoidostomy. One study found a 3.8% incidence of bladder malignancy in a large cohort of enterocystoplasty patients followed for 20–25 years. Patients who have undergone enterocystoplasty in childhood require careful long-term follow-up but protocols no longer include routine periodic cystoscopy since this has not been shown to be effective in screening for bladder cancers.

SPINA BIFIDA – SOCIAL AND SEXUAL DEVELOPMENT

In spite of great advances in the management of infants born with spina bifida they continue to face numerous long-term problems. The mortality rate in the first year is approximately 20%. This

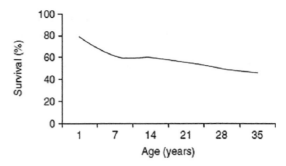

Figure 24.8 Survival curve for all patients born with spina bifida.

is followed by a period of stability in childhood, before mortality increases again from puberty onwards. Only 45% of patients are still alive at the age of 35 (Figure 24.8). Neurological complications related to hydrocephalus are the commonest cause of death in childhood and adolescence, with cardiovascular and pulmonary diseases being the commonest causes in adults. Whereas renal insufficiency was once a major cause of mortality in young adults with spina bifida, death from renal failure now very unusual. Because about 10% of adolescents are unfit for major surgery, reconstructive surgery should be completed in childhood whenever possible.

Spina bifida is associated with a wide spectrum of disability ranging from virtual normality to severe disability characterised by wheelchair dependence and poor executive function. During childhood a heavy burden falls upon the parents, but independent self-care should always be the long-term objective. Achieving this goal depends on:

- Adaptation of daily living to permit self-sufficiency in tasks such as dressing, washing and performing routine household chores
- Effective management of the neuropathic bladder and bowel
- Sexual education
- General education

Bladder

The investigation and management of neuropathic bladder dysfunction in children is considered in detail in Chapter 13. Whenever possible, any major reconstructive surgery should be completed before puberty because there is a natural tendency for continence to deteriorate rather than to improve after this age. Very few adults with spina bifida, especially females, can learn to perform urethral self-catheterisation if they were not taught it in childhood.

Bowel

Even the mildest neurological deficit leads to incompetence of the anal sphincter. Fecal continence is usually dependent on acquiring a pattern of 'controlled constipation'. The concept of the Malone antegrade continence enema (MACE) has been an important advance in the management of the neuropathic bowel. Although this is still widely used, newer alternatives such as transanal irrigation systems are also effective.

Sexual Development – Females

The impact on sexual function is closely related to the level of the spinal cord lesion and the severity of the associated neuropathic bladder dysfunction. Whereas sexual function is likely to be normal in the majority of females with a neurological 'level' below L2 only 20% of those with higher cord lesions or urinary incontinence will have normal sexual function. Nevertheless, two-thirds of women form steady sexual relationships, regardless of the degree of handicap or continence. Pregnancies are complicated by high rates of urinary infection and deterioration in bladder function. The overall risk of neural tube defect in their offspring is 1:23 (1:50 for sons and 1:13 for daughters) although it can be significantly reduced by folic acid supplements for 3 months prior to conception. Few spina bifida patients will accept antenatal screening and termination of affected pregnancies.

Sexual Development – Males

The small minority of males with intact sacral reflexes and preservation of urinary continence will be potent. Of those with absent sacral reflexes, 64% of those whose with a primary neurological level below T10 are potent, but the figure falls to 14% in men with higher neurological lesions. Sildenafil (Viagra) may be helpful in treating erectile dysfunction in some cases. Semen can be obtained from impotent men by electroejaculation. Despite these drawbacks 60% of adult males with spina bifida have a regular sexual partner regardless of their degree of mobility or continence.

FERTILITY AND PREGNANCY IN ADULT PATIENTS WITH MAJOR GENITOURINARY ABNORMALITIES

Most major genitourinary anomalies have the potential to cause sexual and reproductive problems which may affect fertility and pregnancy. Although advances in techniques of assisted conception have improved the outlook considerably, they are nevertheless accompanied by stress and expense.

Impaired male fertility is a feature of bladder exstrophy, prune-belly syndrome, renal failure, DSD and spina bifida. In a recent study of men with bladder exstrophy epispadias complex with a mean age of 32 years, 55% reported objectively 'normal' erections. Despite impaired semen quality in 93% of individuals, one-third of this cohort had achieved parenthood – although this was dependent on assisted reproductive techniques in 50% of cases. Spina bifida, bladder exstrophy, enterocystoplasty and previous ureteric reimplantation all have the potential to cause problems in pregnancy. But despite being counselled on these risks very few women are deterred from wanting to have having a baby. However, women with a GFR below 50 ml/min/1.73 m^2 and a diastolic blood pressure (untreated) above 90 mmHg should be cautioned against embarking on pregnancy because of the very significant risks of irreversible deterioration in renal function and/or hypertension.

KEY POINTS

- Individuals with evidence of renal scarring (reflux nephropathy) should undergo lifetime measurement of blood pressure. Closer monitoring is required for those with severe scarring who are at risk of renal impairment.

- Approximately one-third of boys with posterior urethral valves are destined for renal failure by the time of adolescence or adult life.
- The incidence of new cases of prune-belly syndrome has fallen dramatically following the introduction of antenatal screening.
- Enterocystoplasty may be associated with stones and metabolic disturbances. The full extent of the risk of malignancy in reconstructed bladders may not be apparent for some decades.
- Measures needed to restore urinary continence in patients with spina bifida should be commenced during childhood and completed before adulthood.
- Congenital urinary tract malformations can have a major long-term impact on fertility. Advances in in- vitro fertilisation and improved obstetric care may, however, offer the prospect of fertility to some of those who would previously have been denied parenthood.

FURTHER READING

Bower WF, Christie D, DeGennaro M et al. The transition of young adults with lifelong urological needs from paediatric to adult services: an International Children's Continence Society position statement. Neurourol Urodyn. 2017;36(3):811–819.

Wood H, Wood D. Transition and Lifelong Care in Congenital Urology. Humana Press, Springer International Publishing, 2015.

Woodhouse CRJ. Adolescent Urology and Long-Term Outcomes. Oxford: John Wiley Blackwell, 2015

Woodhouse CRJ. Long-Term Paediatric Urology. Oxford: Blackwell Scientific, 1991.

Pediatric and Adolescent Gynecology

VERONICA I ALANIZ and PATRICIA HUGUELET

Topics covered

Prepubertal lichen sclerosus	Labial hypertrophy
Vulvovaginitis	Hymenal and vaginal anomalies
Labial adhesions	Ovarian masses

PREPUBERTAL LICHEN SCLEROSUS

Introduction

Lichen sclerosus is a chronic inflammatory condition that affects the anogenital skin and typically develops during times of low estrogen production. Although the majority of cases are diagnosed in postmenopausal women, approximately 10–15% of cases occur during childhood. The estimated incidence in prepubertal girls is approximately 1 in 900. The exact pathogenesis of lichen sclerosus is unknown and is likely to be multifactorial. Lichen sclerosus has been associated with conditions such as vitiligo, alopecia, and thyroiditis, suggesting an autoimmune mechanism contributing to the disease.

Presentation

Prepubertal lichen sclerosus typically presents with intense and unrelenting genital itching. Other presenting symptoms may include vulvar discomfort or soreness, genital bleeding, dysuria, or pain with defecation. On examination of the external genitalia, the classic appearance is hypopigmentation in a figure of eight pattern surrounding the vestibule and anus. The vulvar skin is typically thin and akin to "parchment paper". Other examination findings include fissures or superficial breaks in the skin and subepithelial hemorrhages or "blood blisters". For those who are unfamiliar with prepubertal lichen sclerosus the appearances of genital ecchymosis and bleeding can sometimes raise concerns regarding genital trauma (see Figure 25.1). Resorption of labia minora, adhesions of the prepuce resulting in a buried clitoris, and introital narrowing can occur in late stage and untreated cases of lichen sclerosus.

Investigations

Prepubertal lichen sclerosus can almost invariably be diagnosed on the basis of the clinical history and examination of the external genitalia alone. Vulvar biopsy should not be routinely performed and is rarely indicated.

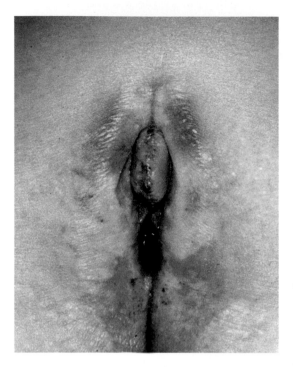

Figure 25.1 Prepubertal lichen sclerosus. (Boms, S., Gambichler, T., Freitag, M., Altmeyer, P., & Kreuter, A. (2004). Pimecrolimus 1% cream for anogenital lichen sclerosus in childhood. *BMC Dermatol, 4*(1), 14. doi:10.1186/1471-5945-4-14.)

Treatment

The goals of treatment are to relieve symptoms and prevent physical changes of the vulva. Girls with acute symptoms are treated with a course of topical steroids over 2–3 months, starting with a high potency steroid ointment, then titrating down to a lower potency steroid (see Table 25.1). Patients treated with topical steroids should be monitored as prolonged treatment can be

associated with thinning of the vulvar skin and superimposed infections. For refractory cases, topical immune modulators, such as pimecrolimus or tacrolimus can also be used, though published data regarding the use of these agents in children is very limited. Recurrent symptoms occur with an average frequency of 1–2 flares (exacerbations) per year. Acute exacerbations of symptoms are treated with further courses of topical steroids which can be modified depending on their severity. Maintenance steroids can be considered for girls who are experiencing more frequent episodes. Surgery is reserved for symptomatic adhesions or scarring.

Prognosis

Prepubertal lichen sclerosus was previously thought to resolve during puberty with the onset of endogenous estrogen production. However, several reports have shown that many patients will experience persistent signs or symptoms in adolescence. Although post-menopausal women with lichen sclerosus are known to be at increased risk of vulvar squamous cell carcinoma, the risk of malignancy associated with prepubertal lichen sclerosus has not been established. Girls with lichen sclerosus should be seen for follow up every 6–12 months.

VULVOVAGINITIS

Introduction

Inflammation of the vulva, vestibule, and vagina occurring in prepubertal girls is of

Table 25.1 Example of lichen sclerosus treatment

Topical steroid	Frequency	Period
Clobetasol propionate 0.5%	Twice daily	2 weeks
Clobetasol propionate 0.5%	Once daily	2 weeks
Triamcinolone acetonide 0.1%	Twice daily	2 weeks
Triamcinolone acetonide 0.1%	Once daily	2 weeks
Triamcinolone acetonide 0.1%	1–2 times weekly	Maintenance

non-specific etiology in the majority of cases. Anatomical factors which predispose to vulvovaginitis in this age group include; close proximity of the vagina to the anus, lack of labial fat pads, and thin vaginal mucosa with an alkaline pH. Behavioral factors such as poor hand washing, incorrect wiping, chronic constipation, and exposure to irritants also contribute to the development of vulvo vaginitis. An infectious etiology is identified up to 25% of cases and when bacteria are isolated they are usually enteric or respiratory in origin. Unless other risk factors are present yeast infection is rarely the cause of vulvovaginitis in toilet trained prepubertal girls because the unestrogenized and alkaline environment of the prepubertal vagina does not permit the growth of candida.

Presentation

The most common symptoms are vulvar redness and soreness. Vaginal discharge, genital itching, and bleeding from irritation or breakdown of mucosal surfaces can also occur. The presenting symptoms are generally chronic in nature, with waxing and waning in their severity. On examination of the external genitalia the findings are varied and may appear normal or erythematous. Bacterial vulvovaginitis is more likely to be accompanied by significant vaginal discharge, severe inflammation, and offensive odor.

Investigations

Vulvovaginitis is diagnosed on the basis of the clinical history and examination of the external genitalia. An aerobic culture can be collected when bacterial vulvovaginitis is suspected or discharge is visible at the vestibule. If an intravaginal specimen is needed, this should be obtained without touching the hymen. A small moistened swab can be inserted gently past the hymen to collect a specimen. Patients with foul smelling, blood tinged, or recurrent vaginal discharge which does not respond to typical treatments may need vaginoscopy to look for a possible vaginal foreign body.

Table 25.2 Vulvar and vaginal hygiene recommendations

- Avoid irritants including bubble bath or scented soaps.
- Wear plain white, cotton underwear.
- Use unscented detergent.
- Wear a nightgown or loose clothing for sleeping. Try sleeping without underwear.
- Change quickly out of wet swimsuits and exercise clothes.
- Take a bath every day and use water only to clean the genitalia.
- Always wipe from front to back after bowel movements.
- Apply a non-medicated barrier cream once to twice daily.

Treatment

The primary treatment for non-specific vulvovaginitis is health education and measures to improve vulvar hygiene (see Table 25.2). Patients with persistent symptoms or suspected bacterial vulvovaginitis can be treated with a course of oral antibiotics, such as amoxicillin.

LABIAL ADHESIONS

Introduction

Agglutination (adhesion) of the labia minora is most common between 3 months and 3 years of age and occurs in response to vulvar irritation and low estrogen levels in this age group. The mucosal surfaces of the labia minora become inflamed and raw from irritation and then adhere together in the midline.

Presentation

For many girls, labial adhesions are asymptomatic and are discovered incidentally during the course of a routine "well child" examination. Symptomatic presentations include; genital discomfort, abnormal urine stream, post void dribbling, and in rare cases, urinary tract infections.

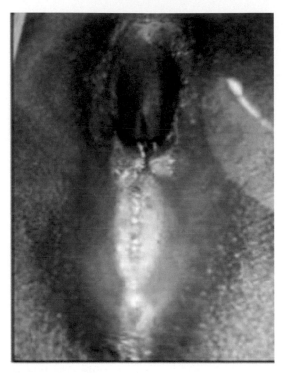

Figure 25.2 Labial adhesion. (Al Jurayyan NAM (2012) Labial agglutination (adhesion) in pre-pubertal girls. What a primary care physician should know? *Primary Health Care* 2:128. doi:10.4172/2167-1079.1000128.)

When gentle lateral traction is applied to the labia majora, a midline area of clear or grey fibrotic tissue is seen covering the vaginal opening. Labial adhesions cause varying degrees of occlusion of the introitus and in severe cases only a pinpoint residual opening may be present (Figure 25.2).

Investigations

Labial adhesions are diagnosed on the basis of the clinical history and examination of the external genitalia.

Treatment

- Nothing
- Topical estrogen
- Topical steroids
- Rarely, surgery

Expectant management is reasonable in patients who are asymptomatic. When the adhesions are extensive or causing symptoms, medical management is indicated. First line treatment consists of the application of a topical estrogen twice daily for 2 weeks. Caregivers should be advised to apply a small (pea-sized) amount of cream to the adhesion using a digit or Q tip. Generally, topical estrogen is well tolerated with minimal systemic effects due to absorption of estrogen. Side effects with prolonged use include vulvar hyperpigmentation or breast budding. An alternative to topical estrogen is a topical steroid, such as betamethasone 0.05% ointment applied twice daily for 4–6 weeks. Division of adhesions can be performed after application of local anesthetic cream in clinic. Manual separation or sharp dissection in the operating room is only indicated for symptomatic cases which are refractory to medical management.

Prognosis

Adhesions may resolve spontaneously and almost always separate during puberty with onset of endogenous estrogen production. Medical management with topical estrogen is effective in 90% of cases, though recurrence is quite common. To prevent recurrence, non-medicated barrier cream and vulvar hygiene is recommended.

LABIAL HYPERTROPHY

Introduction

Labial hypertrophy is poorly defined. Although variability in the appearance of external genitalia is expected, few studies have attempted to define the normal size of labia minora. The width, or protrusion, of the labia minora in adolescent females can range from a few millimeters to several centimeters. In general, a width of greater than 5–6 cm is considered hypertrophied.

Presentation

Enlargement of the labia minora can be unilateral or bilateral. Patients may be asymptomatic and present primarily because of dissatisfaction with the appearance of their genitalia. Functional symptoms also occur and may include irritation, discomfort or pulling with movement, interference with intercourse, and difficulty with menstrual hygiene.

Investigations

The width of the labia minora is measured from the vestibule to the distal/free end of the labia minora with and without stretch (Figure 25.3).

Treatment

Clinicians should first and foremost educate and reassure patients and parents about the normal variation in the appearances of the female genitalia. The use of online resources such as *The Labia Library* (www.labialibrary.org.au) and *Great Wall of Vagina* (www.greatwallofvagina.co.uk) can be helpful in demonstrating the differences in normal anatomy. Measures to alleviate discomfort should be discussed – including supportive undergarments, avoidance of irritants, use of a barrier cream for minor irritation, and arranging or tucking the labia prior to physical activity. In the United States and many European countries female genital surgery in children is legally prohibited unless there are valid medical indications.

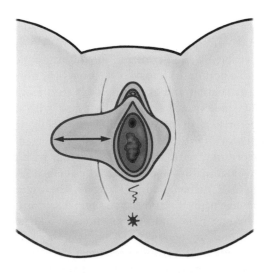

Figure 25.3 Measurement of labial hypertrophy.

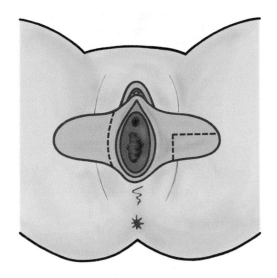

Figure 25.4 Labiaplasty incisions.

Surgical intervention (labiaplasty) should therefore not be performed for cosmetic reasons in patients under 18 years of age. Labiaplasty should only be considered for patients with labial enlargement which is outside the typical range and whose functional symptoms are not relieved with supportive measures. There are several surgical techniques for labiaplasty, of which wedge resection and free edge amputation are the most commonly performed (Figure 25.4). The surgical risks associated with labiaplasty are pain, bleeding, hematoma, infection, would dehiscence, need for reoperation, and dissatisfaction with appearance.

HYMENAL AND VAGINAL ANOMALIES

Introduction

Hymenal and vaginal anomalies are congenital abnormalities of the lower genital tract and can be obstructing or non-obstructing (see Table 25.3).

Hymenal Anomalies

During adolescence, an imperforate hymen typically presents with primary amenorrhea

Table 25.3 Hymenal and vaginal anomalies

Obstructing	Non-obstructing
Hymenal	Hymenal
Imperforate hymen	Septate hymen
Vaginal	Microperforate hymen
Obstructed hemi-vagina	Cribiform hymen
Transverse vaginal septum	Vaginal
Distal or partial vaginal agenesis	Perforated transverse vaginal septum
	Longitudinal vaginal septum
	Mayer Rokitansky Kuster Hauser (MRKH) Syndrome

and cyclic abdominal pain. If significant hematometrocolpos is present, patients may have an abdominal mass and a bulging hymen at the perineum. Patients with partially occlusive hymenal anomalies (septate, cribiform, or microperforate hymen) have normal menstruation but may have difficulty using tampons for menstrual hygiene. The most common hymenal anomaly is a septate hymen (Figure 25.5). Girls with this anomaly may specifically report difficulty removing a tampon, which remains stuck behind a hymenal band. Hymenal anomalies diagnosed in childhood on routine examination

do not require intervention and surgery should be deferred to adolescence. Surgical management consists of hymenectomy in which the obstructing hymenal tissue is excised and the cut edges reapproximated with interrupted absorbable sutures such as 4–0 Vicryl. The risk of genital scarring and recurrent obstruction is minimal after hymenectomy, and therefore, post-operative dilation is not required.

Transverse Vaginal Septum

Transverse vaginal septa are rare anomalies that result from failed fusion of the vaginal plate and Müllerian ducts. A transverse vaginal septum can be located anywhere in the vagina, with or without a perforation. A complete transverse vaginal septum presents in a similar fashion to an imperforate hymen with primary amenorrhea and worsening pelvic pain in early adolescence. However, no bulging hymen or vagina is visible on the perineum. In contrast, patients with a perforated transverse septum have normal menstruation and are more likely to present in later adolescence or early adulthood with dysmenorrhea, dyspareunia, difficulty using tampons or infertility. It is especially important to determine the thickness of the septum with pelvic examination and magnetic resonance imaging (MRI) when planning surgery. The goals for management of a transverse vaginal septum are to relieve pain and other symptoms associated with obstruction and to restore anatomy so that the vagina will permit normal menstruation and sexual intercourse. The management options consist of either primary resection of the septum

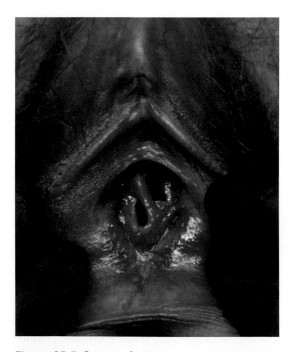

Figure 25.5 Septate hymen.

or, alternatively, menstrual suppression (with or without drainage of hematometrocolpos) followed by delayed septum resection. If drainage is required to relieve pain this should be performed percutaneously because of the high risk of infection with a vaginal drain. Surgical management consists of resection of the entire vaginal septum, with re-approximation of the vaginal mucosa with interrupted stitches. Mobilization of the upper vagina may be required if there is a thick septum or partial vaginal agenesis and on rare occasions the use of a graft material may also be also be necessary. Post-operative dilation is recommended after treatment of a transverse vaginal septum because of the higher risks of stenosis and recurrent obstruction. For this reason, the age and maturity of the patient should be considered before definitive surgical management.

Obstructed Hemi Vagina

A didelphys uterus can be associated with obstructed hemi-vagina and ipsilateral renal anomalies (OHVIRA). Because only half the vagina is obstructed, patients will typically present with normal menarche, but worsening dysmenorrhea. On examination a lateral bulge is palpated in the vagina. Pelvic imaging with MRI confirms the diagnosis. Definitive treatment consists of surgical resection of the obstructing septum. Stenosis and re-obstruction is unlikely unless the septum is high or incompletely excised. In these cases, a hemi-hysterectomy may be indicated.

Longitudinal Vaginal Septum

A longitudinal vaginal septum is a non-obstructing anomaly of the vagina which results from failed fusion of the distal Müllerian ducts. This vaginal anomaly is typically associated with didelphys or septate uterus. Patients may present with inability to use tampons, leaking of menstrual blood despite the use of tampons, dyspareunia, and post coital hemorrhage. On examination, a septum is identified which divides the vagina into two halves (Figure 25.6). The length of the septum may be partially or completely

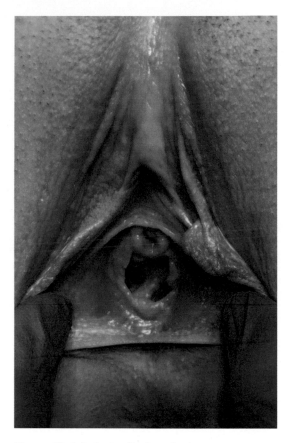

Figure 25.6 Longitudinal vaginal septum.

dividing the vagina. Septum resection should be offered to patients who are symptomatic.

Mayer Rokitansky Kuster Hauser (MRKH) Syndrome

Müllerian agenesis (MRKH) occurs in approximately 1 in 4,500 female births and results from the failure of normal development of the Müllerian ducts. Girls with MRKH have normal pubertal development and usually present with primary amenorrhea. Most girls with MRKH do not experience associated pain, though cyclic pain can occur during ovulation or as a result of an obstructed uterine remnant or endometriosis. On examination, the external genitalia including the hymen are normal but the vagina is underdeveloped. The diagnosis is confirmed with pelvic imaging (usually MRI) in combination with chromosomal analysis and/or measurement of plasma testosterone to rule out complete androgen insensitivity syndrome (CAIS). Associated renal and skeletal anomalies are common and can be screened for with a renal ultrasound scan and spinal X-ray. The loss of fertility is particularly challenging for young patients with MRKH and emotional support is perhaps the most important aspect of their care. All patients should be put in contact with support groups and offered counseling. Surgery to create a neo vagina should only be considered when this is desired by the patient. The first line treatment of vaginal agenesis consists of vaginal dilation – which is successful in up to 90% of those patients who are motivated and committed to achieving a successful outcome. Patients are provided with a set of serial vaginal dilators (Figure 25.7) and instructed to insert the dilator into the vagina and apply pressure to it for 20–30 minutes once to twice daily. The successful creation of a functional vagina usually requires dilation over 6–12 months. Coital dilation can augment the use of serial dilators. Surgical vaginoplasty can be considered in patients in whom vaginal dilation is unsuccessful. A range of different procedures have been described. The Vecchietti procedure is a laparoscopically assisted vaginal dilation. Alternatively, a neo-vagina can be created with bowel, buccal mucosa, skin, or peritoneum.

OVARIAN MASSES

Simple Ovarian Cysts

Unilocular and anechoic ovarian cysts are almost always benign. They can represent a functional ovarian cyst, serous cystadenoma, mucinous cystadenoma, or para tubal cyst. Simple ovarian cysts may be asymptomatic or may present with symptoms such as acute or chronic pelvic pain, increasing abdominal girth, nausea and vomiting. Surgical management, consisting of ovarian cystectomy is indicated for symptomatic cysts and for those which are persistent and enlarging beyond 4–6 cm in diameter. Asymptomatic cysts which are less than 10 cm in diameter can safely be observed and followed with serial pelvic ultrasound scans.

Complex Ovarian Masses

A complex mass with both solid and cystic components may represent a hemorrhagic functional cyst, a benign neoplasm such as a mucinous cystadenoma or mature teratoma, a borderline tumor or, rarely a malignant tumor. Complex masses that do not have classic features of a mature teratoma should be evaluated by measurement of tumor makers which are often elevated in the most common ovarian malignancies occurring in adolescence (see Table 25.4).

Table 25.4 Evaluation of complex ovarian masses

Tumor type	Tumor markers
Germ cell tumors	Alpha-fetoprotein (AFP)
	Lactate dehydrogenase (LDH)
	Human chorionic gonadotropin (HCG)
Sex cord tumors	Inhibin A&B
	Estradiol
	Testosterone
Epithelial tumors	Cancer antigen 125

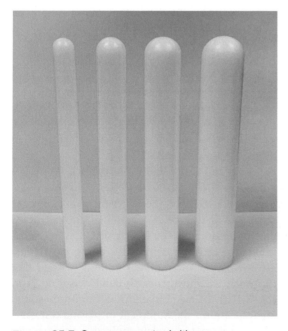

Figure 25.7 Syracuse vaginal dilators.

Functional Ovarian Cysts

These cysts arise during normal and abnormal ovulation. A follicular cyst is a simple thin walled cyst which either develops prior to ovulation or persists and enlarges following failed ovulation. Typically these cysts are 2–3 cm in size, though they can increase in size when due to failed ovulation. A corpus luteum cyst develops after ovulation and has more complex appearances on ultrasound with internal echoes related to hemorrhage. Functional ovarian cysts can be asymptomatic and found incidentally on imaging. Alternatively, they may present with acute pelvic pain secondary to cyst rupture or hemorrhage. Functional ovarian cysts resolve spontaneously within 2–8 weeks and do not require surgical intervention. Hormonal contraception to suppress ovulation can be used to prevent recurrence of physiologic ovarian cysts.

Endometrioma

Endometriomas are rare benign cysts that result from ectopic growth of endometrial tissue within the ovary in adolescents. They may present with an enlarging mass, dysmenorrhea, or generalized pelvic pain. On ultrasound they appear as complex cystic lesions with homongenous low level echoes and may be unilocular or multilocular. Endometriomas do not resolve with hormonal management and should be removed laparoscopically if they are symptomatic or if the cyst is greater than 5 cm.

Mature Teratoma (Dermoid Cysts)

Benign dermoid cysts are the most common germ cell tumor occurring in this age group and are bilateral in in 10–15% of cases. Patients with dermoid cysts may be asymptomatic or may present with an enlarging mass, pelvic pain, or ovarian torsion. The cysts are composed of mature tissue elements and have characteristic appearances on ultrasound due to the presence of sebaceous fluid, hair, and calcifications (see Figure 25.8). Surgical intervention, preferably ovarian cystectomy, is indicated for large and/or symptomatic dermoid cysts. If cyst contents are spilled intraoperatively the abdominal cavity and pelvis should be copiously irrigated to prevent chemical peritonitis.

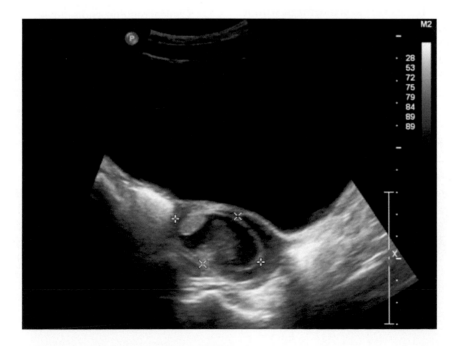

Figure 25.8 Ultrasound appearance of dermoid cyst.

Ovarian and Fallopian Tube Torsion

Adnexal torsion is a surgical emergency. Patients with torsion typically present with an acute onset of pelvic pain, nausea, and vomiting. On examination, the abdomen is markedly tender and there may be rebound and guarding. The diagnosis of torsion should be suspected on the basis of the clinical history and examination findings. Ultrasound is not a reliable investigation for confirming or excluding the diagnosis of ovarian torsion, though it might show enlarged adnexa, peripheral ovarian cysts with centralized edema, "whirlpool" sign, or absence of arterial blood flow on Doppler. However, the presence of arterial blood flow does not rule out ovarian torsion. Regardless of the ultrasound findings the clinician should therefore have a "low threshold" for proceeding to diagnostic laparoscopy if the clinical history and examination findings are suggestive of ovarian torsion. Because the intraoperative appearance of the adnexa is not a reliable predictor of irreversible ischemic damage, ovarian preservation is the recommended management of acute ovarian torsion. The surgical approach consists of detorsion (untwisting the adnexa) followed by cystectomy if a mass or cyst is easily identified. If the ovary is hemorrhagic without any identifiable lesion, detorsion with or without drainage should be performed followed by a postoperative ultrasound at 4–6 weeks to assess for an occult ovarian cyst. Oophorpexy is only indicated for cases of recurrent ovarian torsion.

KEY POINTS

- Vulvar complaints in pre pubertal girls are evaluated with history and physical examination only.
- Labiaplasty in adolescents <18 years of age should only be offered to those with significant labial enlargement or those whose symptoms are not relieved by supportive care.
- Obstructive vaginal anomalies typically present during adolescence with primary amenorrhea and pelvic pain. The management options include; menstrual suppression, percutaneous drainage, resection of the septum or vaginoplasty.
- Mayer Rokitansky Kuster Hauser Syndrome (MRKH) is characterized by agenesis of the uterus and upper vagina. Patients should be offered emotional support and counseling regarding fertility options. Vaginal dilation is the first line method to create a vagina.
- Ovarian preservation is recommended in the management of ovarian torsion and for ovarian cysts which appear to be benign.

FURTHER READING

1. Bacon JL, Romano ME, Quint EH. Clinical recommendation: labial adhesions. J Pediatr Adolesc Gynecol. 2015;28(5):405–409.
2. Zuckerman A, Romano M. Clinical recommendation: vulvovaginitis. J Pediatr Adolesc Gynecol. 2016;29(6):673–679.
3. Breech LL, Laufer MR. Obstructive anomalies of the female reproductive tract. J Reprod Med. 1999;44(3):233–240.
4. Dietrich JE, Millar DM, Quint EH. Non-obstructive Müllerian anomalies. J Pediatr Adolesc Gynecol. 2014;27(6):386–395.
5. Bercaw-Pratt JL, Boardman LA, Simms-Cendan JS. Clinical recommendation: pediatric lichen sclerosus. J Pediatr Adolesc Gynecol. 2014;27(2):111–116.

Appendix I

Self-Assessment Section: Questions

This section is intended to provide readers with an opportunity to test their understanding of the content of individual chapters by answering a series of multiple choice questions (MCQs).

- **All questions have been set using the 'single best answer' or 'single correct answer' format.**
  - Five answers are provided after each question – of which only one answer is correct. There is no negative marking for incorrect answers.
- **All the information needed for the reader to answer the MCQs correctly is provided within the relevant chapter.**
  - Where percentages are quoted (for example, to incidence, complication rates, etc.), the 'correct' answer is the figure quoted in the chapter. It is recognised that there is sometimes considerable variation in quoted incidences of different conditions in the published literature. However, the authors have, as far as possible, cited figures for incidence, complication rates, etc., which are evidence-based and derived from a range of sources.

CHAPTER 1: EMBRYOLOGY

1 **Which of the following mechanisms is primarily responsible for initiating early development of the kidney?**

   a) Differentiation of the pronephros
   b) Interaction between the mesonephric ducts and metanephros
   c) Interaction between the ureteric bud and the mesonephros
   d) Interaction between the paramesonephric ducts and metanephros
   e) Interaction between the ureteric bud and metanephros

2 **Which of the following is a recognised function of anti-Müllerian hormone (Müllerian Inhibitory Substance)?**

   a) Causes regression of the mesonephric ducts
   b) Causes regression of the paramesonephric ducts
   c) Converts testosterone to dihydrotestosterone
   d) Stimulates the second phase of testicular descent
   e) None of the above

3 **Which of the following statements does *not* apply to the paramesonephric ducts?**

a) They are present from the 6th week of gestation

b) They give rise to the fallopian tubes, uterus and upper vagina

c) They regress in response to exposure to fetal MIS

d) Their development is dependent upon exposure to fetal oestrogens

e) They may persist in some individuals with a 46XY karyotype

4 **Which of the following common conditions have been shown to be linked to single gene mutations?**

a) Adult polycystic kidney disease

b) Vesico ureteric reflux

c) Hypospadias

d) Ureteric duplication

e) All of the above

5 **Klinefelter's syndrome is most commonly associated with which of the following karyotypes?**

a) 46XY

b) 47XYY

c) 45Y

d) 47XXY

e) 45X

CHAPTER 2: RENAL DEVELOPMENT AND DYSFUNCTION

1 **Which of the following patterns of physiological disturbance is most commonly encountered in neonates?**

a) Metabolic alkalosis

b) Respiratory alkalosis

c) Compensatory hypernatraemia

d) Hypervolaemic hyponatraemia

e) Compensatory hypokalaemia

2 **Which of the following statements is most applicable to chronic kidney disease – mineral and bone disorder (renal osteodystrophy)?**

a) It is caused by primary hyperprathyroidism

b) It results in increased bone deposition

c) It is a response to abnormally elevated levels of calcitriol (vitamin D3)

d) It is not associated with radiological abnormalities in children

e) Cinacalcet can be used for treatment of severe cases

3 **Which of the following statements best describes the use of Erythropoietin in children with chronic renal failure or end-stage renal disease?**

a) It is usually administered orally

b) It can be administered subcutaneously

c) The dosage is increased until a target haemoglobin of 15.5g/dl is achieved

d) It is unsafe for use in children on dialysis

e) Erythropoietin avoids the need for iron supplements

4 **Which of the following is most applicable to renal replacement therapy in children and young people?**

a) It is routinely required in cases of Stage 4 CKD

b) The use of home haemodialysis has been largely discontinued because of the high incidence of complications

c) Continuous ambulatory peritoneal dialysis is the most widely used form of peritoneal dialysis in children

d) Immunization with live vaccines is contraindicated following renal transplantation

e) Peritoneal dialysis is more effective than haemodialysis for removing fluid in patients with pulmonary edema

5 **A young child has a GFR of 40 mL/min/ 1.73 m². What is the probability that they will require renal replacement therapy by the age of 20 years of age?**

a) <5%
b) 15%
c) 55%
d) 70%
e) >90%

CHAPTER 3: IMAGING

1 **Which of the following statements best describes indirect isotope cystography in children?**

a) No oral fluids should be given to the child for 4 hours preceding the study
b) The agent used is intravenous Tc^{99m} dimercapto-succinic acid
c) The agent used is intravenous Tc^{99m} mercapto-acetyltriglycine
d) It is more sensitive than MCUG for the detection of Grades I and II VUR
e) It is suitable for the investigation of VUR in children of all ages

2 **On initial postnatal ultrasound which of the following measurements of renal pelvic antero posterior diameter is regarded as an abnormal finding?**

a) Any degree of renal pelvic dilatation
b) Renal pelvic AP diameter 5 mm
c) Renal pelvic AP diameter 7 mm
d) Renal pelvic AP diameter >10 mm
e) None of the above

3 **Which of the following statements best describes the use of ultrasonography in the evaluation of the urinary tract in children?**

a) Anatomical resolution is generally better in children than adults
b) Contrast-enhanced ultrasound (CEUS) is a simple technique which can be reliably performed with basic equipment
c) Ultrasound is a sensitive modality for visualising non dilated ureters
d) Ultrasound is a sensitive modality for visualising mid ureteric calculi
e) A significant post void residual volume is defined as one exceeding 25% of normal age-adjusted bladder capacity

4 **Which of the following statements most accurately describes the role of MRI in for urological investigation in children?**

a) MRI is not suitable for use with contrast media
b) T2-weighted images provide better anatomical detail than T1–weighted images
c) Modern MRI scanners no longer require sedation or anaesthesia in infants or young children
d) MRI has largely replaced CT for the urgent assessment of acute abdominal trauma
e) MRI can be used to visualise tumour vasculature and 'crossing vessels' associated with PUJ obstruction

5 **Which of the following statements most accurately describes the role of CT in urological investigation in children?**

a) Scan times are typically 30–40 minutes
b) Evaluation of major trauma is now the main indication in children
c) With modern scanners the radiation dose is lower than a chest X ray
d) CT generates multiplanar images
e) It is better than MRI for the assessment of malignant tumours

CHAPTER 4: PRENATAL DIAGNOSIS

1 **Which statement best applies to Grade 1 hydronephrosis (as classified by the Society for Fetal Urology)?**

a) It is a common finding, which is present in 1 in 30 pregnancies
b) This finding demands further investigation with a MAG3 renogram in the first 3 months of life
c) It Is defined as dilatation of the renal pelvis and major calyces
d) It is defined as dilatation confined to the renal pelvis
e) This finding routinely requires further investigation with a VCUG

2 **Which of the following antenatal ultrasound findings would *not* routinely require further investigation with a VCUG?**

a) Duplex kidney with upper and lower pole hydronephrosis
b) Thick walled bladder
c) Unilateral pelvi calyceal dilatation (AP diameter renal pelvis 15 mm) without ureteral dilatation
d) Bilateral hydronephrosis in a male infant
e) Unilateral pelvi calyceal dilatation AP diameter renal pelvis 25 mm with ureteral dilatation

3 **At 24 weeks gestation a male fetus is found to have dilatation of the left renal pelvis and calyces (AP diameter renal pelvis of 16 mm), the right kidney is normal. Which of the following would be the most appropriate advice to the parents regarding management at this stage in the pregnancy?**

a) Vesico amniotic shunt procedure
b) Ultrasound guided nephrostomy to decompress the left kidney
c) Fetoscopic pyeloplasty
d) No intervention, re scan during the third trimester
e) Elective pre term delivery at 34 to 36 weeks followed by urgent neonatal pyeloplasty

4 **Which of the following would *not* be regarded as a predictor of poor outcome for renal function in a fetus with outflow obstruction?**

a) Fetal urine sodium <100 mEq/L
b) Recent onset oligohydramnios
c) Echogenic kidneys on ultrasound
d) Fetal urinary osmolality >300 mOsm/L
e) Fetal urinary β_2-microglobulin >20 mg/L

5 **Which of the following are *not* indications for a radionuclide scan (MAG3 or DMSA) in the first 6–8 weeks of life?**

a) Grade III–IV hydronephrosis in the SFU classification
b) Poorly functioning kidney prior to nephrectomy
c) Crossed renal ectopia
d) Grade I hydronephrosis in the SFU classification
e) Ureterovesical obstruction (megaureter) prior to surgery

CHAPTER 5: URINARY TRACT INFECTION

1 A 7-year-old girl is admitted acutely with a temperature of 39.5°C and left loin pain. What is the most appropriate method of collecting urine to confirm the presumed diagnosis of pyelonephritis?

 a) Suprapubic puncture
 b) Clean catch mid-stream specimen
 c) Catheter urine specimen
 d) Adhesive collection bag applied to the genitalia
 e) Percutaneous renal aspiration

2 Which of the following is *not* regarded as an indication to proceed to some form of diagnostic imaging. ?

 a) Family history of vesico ureteric reflux
 b) Palpable bladder
 c) Proteinuria (+) on reagent stick testing)
 d) Infection with an organism other than *E. coli*
 e) Elevated plasma creatinine

3 A 4-year-old girl presents with symptoms of dysuria, urgency and 'smelly' urine but is otherwise well. A urine dipstick test is negative for leucocyte esterase negative but positive for nitrite. What is the most appropriate course of action?

 a) Send urine sample for microscopy and culture but await result before commencing antibiotics
 b) Commence antibiotic treatment. It is not necessary to send urine for microscopy and culture
 c) Do not commence antibiotics and do not send urine for microscopy and culture
 d) Advise increased oral fluid intake and repeat dipstick test in 48 hours
 e) Commence antibiotic and send urine for culture

4 Which of the following is regarded as diagnostic of infection in a clean catch midstream specimen of urine?

 a) Pure growth of >10^7 bacterial colony forming units (CFU) per ml
 b) Mixed growth of >10^7 bacterial colony forming units (CFU) per ml
 c) Pure growth of >10^2 bacterial colony forming units (CFU) per ml if pyuria is also present
 d) Pure growth of >10^4 bacterial colony forming units (CFU) per ml if nitrites positive on dipstick
 e) Pure growth of >10^5 bacterial colony forming units (CFU) per ml

5 A 6-month-old male infant has made a full recovery following a non-specific febrile illness which proved to be a urinary infection. Ultrasound demonstrates bilateral upper tract dilatation (collecting systems and ureters). Which of the following is the most appropriate next investigation?

 a) Intravenous urogram (IVU)
 b) Micturating cystourethrogram (MCUG)
 c) Indirect MAG3 isotope cystogram
 d) Direct MAG3 isotope cystogram
 e) MRI

CHAPTER 6: VESICOURETERAL REFLUX

1 The injectable implant material deflux consists of which of the following materials?

 a) Dextranomer/hyaluronic acid copolymer
 b) Polytetrafluoroethylene (PTFE)
 c) Polydimethylsiloxan (PDMS)
 d) Deactivated bovine collagen
 e) Deactivated bovine collagen/hyaluronic acid copolymer

2 **Which of the following statements best describes the familial basis of vesico ureteral reflux?**

   a) VUR can be demonstrated in approximately 55% % of siblings of children with known VUR
   b) VUR can be demonstrated in approximately 30% of siblings of children with known VUR
   c) VUR can be demonstrated in 10% to 20% of the offspring of parents with known VUR
   d) 40–45% of children with non syndromic VUR have an associated mutation of the PAX2 gene
   e) None of the above

3 **Which of the statements best describes the optimal diagnostic pathway for the diagnosis and assessment of VUR?**

   a) Radionuclide cystography is the 'gold standard' investigation in small infants
   b) The same diagnostic protocol should be used for children with febrile UTIs as those with afebrile UTIs
   c) A contrast-enhanced ultrasound scan (CEUS) is the most sensitive test for demonstrating renal scarring
   d) A Technetium-99m DMSA radionuclide scan is the most sensitive test for demonstrating renal scarring
   e) Sibling screening has been shown to reduce the incidence of end-stage renal disease in siblings by 35%

4 **Which of the following statements best describes the Cohen technique of ureteric reimplantation?**

   a) It is an extravesical procedure
   b) The overall success rate for the complete correction of VUR exceeds 90%
   c) It is the operation of choice when reimplanting grossly dilated mega ureters
   d) When re implanting the refluxing lower pole ureter of a duplex kidney the ureter should first be completely mobilized from the upper pole ureter
   e) All of the above

5 **Which of the following statements most accurately describes the etiology of reflux nephropathy?**

   a) Focal scarring seen on a DMSA scan is more likely to be due to congenital renal dysplasia than pyelonephritis
   b) Ongoing reflux of sterile urine results in progressive renal damage
   c) Pyelonephritis can only occur when VUR is present
   d) Reflux nephropathy accounts for >50% of children on end-stage renal failure programs
   e) Children under 4 years of age are at greater risk of pyelonephritic scarring

CHAPTER 7: UPPER TRACT OBSTRUCTION

1 **Unilateral upper tract dilatation has been detected antenatally in a male infant. Postnatal imaging is as follows; *Ultrasound* ureteric dilatation (diameter 1.1 cm) and pelvi calyceal dilatation with a renal pelvic AP diameter of 1.3 cm. *MAG3* at 6 weeks – ipsilateral differential function 49%, minimal washout with diuretic (type 3 B curve). *MCUG* – no reflux, normal bladder and urethra. Which of the following would be the most appropriate management in this case?**

   a) Cutaneous ureterostomy
   b) Leadbetter Politano ureteric reimplantation
   c) Cohen ureteric reimplantation
   d) Percutaneous nephrostomy
   e) Antibiotic prophylaxis, follow-up ultrasound at 3–6 months

2 **Which of the following statements best describes pyeloplasty in children?**

a) The Anderson-Hynes pyeloplasty has been superseded by newer techniques
b) The overall long-term success rate of Anderson-Hynes pyeloplasty is greater than 95%
c) Randomised controlled studies have consistently shown a statistically significant reduction in post operative complications with the use of JJ stents
d) The lumbotomy incision offers greater flexibility to deal with unexpected operative findings
e) Redo pyeloplasty has a failure rate of 50–60%

3 **A 6-year-old girl is referred following an episode of left abdominal/loin pain which has now resolved. Ultrasound demonstrates moderate dilatation of the pelvis (AP diameter 30 mm) and calyces. Which of the following would be the most appropriate next investigation?**

a) Intravenous urogram
b) 99^{m}Tc MAG3 isotope renogram
c) Micturating cystourethrogram
d) CT scan
e) Antegrade pyelogram

4 **Which of the following statements best describes the aetiology of pelvi ureteric junction obstruction?**

a) It has a familial basis in 30–35% of cases
b) It is inherited as an autosomal recessive condition in 10–15% of cases
c) Aberrant 'crossing vessels' are present in 30–35% of infants with prenatally detected PUJ obstruction
d) It occurs more commonly in boys than girls by a ratio of 3–1
e) It affects the left kidney more commonly than the right by a ratio of 2–1

5 **Which of the following statements apply to obstructed mega ureter?**

a) Obstruction can always be reliably diagnosed from drainage curve data on a MAG3 scan
b) A MCUG should always be performed in the work up to exclude vesico ureteric reflux as the cause of the dilatation
c) Surgical intervention is mandatory in cases where the diameter of the ureter exceeds 10mm
d) A period of external cutaneous ureterostomy drainage is required in 25% of infants with prenatally detected mega ureter
e) The occurrence of an afebrile urinary tract infection should be routinely regarded as an indication for surgery

CHAPTER 8: DUPLICATION ANOMALIES, URETEROCELES AND ECTOPIC URETERS

1 **According to the Meyer-Weigart Law,**

a) The ureter draining the upper renal moiety always enters the urinary tract below the bladder neck in females
b) The ureter draining the upper renal moiety always joins the ejaculatory ducts in males
c) The upper and lower pole ureters may both drain into the bladder
d) The ureter draining the lower pole enters the urinary tract in a more caudal position than the ureter draining the upper renal pole
e) The ureter draining the lower renal pole drains ectopically into the vagina in 10–15% of cases

2 **During investigation of urinary tract infection a 4-year-old boy is found to have a unilateral right-sided single system (orthotopic) ureterocele. A MAG3 study demonstrates obstruction with 32% differential function in the affected kidney. Which of the following would be the most appropriate management in this case?**

a) Endoscopic incision
b) Heminephroureterectomy
c) Vesicostomy
d) Trans uretero ureterostomy
e) Pyelopyelostomy

3 **What is the overall incidence of upper tract duplication in the general population (as determined by autopsy and radiological data)?**

a) 0.05% to 0.1%
b) 0.5% to 1%
c) 1% to 3%
d) 2.5% to 5%
e) 5% to 10%

4 **A 7-year-old girl is referred with diurnal enuresis. Although the history is suggestive a duplex kidney with an ectopic ureter the ultrasound findings are reported to be normal. Which of the following investigations would probably be the most helpful in pursuing the presumed diagnosis further?**

a) IVU
b) MRI
c) 99ᵐTc MAG3 scan
d) Cystoscopy and retrograde ureterogram
e) Careful examination of the perineum under anaesthesia

5 **Which of the following statements best describes the occurrence and management of vesico ureteric reflux (VUR) in duplex systems?**

a) VUR typically affects the lower pole ureter in cases of complete duplication
b) VUR typically affects the upper pole ureter in cases of complete duplication
c) VUR in duplex systems is more likely to resolve spontaneously than VUR in single systems
d) Lower pole VUR should never be managed by ureteric reimplantation
e) Severe loss of function in the lower pole is due to pyelonephritis in > 80% of cases

CHAPTER 9: POSTERIOR URETHRAL VALVES AND OTHER URETHRAL ABNORMALITIES

1 **Which of the following is *not* a recognised predictor of long-term renal impairment?**

a) Maternal oligohydramnios
b) Proteinuria
c) Clinical presentation after 7 years of age
d) Bilateral vesico ureteric reflux
e) Impaired daytime urinary continence after the age of 5 years

2 **A 3.5 kg term infant is born with an antenatal diagnosis of posterior urethral valves which is confirmed postnatally on MCUG. His plasma creatinine on the second day of life is 46 μmol/L Which of the following would be the most appropriate form of intervention at this stage?**

a) Vesicostomy
b) Endoscopic valve ablation
c) Bilateral nephrostomies
d) Bilateral loop ureterostomies
e) Bilateral end ureterostomies

3 **Which of the following statements best applies to refluxing ureterostomy?**

a) Promotes better drainage from the ipsilateral kidney
b) Protects both kidneys from elevated intravesical pressure
c) Maintains bladder filling and emptying (cycling)
d) Is usually closed at 2–3 years of age
e) All of the above

4 **Which of the following statements best describes the current status of vesico amniotic shunting for fetuses with prenatally detected posterior urethral valves?**

a) The long-term benefits of shunting have been confirmed by the United Kingdom's PLUTO trial
b) It is performed percutaneously under ultrasound guidance
c) It should be performed routinely if bilateral upper tract dilatation is present in a male fetus at 20 weeks gestation
d) Shunting may increase the severity of pulmonary hypoplasia
e) The long-term results of intra uterine valve ablation are superior to vesico amniotic shunting

5 **An 11-year-old boy is referred with a 4-month history of dysuria and occasional spotting of blood from the urethral meatus. Which of the following is the most likely diagnosis?**

a) Cobbs collar
b) Posterior urethral polyp
c) Urethral calculus
d) Urethritis
e) Rhabdomyosarcoma involving the posterior urethra

CHAPTER 10: CYSTIC RENAL DISEASE

1 **Which of the following statements best describes the features of autosomal recessive polycystic kidney disease?**

a) The kidneys typically appear small and cystic on antenatal ultrasound
b) The disorder typically presents with hypertension, abdominal pain, abdominal mass, etc., in late childhood or adult life
c) Mutations of the PK2 gene are present in 85 to 90% of cases
d) This form of polycystic disease may be associated with maternal oligohydramnios
e) Percutaneous cyst drainage reduces the incidence of pain and infection

2 **Which of the following statements most accurately describes the inheritance of multicystic dysplastic kidney (MCDK)?**

a) MCDK is most commonly inherited as an autosomal recessive disorder
b) MCDK is most commonly inherited as an X-linked recessive disorder
c) MCDK is most commonly inherited as an autosomal dominant disorder
d) MCDK is most commonly a sporadic anomaly
e) MCDK is associated with mutation of the PK1 gene on chromosome 16 in 65–70% of cases

3 **Approximately what percentage of adults on end-stage renal replacement programmes has autosomal dominant polycystic kidney disease?**

a) 5%
b) 10%
c) 35%
d) 40%
e) 55%

4 **A female infant has an antenatally detected unilateral MCDK. Her contralateral kidney is normal and she is otherwise healthy. What is her approximate risk of developing a Wilms tumour in the MCDK?**

a) Less than 0.1%
b) 0.5% to 1%
c) 1% to 1.5%
d) 1.5% to 2%
e) Greater than 2%

5 **A postnatal ultrasound in a newborn infant reveals findings consistent with a diagnosis of unilateral multicystic dysplastic kidney. Which of the following would be the most appropriate next investigation?**

a) 99^mTC DMSA scan
b) IVU
c) Measurement of glomerular filtration rate (GFR)
d) CT scan
e) MRI

CHAPTER 11: URINARY TRACT CALCULI

1 **A 9-year-old boy presents with a 1.1 cm stone in the distal left ureter. There is moderate dilatation of the ureter and collecting systems on ultrasound. He is pain free but the appearances on further imaging after 2 weeks are unchanged. Which of the following is now the optimal management of this young patient?**

a) External shockwave lithotripsy (ESWL)
b) Conservative – re-assess with further imaging after 12 months
c) Open ureterolithotomy
d) Basket extraction
e) Ureteroscopy and laser lithotripsy

2 **Which of the following statements best describes the role of percutaneous nephro lithotomy (PCNL) in children?**

a) PCNL is unsuitable for the treatment of staghorn calculi
b) PCNL can be performed under sedation in older children
c) Stones are most commonly disintegrated with an ultrasound probe
d) Stones are most commonly extracted intact from the kidney using a modified stone basket
e) None of the above

3 **A 10-year-old girl is referred with a provisional diagnosis of xanthogranulomatous pyelonephritis? Which of the following features of her presentation and investigation is *not* consistent with this diagnosis?**

a) Differential function 20% on DMSA scan
b) Elevated inflammatory markers
c) Haemoglobin 8.5 g/dl
d) Palpable mass
e) Presence of calculi on CT scan

4 **Which of the following is the most common cause of metabolic stones in children?**

a) Hyperoxaluria
b) Cystinosis
c) Hypercalciuria
d) Uric acidaemia
e) Xanthine oxidase deficiency

5 **A 2-year-old boy presents with haematuria. An ultrasound scan on admission demonstrates a 'staghorn' calculus in the left kidney. Urine culture is positive. Which of the following is most likely to be the infecting organism in this case?**

a) *E. coli*
b) Bacteroides
c) Enterococcus
d) *Staph aureus*
e) *Proteus mirabilis*

CHAPTER 12: URINARY INCONTINENCE

1 **During the process of normal voiding, detrusor contraction is initiated in response to stimulation via which of the following pathways?**

   a) Voluntary somatic S2-4 pathways
   b) Parasympathetic S 2 to 4 pathways
   c) T 10 to 12 lumbar sympathetic pathways
   d) T 10 to 12 lumbar parasympathetic pathways
   e) None of the above

2 **A 6-year-old girl is referred with a history of diurnal and nocturnal incontinence. She came out of nappies at 2½ years of age and was dry during the daytime (but not at night), until around 3 years of age. Since then, she has been wetting on an almost daily basis. Which of the following is the most likely diagnosis based upon this history?**

   a) Occult spinal dysraphism
   b) Dysfunctional voiding
   c) Sacral agenesis
   d) Pelvic floor weakness (stress incontinence)
   e) Ectopic ureter

3 **A 5-year-old boy is referred with a lifelong history of nocturnal enuresis. He wets the bed virtually every night but has been consistently dry during the daytime since the age of three. Physical examination is normal. What should be done next?**

   a) Commence treatment with oxybutynin
   b) Check urine osmolality on early morning urine sample
   c) Videourodynamics
   d) MRI scan of the spine
   e) None of the above

4 **A 12-year-old girl is referred with a history of incontinence which only occurs when she is laughing and joking with friends. She is dry at other times. Which of the following forms of treatment would have the highest chance of providing symptomatic relief in this patient?**

   a) Pelvic floor exercises
   b) Treatment with Methylphenidate
   c) Referral to a child psychologist
   d) Treatment with Desmopressin
   e) Avoiding soft drinks which contain caffeine

5 **Which of the following anatomical causes of urinary incontinence in girls is *least* likely to be detected on visual examination of the perineum?**

   a) Congenital cloacal anomaly
   b) Urogenital sinus anomaly
   c) Primary epispadias
   d) Ectopic ureter
   e) Labial adhesions

CHAPTER 13: NEUROGENIC BLADDER

1 **Which of the following statements are most applicable to the neurology and pathophysiology of neurogenic bladder dysfunction?**

   a) Neurologic lesions in the lumbosacral region account for 80% of cases
   b) The neurologic picture (upper or lower motor) in children with myelomeningocele is closely correlated with the level of the spinal abnormality
   c) The urodynamic finding of detrusor/sphincter dyssynergia denotes a 'safe' type of neurogenic bladder
   d) Sphincter weakness incontinence is usually a feature of a lower motor neuron lesion
   e) Sacral agenesis is accompanied by the presence of a cutaneous lesion in 80% of cases

2 **Which of the following structures is usually used to create the Monti continent catheterisable channel?**

   a) Ileum
   b) Caecum
   c) Colon
   d) Appendix
   e) Rectus sheath

3 **Using the formula provided in the chapter, what is the calculated functional bladder capacity of a normal 6-year-old child?**

   a) 110 to 130 ml
   b) 150 to 170 ml
   c) 230 to 250 ml
   d) 280 to 300 ml
   e) 350 to 370 ml

4 **Which of the following is *not* a recognised form of treatment for detrusor over activity?**

   a) Ileocystoplasty
   b) Botulinum toxin A
   c) Sigmoid colocystoplasty
   d) Medication with Alpha adrenergic blocking agents
   e) Medication with anticholinergic agents

5 **What is the most common cause of neurogenic bladder in children?**

   a) Spinal injury
   b) Myelomeningocele
   c) Transverse myelitis
   d) Sacral agenesis
   e) Lipomyelomeningocele

CHAPTER 14: UROLOGIC ANOMALIES IN ANORECTAL MALFORMATIONS AND RENAL ECTOPIA

1 **What percentage of children with anorectal malformations have anomalies of the urinary tract?**

   a) 25% to 35%
   b) 35% to 45%
   c) 45% to 55%
   d) 55% to 65%
   e) 65% to75%

2 **A newborn male infant has a low anorectal anomaly. What imaging modality is currently recommended for initial imaging of his spine?**

   a) MRI
   b) CT
   c) Spinal x-ray and ultrasound
   d) Bone scan
   e) Contrast myelography

3 **Which of the following is *not* a recognised feature of the VACTERL association?**

   a) Limb anomalies
   b) Vertebral anomalies
   c) Anorectal anomalies
   d) Optic anomalies (coloboma)
   e) Renal anomalies

4 **A healthy newborn female infant is born with a presumed diagnosis of unilateral renal agenesis – based on antenatal ultrasound. Only one (normal) kidney is seen on the postnatal ultrasound scan. What investigation (if any) is indicated next?**

   a) None. The diagnosis of renal agenesis had been confirmed by ultrasound.
   b) CT
   c) Laparoscopy d
   d) Mag 3 renogram
   e) Isotope renography (DMSA)

5 **Which of the following statements does *not* apply to horseshoe kidneys**

a) Horseshoe kidneys are well visualised on DMSA renography
b) Horseshoe kidneys occur more commonly in children with Turners syndrome
c) The autopsy incidence of horseshoe kidney is reported to lie between 1:400 and 1:1800
d) 35% to 45% of horseshoe kidneys are associated with fusion of the upper pole renal parenchyma
e) Horseshoe kidney is associated with an increased incidence of PUJ obstruction

CHAPTER 15: BLADDER EXSTROPHY AND EPISPADIAS

1 **What is the approximate incidence of bladder exstrophy?**

a) 1 in 5000 live births
b) 1 in 25,000 live births
c) 1 in 50,000 live births
d) 1 in 150,000 live births
e) 1 in 300,000 live births

2 **Which of the following is *not* a common feature of primary epispadias?**

a) Sphincteric weakness
b) Pubic diastasis
c) Normal calibre ureteric orifices
d) Urethra sited on the dorsal aspect of the penis
e) Anterior ectopic anus

3 **A 3.5 kg male infant with classic bladder exstrophy is transferred to a specialist centre at 6 hours of age. He is otherwise well with no evidence of cardiac or other anomalies. What is now regarded as the optimal management of this infant?**

a) Primary closure with pelvic osteotomy in the first 48 hours of life
b) Primary closure without pelvic osteotomy in the first 2–3 weeks of life
c) Parentral nutrition for one month followed by closure with pelvic osteotomies
d) Temporary urinary diversion with ureterostomies following by primary closure and undiversion at 6 months
e) Delayed closure with augmentation cystoplasty at 12 months

4 **Which of the following statements best describe the surgical closure of bladder exstrophy?**

a) The complete primary repair described by Mitchell is the simplest procedure and the one best suited to non-specialists
b) The Kelly operation is performed without osteotomy in the first 2–3 weeks of life
c) The Kelly operation is suitable for use in girls as well as boys
d) The Modern Staged Reconstruction was devised by Ransley and Gearhart
e) Use of the international standardised continence grading system (ISCGS) ensures consistent reporting of continence rates

5 **Which of the following statements best describes the features of primary epispadias in females?**

a) Normal continence occurs spontaneously in 85% of cases by 7 years of age
b) Sphincter weakness incontinence is invariably present
c) The external genitalia are usually normal
d) The clitoris is usually absent
e) The overall chances of achieving pregnancy are less that 10%

CHAPTER 16: HYPOSPADIAS

1 **Which of the following statements is most applicable to chordee?**

   a) It is present in 75% of cases of distal hypospadias
   b) Successful correction in childhood may not prevent recurrence after puberty
   c) A 2 stage repair is always required
   d) Chordee can usually be successfully corrected with a ventral tunica plication
   e) The tubularized incised plate (Snodgrass) technique has the highest success rate for the correction of moderately severe chordee

2 **What is the overall incidence of co-existing upper urinary tract anomalies in boys with distal hypospadias?**

   a) 1% to 5%
   b) 5% to 10%
   c) 10% to 15%
   d) 15% to 20%
   e) 20% to 25%

3 **Which of the following graft materials is most widely used in the first stage of a two stage repair of proximal hypospadias?**

   a) Post auricular skin
   b) Buccal skin
   c) Bladder mucosa
   d) Porcine dermis
   e) Inner preputial skin

4 **Which if the following statements best describes the aetiology and epidemiology of hypospadias?**

   a) Environmental factors (endocrine disruptors) have been demonstrated to account for >20% of cases
   b) The incidence of hypospadias in first degree relatives is approximately 10%
   c) Genetic factors are more likely be implicated in distal hypospadias
   d) Co existing abnormalities of the upper urinary tract are present in 15–20% of cases
   e) The incidence is lower in the offspring of older mothers

5 **Which of the following statements is most applicable to the urethrocutaneous hypospadias fistulae?**

   a) The overall incidence for all types of hypospadias repair is 5–7%
   b) The optimal time for fistula repair is within 6 weeks of the original surgery
   c) Success rates for flap based techniques are no higher than simple closure
   d) The reported recurrence rate in some published series is 50%
   e) Suprapubic catheter drainage is mandatory to reduce the risk of recurrence

CHAPTER 17: THE PREPUCE

1 **Which of the following statements best describes the aetiology and management of balanitis xerotica obliterans (BXO) in children**

   a) BXO carries a 1% to 3% risk of penile carcinoma before the age of 20 years
   b) Treatment with topical steroids avoids the need for surgery in 80% to 85% of cases
   c) Preputioplasty is preferable to circumcision for the treatment of BXO in boys over 10 years of age.
   d) Glans involvement is present in 5 to 7% of cases
   e) BXO is rare in children under 5 years of age

2 **The parents of a 4-year-old boy are concerned because they have observed obvious ballooning of his prepuce during micturition. Which of the following is most applicable in this case?**

   a) The ballooning probably denotes the presence of BXO
   b) Measurement of his urine flow rate is likely to show partial obstruction.
   c) The most likely diagnosis is congenital mega prepuce
   d) The parents can be reassured that ballooning is a self-limiting phenomenon of no pathological significance
   e) The presence of ballooning is a strong indication for circumcision

3 **Which of the following statements best describes the features of congenital mega prepuce?**

   a) The condition is characterised by an excessively long, redundant prepuce
   b) The overall appearances may resemble a 'buried' penis
   c) A standard circumcision usually gives satisfactory cosmetic results
   d) Any male siblings will also have a 1:10 chance of being born with this condition
   e) Voiding is usually normal despite the megaprepuce

4 **Which of the following statements is most applicable to preputioplasty?**

   a) Preputioplasy can be used as an effective alternative to circumcision in 70% to 80% of boys with BXO
   b) Retraction of the prepuce should be avoided for three to six months after the procedure
   c) Regular retraction of the prepuce should be advised in the early post operative period
   d) Preputioplasty is equally successful in all age groups
   e) None of the above

5 **A 5-year-old boy is referred with a non retractile prepuce. The prepuce is healthy but cannot be retracted beyond the tip of the glans because of preputial adhesions. What management should be advised?**

   a) Reassurance, see again only if symptoms arise
   b) Circumcision
   c) Preputioplasty
   d) Surgical release of adhesions under general anaesthesia
   e) Surgical release of adhesions under general anaesthesia if the prepuce is still partially adherent to the glans at 6 years of age

CHAPTER 18: TESTIS, HYDROCOELE AND VARICOCOELE

1 **Which of the following statements best apply to the aetiology and pathophysiology of the undescended testis?**

   a) The incidence of undescended testis is 0.5–1% in term infants
   b) Transformation from fetal gonocytes to Ad dark spermatogonia occurs at around 36–38 weeks of gestation
   c) Following meiotic divisions primary spermatocyte gives rise to 8 spermatozoa
   d) Gonocyte transformation is impaired in undescended testes
   e) The histological appearances of ascending testes are normal

2 **A 3-year-old boy is referred with a unilateral impalpable testis. Which of the following is the most reliable means of confirming the presence or absence of the testis?**

   a) Abdominal ultrasonography
   b) MRI
   c) CT scan
   d) Retrograde venography
   e) Laparoscopy

3 **Which of the following statements best apply to the management of the undescended and retractile testes?**

   a) Orchidopexy should be performed for ascending testes at the time of presentation
   b) Double blind studies have demonstrated that hormonal treatment for congenitally undescended testes has a success rate of 25–30%
   c) The Fowler-Stephens procedure is operation of a choice for high inguinal testes
   d) The optimal age for orchidopexy for a congenitally undescended testis is currently thought to be 2 years of age
   e) The parents of boys with retractile testes can be reassured that no treatment or follow up are required

4 **An 11-year-old boy presents with a painless grade III left sided varicocele. What advice should be given to his parents?**

a) Infertility is inevitable unless some form of intervention is undertaken
b) Treatment of the varicocele is likely to carry a 50% failure rate regardless of the mode of treatment
c) A CT renal scan should be performed in view of the 2% risk of Wilms tumour
d) An ultrasound scan of the testes and kidneys is all that is required at this stage
e) A semen sample should be analysed before determining further management

5 **Testicular ultrasound in a 14-year-old boy demonstrates bilateral microcalcification. This is an incidental finding following a sporting injury. What action should be advised in the light of these findings?**

a) Reassurance, no further follow up unless symptomatic
b) Urgent testicular biopsy
c) Testicular biopsy around the age of 19 or 20 years
d) Bilateral prophylactic testicular fixation in view of the high risk of testicular torsion
e) Six monthly ultrasound review for 5 years with annual ultrasound examination thereafter

CHAPTER 19: THE ACUTE SCROTUM

1 **Scrotal exploration is being performed in a 14-year-old boy for a presumed diagnosis of right testicular torsion. He has a 10-hour history of symptoms. The diagnosis is confirmed but despite detorsion, the testis remains dark blue in colour with no evidence of perfusion. What action should the surgeon take?**

a) Right orchidectomy. Defer fixation of the left testis for at least 3 months second because of the risk of infection
b) Leave the right testis in situ because it might contribute to endocrine function. Defer fixation of the left testis until the fate of the right testis is known
c) Right orchidectomy combined with simultaneous fixation of the left testis
d) Leave the right testis in situ because it might contribute to endocrine function. Simultaneous suture fixation of the left testis
e) Right orchidectomy and implantation of silicone gel prosthesis, simultaneous suture fixation of the left testis

2 **A 5-year-old boy presents with diffuse swelling involving both sides of the scrotum He is afebrile and has only minimal discomfort. What action should be taken next?**

a) Urgent surgical exploration to exclude an atypical presentation of bilateral synchronous testicular torsion.
b) Commence intravenous antibiotics
c) Take blood for alpha feto protein and other tumour markers
d) Oral Prednisilone
e) No specific treatment

3 **A 13-year-old boy presents with severe right iliac fossa pain of sudden onset 4-hours earlier. No abnormality is detected on abdominal palpation. His right testis is tender but there is no erythema of the overlying scrotal skin. How should he be investigated and managed?**

a) Scrotal ultrasound
b) Admit for observation, re-assess clinical findings after 4 hours
c) Doppler ultrasound
d) Radionuclide scan
e) No investigation, advise patient and parents of risk of torsion and proceed directly to surgical exploration.

4 **A 17-year-old patient with testicular torsion has undergone unilateral orchidectomy for a non-viable testis. What advice should be given in response to questions regarding the prognosis for endocrine function and fertility?**

a) Testosterone levels should be checked annually since endocrine replacement treatment may be required
b) There is a risk that semen quality will be reduced but his prospects of achieving paternity will probably be normal
c) He has a 20% chance of being infertile but could probably achieve paternity with assisted conception techniques
d) He may experience erectile dysfunction due to low testosterone levels but this could be treated with sildenafil.
e) None of the above

5 **Which of the following statements does *not* apply to torsion of the Hydatid of Morgagni?**

a) The 'blue dot' sign is present in 50% to 60% of cases
b) The peak incidence is between 10 to 12 years of age
c) It can usually be diagnosed on clinical grounds
d) The pain is usually more gradual in onset than testicular torsion
e) Conservative management can be safely considered if symptoms are mild or resolving

CHAPTER 20: DISORDERS OF SEX DEVELOPMENT

1 **Which is the commonest disorder of sex development encountered in North America and Europe?**

a) Ovotesticular DSD
b) 5 Alpha reductase deficiency
c) 46XX DSD due to congenital adrenal hyperplasia
d) Mixed gonadal dysgenesis
e) 46XY DSD (male pseudo hermaphroditism)

2 **Which of the following statements best describes the features of children with Turner syndrome?**

a) Clitoral hypertrophy is present in 80–90% of patients
b) Normal ovarian tissue is present in 55% to 75% of patients
c) The lifetime risk of gonadal malignancy is significantly increased
d) The lifetime risk of gonadal malignancy is not significantly increased
e) The diagnosis is most commonly made during investigation of ambiguous genitalia in infancy

3 **Which of the following statements best describes the aetiology and epidemiology of congenital adrenal hyperplasia (CAH)?**

a) CAH accounts for 20 to 25% of all infants with ambiguous genitalia
b) The most common underlying endocrine defect is 11 Beta hydroxylase deficiency
c) CAH is an autosomal dominant disorder with variable expression
d) CAH is an X linked recessive disorder
e) CAH is an autosomal recessive disorder

4 **As a consequence of the findings during a hernia operation, Sarah, aged 5, is diagnosed with complete androgen insensitivity syndrome. Which of the following statements best describes the other features and the karyotype?**

a) The most likely karyotype is 47XXY
b) The most likely karyotype is 46XY
c) The most likely karyotype is 47XYY
d) The gonads identified in the hernial sacs are most like to be dysgenetic streak gonads
e) The internal genitalia are most likely to comprise a vestigial uterus and fallopian tubes.

5 **Which disorder of sex development is characterised by an elevated plasma level of 17 OH progesterone?**

a) Mixed gonadal dysgenesis
b) Ovotesticular DSD (true hermaphroditism)
c) 46XY DSD (male pseudohermaphroditism)
d) Müllerian inhibitory substance receptor insensitivity
e) 46XX DSD due to congenital adrenal hyperplasia

CHAPTER 21: GENITOURINARY MALIGNANCIES

1 **Which of the following statements most accurately refers to the epidemiology and aetiology of rhabdomyosarcoma?**

a) The prognosis in not influenced by the site of origin within the genitourinary tract
b) Tumours with embryonal histology have a higher survival rate
c) Rhabdomyosarcomas of the bladder and prostate most commonly present as Stage 1 tumours
d) Approximately 50% of all rhabdomyosarcomas in children arise within the genitourinary tract
e) Paratesticular rhabdomyosarcoma is usually treated with chemotherapy prior to surgery

2 **Which of the following statements best describes evaluation of primary testicular tumours in prepubertal boys?**

a) A CT scan should be performed routinely because of the high incidence of occult metastatic disease
b) CT scans can be performed selectively because of the low incidence of metastatic disease
c) Serum alpha fetoprotein is the most reliable marker of malignancy in the first 6 months of life
d) Painful swellings are of greatest concern
e) The presence of retroperitoneal lymph nodes is classified as Stage IV

3 **What is the approximate current overall 5-year survival rate for children with Stage I–II nephroblastoma (Wilms tumour)?**

a) 20%–30%
b) 40%–50%
c) 50%–60%
d) 80%–90%
e) >95%

4 **Which of the following statements best apply to the histology and staging of nephroblastoma (Wilms tumour)?**

a) The histology is classified as unfavourable in 20%–25% % of cases
b) Bilateral tumours are classified as Stage 4b
c) Metastatic spread is present in 25% of cases at presentation
d) Wilms tumours classically have a biphasic histological appearance comprised of blastemal and epithelial components
e) Abnormalities of chromosome 16 are associated with poorer survival

5 **Which of the following statements is most applicable to Congenital Mesoblastic Nephroma?**

a) Complications of treatment are the commonest cause of death
b) It accounts for 15% of all pediatric renal tumours
c) Stage III tumours with mixed histologic subtype a higher risk of local recurrence
d) The mortality rate is lower when it presents in the first month of life
e) It is a benign tumour which never metastasizes

CHAPTER 22: PEDIATRIC GENITOURINARY TRAUMA

1 **A 7-year-old boy was admitted to hospital 4 hours previously following a fall from a climbing frame. On admission he was haemodynamically stable but is tender in the left upper quadrant. An ultrasound scan on admission demonstrated a small haematoma in the region of the upper pole. He is complaining of increasing pain. He now has tachycardia and his systolic blood pressure blood is 105 mm. Which of the following would be most appropriate?**

a) Urgent DMSA scan
b) Increased dose of analgesia and repeat ultrasound scan if no improvement after 12 hours.
c) Intravenous urogram
d) CT scan
e) Proceed directly to urgent surgical exploration

2 **Which of the following statements is most applicable to bladder injuries in children?**

a) They are most commonly caused by falls and sporting injuries
b) CT Cystography should be routinely performed at the time of presentation to assess the severity of the injury
c) Localized peri vesical extravasation can usually be managed by catheter drainage
d) Any degree of peri vesical extravasation is an indication for urgent surgical exploration
e) The bladder is less prone to injury in children than adults because of its smaller size

3 **What is the long-term risk of hypertension arising from a renal injury in childhood?**

   a) Less than 5%
   b) 5% to 10%
   c) 10% to 15%
   d) 15% to 20%
   e) 20% to 25%

4 **Which of the following statements is most applicable to renal injuries in children?**

   a) Contact sports are the commonest cause
   b) Haematuria is a reliable indicator of the severity of injury in this age group
   c) Grade I injuries account for 45% of case
   d) Urinary extravasation always requires either extrarenal and/or intrarenal drainage
   e) The outcomes of penetrating injuries are worse than those of blunt injuries

5 **A 2½-year-old girl is brought by her mother to the accident and emergency department following an accident which occurred whilst being looked after overnight by a neighbour. No one saw the accident occur. Examination reveals bruising of the perineum and labia, contusion of the introitus and a superficial laceration of the vaginal mucosa. What measures should be taken next?**

   a) Admit to hospital, proceed to urgent cystoscopy
   b) Admit to hospital. Contact the duty pediatrician to investigate the circumstances of the injury
   c) Prescribe antibiotic cream and regular baths. Arrange further review in the outpatient clinic in 2 days
   d) Prescribe oral antibiotics and regular baths. Arrange further review in 2 days
   e) Reassure, no antibiotics prescribed but advise regular baths. No arrangement for follow up

CHAPTER 23: LAPAROSCOPIC PAEDIATRIC UROLOGY

1 **Which of the following statements best describes the use of robotic laparoscopic surgery in children?**

   a) Excellent tactile feedback is one of the advantages of the Da Vinci Robot
   b) It is unsuitable for use in neonates
   c) Comparative studies have found that success rates for Robotic-Assisted Laparoscopic Pyeloplasty are 20% lower than for open and conventional laparoscopic pyeloplasty
   d) The system has two major components: the robot and the cart containing image processing equipment and light source
   e) The ports should be placed no more than 8 cm apart

2 **Which of the following is *not* regarded as an absolute contraindication to laparoscopic adrenalectomy in children?**

   a) Phaeochromocytoma
   b) Cardiac failure due to severe congenital heart disease
   c) Respiratory insufficiency due to cystic fibrosis
   d) Uncorrectable coagulopathy
   e) Systemic sepsis

3 **Which of the following statements are most applicable to the technical aspects of laparoscopic urological surgery in children?**

   a) Anaesthesia does not routinely require endotracheal intubation
   b) Cooling mats are used routinely because of the increased risk of hyperthermia
   c) A 5mm cannula is required when using an Endopouch retrieval device for specimen extraction
   d) Children absorb relatively less CO_2 than adults
   e) The Hasson technique is preferable for establishing a pneumoperitonem

4 Which of the following is *not* currently a well-recognised indication for Minimally Invasive Surgery in Paediatric Urology laparoscopic?

a) Nephrectomy for dysplastic kidney
b) Nephrectomy for Stage IV Wilms tumour
c) Adrenalectomy
d) Gonadal biopsy
e) Excision of ureteric stump

5 What was the first laparoscopic procedure to gain widespread acceptance in Paediatric Urology?

a) Laparoscopic nephrectomy
b) Diagnostic laparoscopy for impalpable testes
c) Laparoscopic pyeloplasty
d) Laparoscopic excision of Müllerian remnants
e) Laparoscopic hemi nephrectomy

CHAPTER 24: ADOLESCENT UROLOGY

1 What is the commonest cause of death in adult spina bifida patients?

a) Renal failure
b) Uncontrolled hydrocephalus
c) Bladder cancer
d) Cardiovascular and respiratory disease
e) Suicide

2 What is the approximate risk of bladder cancer associated with enterocystoplasty after a latency period of 20 to 25 years?

a) 2% to 5%
b) 5% to 7%
c) 7% to 10%
d) 10% to 12%
e) 12% to 15%

3 Which of the following is *not* a well recognised feature of Prune-Belly syndrome?

a) Renovascular malformations
b) Bilateral undescended testes
c) Absent abdominal wall musculature
d) Kyphoscoliosis
e) Dilatation of the upper urinary tract

4 Which of the following statements best describes the prognosis for sexual and reproductive function in female bladder exstrophy patients?

a) Substitution vaginoplasty is usually required to permit normal intercourse
b) Uterine prolapse occurs in up to 50% of women
c) Fewer than 15% of women with a history of bladder exstrophy can achieve pregnancy
d) Genital sensation is severely impaired as a result of clitoral agenesis
e) Infertility is inevitable because of the association between bladder exstrophy and uterine agenesis

5 Which of the following is well-documented prognostic indicators of long-term renal impairment in patients with posterior urethral valves?

a) GFR 70 mls/min/1.73 m^2 at 11 years of age
b) Daytime incontinence after 5 years of age
c) Diagnosis after 5 years of age
d) Non-refluxing upper tracts
e) High urine osmolality

CHAPTER 25: PEDIATRIC AND ADOLESCENT GYNECOLOGY

1 **Which of the following statements is most applicable to labial adhesions?**

a) They present most commonly between 5 and 7 years of age
b) Separation of the adhesions with a blunt surgical instrument is required in 30%– 40% of cases.
c) Labial adhesions can be treated with application of a topical steroid ointment
d) The adhesions usually persist into adolescence
e) Labial adhesions are usually congenital rather than acquired in etiology

2 **Which of the following statements do *not* apply to Mayer Rokitansky Kuster Hauser (MRKH) Syndrome?**

a) MRKH syndrome has an incidence of approximately 1: 4500
b) MRKH results from failure of normal embryological development of the urogenital sinus
c) The condition usually presents with painless amenorrhea
d) Vaginal dilatation is the first line of treatment for patients wishing to become sexually active
e) The external appearances of the genitalia are usually normal

3 **A 14-year-old girl has undergone a non urgent ultrasound scan to investigate upper abdominal pain occurring over several months. The scan demonstrates the presence of a complex mass 10 mm in diameter in the left ovary. The appearances are not those of a typical mature teratoma. Which of the following would be most appropriate?**

a) Rescan with ultrasound in 1 month
b) Arrange for laparoscopy within the next week
c) Urgent CT scan
d) Pregnancy test
e) Send blood for tumour markers

4 **Which of the following statements are most applicable to Lichen Sclerosus?**

a) The incidence is approximately 1 in 200
b) It occurs more commonly in children than adults
c) Biopsy is required to confirm the diagnosis
d) A single 2–3 month course of topical steroids will prevent recurrence in > 90% of cases
e) The appearances can be mistaken for genital trauma

5 **Which of the following may present with obstructed menstruation?**

a) Lichen sclerosis
b) Labial adhesions
c) Imperforate hymen
d) Longitudinal vaginal septum
e) Labial hypertrophy

Appendix II

Self-Assessment Section: Answers

CHAPTER 1 – EMBRYOLOGY

Question 1   -   e
Question 2   -   b
Question 3   -   d
Question 4   -   a
Question 5   -   d

Question 4 Comment. Although conditions such as vesico ureteric reflux, hypospadias and ureteric duplication have a well documented familial basis, attempts to implicate individual gene mutations have been unfruitful and it is generally believed that they result from the interaction of multiple genes. By contrast, specific mutations have been identified in autosomal dominant polycystic kidney disease – see Chapter 10, 'Cystic Renal Disease'.

CHAPTER 2 – RENAL DEVELOPMENT AND DYSFUNCTION

Question 1   -   d
Question 2   -   e
Question 3   -   b
Question 4   -   d
Question 5   -   d

Question 1 Comment. Hyponatremia (plasma sodium less than 130 mmol/L), due to water retention and sodium depletion is a common feature of sick and premature newborn infants. Monitoring of sodium and fluid balance in such infants is particularly important in the early weeks of life.

CHAPTER 3 – IMAGING

Question 1   -   c
Question 2   -   d
Question 3   -   a
Question 4   -   e
Question 5   -   b

Question 2 Comment. A renal pelvic AP diameter of greater than 10 mm is regarded as abnormal but is not necessarily indicative of clinically significant pathology.

CHAPTER 4 – PRENATAL DIAGNOSIS

Question 1   -   d
Question 2   -   c
Question 3   -   d
Question 4   -   a
Question 5   -   d

CHAPTER 5 – URINARY TRACT INFECTION

Question 1 - b
Question 2 - c
Question 3 - e
Question 4 - e
Question 5 - b

Question 1 Comment. A child of this age should be able to cooperate in the correction of a 'clean catch' midstream sample – the least invasive, reliable method of collecting an uncontaminated specimen.

Question 3 Comment. Leucocyte esterase negative, nitrite positive. This finding represents presumptive evidence of UTI. Antibiotic treatment should be commenced and a urine sample sent for culture.

CHAPTER 6 – VESICO-URETERAL REFLUX

Question 1 - a
Question 2 - b
Question 3 - d
Question 4 - b
Question 5 - e

CHAPTER 7 – UPPER TRACT OBSTRUCTION

Question 1 - e
Question 2 - b
Question 3 - b
Question 4 - e
Question 5 - b

Question 1 Comment. The imaging points to a diagnosis of obstructed megaureter with good preservation of function. In most cases the natural history is one of gradual spontaneous resolution. In this case, conservative management would be more appropriate than any form of surgical intervention at this stage.

CHAPTER 8 – DUPLICATION ANOMALIES, URETEROCELES AND ECTOPIC URETERS

Question 1 - c
Question 2 - a
Question 3 - c
Question 4 - b
Question 5 - a

CHAPTER 9 – POSTERIOR URETHRAL VALVES AND OTHER URETHRAL ABNORMALITIES

Question 1 - c
Question 2 - b
Question 3 - e
Question 4 - b
Question 5 - d

Question 4 Comment. There are no long-term data from comparative studies which demonstrate that vesico amniotic shunting improves the prognosis for renal function.

CHAPTER 10 – CYSTIC RENAL DISEASE

Question 1 - d
Question 2 - d
Question 3 - b
Question 4 - a
Question 5 - a

CHAPTER 11 – URINARY TRACT CALCULI

Question 1 - e
Question 2 - e
Question 3 - a
Question 4 - c
Question 5 - e

Question 3 Comment. By the time the diagnosis of xanthogranulomatous pyelonephritis comes to light the kidney is usually non-functioning or contributing only a very small percentage of differential function.

CHAPTER 12 – URINARY INCONTINENCE

Question 1   -   b
Question 2   -   b
Question 3   -   e
Question 4   -   b
Question 5   -   d

Question 3 Comment. This boy has monosymptomatic nocturnal enuresis. In the absence of daytime wetting or any other unusual features the yield from investigation is minimal and the parents can be reassured that he will become dry. Nevertheless some active treatment such as an alarm or Desmopressin may be considered if he does not improve spontaneously.

Question 4 Comment. Giggle incontinence is a rare but distinctive disorder. Treatment with anticholinergics is usually unhelpful, but Methylphenidate (Ritalin) can sometimes be dramatically effective.

CHAPTER 13 – NEUROGENIC BLADDER

Question 1   -   d
Question 2   -   a
Question 3   -   c
Question 4   -   d
Question 5   -   b

Question 1 Comment. Far from denoting a 'safe' pattern of neurogenic bladder dysfunction, the finding of detrusor/sphincter dyssynergia indicates an 'unsafe' or 'hostile' neurogenic bladder which should be actively managed to protect renal function.

CHAPTER 14 – UROLOGIC ANOMALIES IN ANORECTAL MALFORMATIONS AND RENAL ECTOPIA

Question 1   -   d
Question 2   -   c
Question 3   -   d
Question 4   -   e
Question 5   -   d

Question 4 Comment. A pelvic kidney can be missed on ultrasound. A DMSA scan is indicated to identify any ectopic function in renal tissue – principally to look for a pelvic kidney.

CHAPTER 15 – BLADDER EXSTROPHY AND EPISPADIAS

Question 1   -   c
Question 2   -   e
Question 3   -   b
Question 4   -   c
Question 5   -   b

Question 3 Comment. Practice varies between different specialist centres with regard to the timing of primary closure. The authors' preference is to defer primary closure until 2–3 weeks of age, to allow time for the establishment of breast feeding and maternal bonding.

CHAPTER 16 – HYPOSPADIAS

Question 1   -   b
Question 2   -   a
Question 3   -   e
Question 4   -   b
Question 5   -   d

Question 1 Comment. Minor to moderate degrees of chordee can usually be corrected during a single-stage closure. However, severe degrees of chordee are usually associated with proximal hypospadias – for which better long-term results are achieved with a two stage procedure. Despite apparently successful correction in childhood, residual or recurrent chordee may sometimes become apparent again after puberty.

CHAPTER 17 – THE PREPUCE

Question 1   -   e
Question 2   -   d
Question 3   -   b
Question 4   -   c
Question 5   -   a

Question 5 Comment. No form of intervention is usually required is such cases (apart, perhaps from a short course of topical steroid ointment combined with gentle retraction of the foreskin). Division of preputial adhesions under general anaesthesia is of largely historic interest and is rarely performed by Paediatric Urologists.

CHAPTER 18 – TESTIS, HYDROCOELE AND VARICOCOELE

Question 1   -   d
Question 2   -   e
Question 3   -   a
Question 4   -   d
Question 5   -   a

Question 3 Comment. Conservative management of ascending testes has been described but there are concerns regarding temperature – related histological damage during the period the testis remains outside the scrotum. The safest option is to proceed to orchidopexy in any boy with either a congenital or acquired undescended testis.

CHAPTER 19 – THE ACUTE SCROTUM

Question 1   -   c
Question 2   -   e
Question 3   -   e
Question 4   -   b
Question 5   -   a

Question 2 Comment. The diagnosis is idiopathic scrotal oedema – for which no specific treatment is required.

Question 3 Comment. There is a high probability of torsion in this 13 year old. The history is relatively short and there is a reasonable prospect of conserving a viable testis with urgent surgical exploration. Performing an ultrasound scan will lead to inevitable delay which is likely to compromise potential viability of the testis.

CHAPTER 20 – DISORDERS OF SEX DEVELOPMENT

Question 1   -   c
Question 2   -   c
Question 3   -   e
Question 4   -   b
Question 5   -   e

CHAPTER 21 – GENITOURINARY MALIGNANCIES

Question 1   -   b
Question 2   -   b
Question 3   -   d
Question 4   -   e
Question 5   -   a

Question 4 Comment. Wilms tumours classically have triphasic histology with stromal, blastemal, and epithelial components.

CHAPTER 22 – PEDIATRIC GENITOURINARY TRAUMA

Question 1   -   d
Question 2   -   c
Question 3   -   a
Question 4   -   e
Question 5   -   b

CHAPTER 23 – LAPAROSCOPIC PAEDIATRIC UROLOGY

Question 1   -   b
Question 2   -   a
Question 3   -   e
Question 4   -   b
Question 5   -   b

Question 3 Comment. Contrary to answer b, the main risk is of intraoperative hypothermia. For this reason a warming blanket is commonly used during longer procedures.

CHAPTER 24 – ADOLESCENT UROLOGY

Question 1   -   d
Question 2   -   a
Question 3   -   a
Question 4   -   b
Question 5   -   b

Question 1 Comment. Renal failure was historically the commonest cause of death in young adults with spina bifida. However, the long-term outlook for renal function has been transformed in recent decades by advances in management of the neuropathic bladder

CHAPTER 25 – PEDIATRIC AND ADOLESCENT GYNECOLOGY

Question 1   -   c
Question 2   -   b
Question 3   -   e
Question 4   -   e
Question 5   -   c

Index